£29.97

D0537448

Hot Topics

in General Practice 8e

Hot Topics
in General Practice 8e

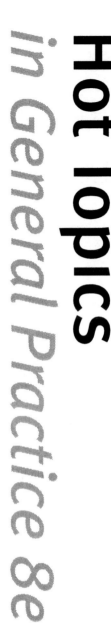

J. Kilburn MRCGP, FRCS(A&E), DA

Newcastle-upon-Tyne

Scion **2007 Edition**

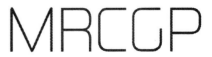

Eighth Edition © Scion Publishing Ltd, 2007

ISBN 978 1 904842 37 8

Seventh Edition 2006 (ISBN 1 904842 35 6)
Sixth Edition 2005 (ISBN 1 904842 05 4)
Fifth Edition first published by Scion Publishing Ltd, 2004 (ISBN 1 904842 00 3)
Fourth Edition 2002 (ISBN 1 85996 073 1); reprinted 2003
Third Edition 2000 (ISBN 1 85996 129 0); reprinted 2001
Second Edition 1998 (ISBN 1 85996 251 3); reprinted 1999
First Edition published by BIOS Scientific Publishers Ltd, 1996 (ISBN 1 85996 210 6); reprinted 1997

A CIP catalogue record for this book is available from the British Library.

Scion Publishing Limited

610.65
KIL

Bloxham Mill, Barford Road, Bloxham, Oxfordshire OX15 4FF
www.scionpublishing.com

Important Note from the Publisher

The information contained within this book was obtained by Scion Publishing Limited from sources believed by us to be reliable. However, while every effort has been made to ensure its accuracy, no responsibility for loss or injury whatsoever occasioned to any person acting or refraining from action as a result of information contained herein can be accepted by the authors or publishers.

The reader should remember that medicine is a constantly evolving science and while the authors and publishers have ensured that all dosages, applications and practices are based on current indications, there may be specific practices which differ between communities. You should always follow the guidelines laid down by the manufacturers of specific products and the relevant authorities in the country in which you are practising.

Typeset by Phoenix Photosetting, Chatham, Kent, UK
Printed by Biddles Ltd, King's Lynn, UK, www.biddles.co.uk

CONTENTS

PRACTICE ISSUES

CLINICAL ISSUES

ABBREVIATIONS

A&E	accident and emergency
AAA	abdominal aortic aneurysm
ACE	angiotensin-converting enzyme
AF	atrial fibrillation
ARB	angiotensin II receptor blocker
BMA	British Medical Association
BMI	body mass index
BNP	B-type natriuretic peptide
BP	blood pressure
BPH	benign prostatic hypertrophy
CAD	coronary artery disease
CBT	cognitive behaviour therapy
CFS	chronic fatigue syndrome
CHD	coronary heart disease
CHF	chronic heart failure
CK	creatine kinase
COPD	chronic obstructive pulmonary disease
COX	cyclo-oxygenase
CRP	C-reactive protein
CT	computed tomography
DEXA	dual energy X-ray absorptiometry
DMSA	dimercaptosuccinic acid
DVT	deep venous thrombosis
ECG	electrocardiogram
FOB	faecal occult blood
FPG	fasting plasma glucose
GGT	gamma glutamyl transferase
GI	gastro-intestinal
GMC	General Medical Council
GORD	gastro-oesophageal disease
GP	general practitioner
GUM	genitourinary medicine
HDL	high density lipoprotein
HIV	human immunodeficiency virus
HPV	human papillomavirus
IBS	irritable bowel syndrome
ICD	International Classification of Diseases
IGT	impaired glucose tolerance
IHD	ischaemic heart disease
LDL	low density lipoprotein
LVH	left ventricular hypertrophy
LVSD	left ventricular systolic dysfunction
MCV	mean corpuscular volume
ME	myalgic encephalomyelitis
MI	myocardial infarction

MMR	measles mumps rubella vaccine
MPA	medroxyprogesterone acetate
MRI	magnetic resonance imaging
NHS	National Health Service
NICE	National Institute for Clinical Excellence
NSAID	non-steroidal anti-inflammatory drug
NSF	national service framework
NYHA	New York Heart Association
OGTT	oral glucose tolerance test
POEM	patient orientated evidence that matters
PPI	proton pump inhibitor
PSA	prostate specific antigen
QALY	quality adjusted life year
RA	rheumatoid arthritis
RCGP	Royal College of General Practitioners
RCT	randomised controlled trial
SHO	senior house officer
SMT	spinal manipulative therapy
SSRI	selective serotonin reuptake inhibitor
TNF	tumour necrosis factor
US	ultrasound
UTI	urinary tract infection
VC	virtual colonoscopy

JOURNAL ABBREVIATIONS

Am Heart J	*American Heart Journal*
Am J Cardiol	*The American Journal of Cardiology*
Am J Epidemiol	*American Journal of Epidemiology*
Am J Gastroenterol	*The American Journal of Gastroenterology*
Am J Med	*The American Journal of Medicine*
Ann Intern Med	*Annals of Internal Medicine*
Ann Rheum Dis	*Annals of the Rheumatic Diseases*
Arch Dis Child	*Archives of Disease in Childhood*
Arch Gen Psychiatry	*Archives of General Psychiatry*
Arch Intern Med	*Archives of Internal Medicine*
Arch Neurol	*Archives of Neurology*
Arch Pediatr Adolesc Med	*Archives of Pediatrics and Adolescent Medicine*
Arthritis Rheum	*Arthritis and Rheumatism*
BJU Int	*British Journal of Urology International*
BMJ	*British Medical Journal*
Br J Cancer	*British Journal of Cancer*
Br J Gen Pract	*British Journal of General Practice*
Br J Psychiatry	*The British Journal of Psychiatry*
Clin Infect Dis	*Clinical Infectious Diseases*

Eur Heart J	*European Heart Journal*
Eur Respir J	*European Respiratory Journal*
Fam Pract	*Family Practice*
J Am Coll Cardiol	*Journal of the American College of Cardiology*
J Am Geriatr Soc	*Journal of the American Geriatrics Society*
J Epidemiol Community Health	*Journal of Epidemiology and Community Health*
J Infect Dis	*The Journal of Infectious Diseases*
J Natl Cancer Inst	*Journal of the National Cancer Institute*
J Neurol Neurosurg Psychiatry	*Journal of Neurology, Neurosurgery, and Psychiatry*
J Rheumatol	*The Journal of Rheumatology*
J Urol	*The Journal of Urology*
JAMA	*The Journal of the American Medical Association*
Mayo Clin Proc	*Mayo Clinic Proceedings*
Med J Aust	*The Medical Journal of Australia*
N Engl J Med	*The New England Journal of Medicine*
Nat Med	*Nature Medicine*
Postgrad Med J	*Postgraduate Medical Journal*
Qual Saf Health Care	*Quality and Safety in Health Care*

PREFACE

This hottest update of *Hot Topics* assesses the current temperature and pulse of the latest doings pertinent to primary care.

Exciting new techniques such as those for preventing cervical cancer lie shoulder to shoulder with all too familiar zones of inertia such as the delay in screening for colorectal neoplasia.

Emerging possibilities such as Google's clout as a diagnostician sit alongside updates on well-known uncertainties such as the pros and cons of prostate screening and new worries such as the mortality associated with long-acting beta agonists.

There is a youthful but burgeoning evidence base regarding the multi-billion pound industry that is complementary therapy, no longer able to hide from new regulatory interference.

And we leave old acquaintances behind. It turns out that folic acid is not as useful as we had hoped, but at least the good old statins seem to be becoming more cost-effective by the day.

Primary care doctors are specialists in managing multisystem disease. They are specialists in risk assessment. If you look for haematuria in your patients, what do you do with the result? How will you screen for chlamydia cost-effectively in the population you serve? How can you help to flatten out the inequalities in care of the elderly in your catchment area?

A shared plan is informed consent for every prescription, referral and review plan. That informed consent is the implied goal of all patient encounters. Each paper in this updated digest is carefully selected for what it can contribute to the discussion of current philosophies and controversies. By identifying areas of uncertainty, we can be less hesitant in our contribution to the negotiation that is the modern consultation. This book will help you to manage that uncertainty. And if you happened to use the information to pass a certain evolving Royal College exam, well... who would blame you?

Julian Kilburn
January 2007

THE CONSULTATION

What we know already:

- Uninterrupted, patients conclude their opening monologue in less than 30 seconds in primary care
- Consultations are more successful where they are perceived to have lasted longer but were not longer. They may be more about quality time as actual time
- Longer consultations lead to more preventative health care, better recognition of psychosocial problems and less prescribing
- Patients forget up to 80% of the information from the consultation. Of the information they do recall, half of it is remembered incorrectly
- Communications skills can be taught but this does not always improve patients' experiences
- Doctors tend not to elicit patients' expectations or unvoiced agendas. They misconstrue patient pressure resulting in more prescribing and less compliance
- Using medical terminology can help patients validate their sick role and bestow a sense of greater professionalism on their doctor. Lay labels can result in a greater sense of ownership of the problem which some perceive as blame
- The GMC advise that doctors should always offer a chaperone for intimate examinations

Recent Papers

COMMUNICATION

Involve the patient and pass the MRCGP: investigating shared decision making in a consulting skills examination using a validated instrument
Siriwardena AN, Edwards A, Campion P et al.
Br J Gen Pract, 2006; **56**: 857–862

This study looked at consultation videos from fail, pass and merit candidates for the MRCGP and validated them against an instrument for shared decision making called OPTION – observing patient involvement.

Those who demonstrated sharing management options better scored higher. Scores decreased with age but had no association with gender of either doctor or patient or the length of consultation.

Shared decision making and the experience of partnership in primary care
Saba GW, Wong ST, Schillinger D et al.
Ann Fam Med, 2006; **4**: 54–62

This study in US primary care showed that relationship factors such as trust and perceived respect influence communication as much as style and behaviour. We have to work on relationship dynamics for effective consultation as this study found that shared decision making between patient and physician is frequently a negative experience for the patient.

It can 'look good,' but when it does not also 'feel good', we need to recognise that a purely behavioural model for teaching communication skills appears inadequate

Doctors' communication of trust, care, and respect in breast cancer: qualitative study
Burkitt Wright E, Holcombe C, Salmon P
BMJ, 2004; **328**: 864

This series of interviews with women with breast cancer eases communication research in a slightly different direction.

Most important to patients was not so much the communication skills of their doctors as their enduring characteristics. They wanted to feel their doctor had expertise. An efficient air and open manner helped. A word of recommendation from a nurse was very useful. Even just being a doctor was often enough.

They wanted a unique relationship with their doctor which made them feel unique and special. Enhanced eye contact, smiling, touching, a sense of humour or display of the odd idiosyncrasy were characteristics which helped them lock in on this. These forms of communication differ from those usually taught.

Consulting at eye level and giving patients 'the option' was valued but interestingly no patients described a process of decision-making. This was just their part of accepting the clinician's recommendation and an important part of having their autonomy as an individual respected.

Patients wanted to be left on a positive note. Saying that the cancer was not as bad as it might have been seemed to be a good ruse.

The authors argue that clinical communication should begin with assessment of patients' vulnerability and dependence on doctors. Relationships may be influenced more by attachment need than communication skills.

The teaching of communication skills may be misguided
Smith R
BMJ, 2004; 328

Richard Smith's accompanying 'Editor's choice' article deserves inclusion here for the title alone. He summarises that patients were more concerned about doctors' expertise than their communication skills. Patients appear to start by trusting doctors. Trust does not have to be won but can be lost. Doctors can live up to this by appearing confident and answering questions without hesitation. But are these breast cancer patients truly representative of a wider group? And how do you share the uncertainty that is ubiquitous in medicine?

How can doctors communicate information about risk more effectively?
Alaszewski A, Horlick-Jones T
BMJ, 2003; **327**: 728–731

We do not think rationally about risk.

There is little evidence that knowledge of risk alone has altered public behaviour. The well-known harmful consequences of smoking, alcohol consumption, drug misuse and unsafe sex are a testament to this. By the same token, the beneficial consequences of a healthier lifestyle are largely ignored. The concept that individuals rationally review the available evidence is therefore flawed and explains the lack of impact of mass health campaigns.

However, putting the problem in its proper social context can make it relevant to the individual. Trust in the source of the information given is crucial and means that working on the doctor–patient relationship is worthwhile.

How information fits with previous knowledge, experience and everyday life may decide whether it is acted upon. For example, the threat of social stigma and loss of sexual partners meant that many HIV patients chose to delay seeking diagnosis and treatment.

We also overstate the likelihood of low probability or high consequence risks, e.g. getting killed in a train crash. This happens more if the risk is involuntary, inescapable or poorly understood by science and subject to contradictory statements. Conversely, we underestimate common risks such as smoking.

Technological progress creates new hazards that are 'virtual risks' as there is a dearth of evidence or experience on which to base judgements. Expert opinion is especially important here but individuals still choose which opinion to go with. New evidence added to this pot can distort risk, e.g. the food panics surrounding mad cow disease.

The media plays a big part. News articles may inflate risks in foodstuffs while soap operas overdramatise consequences of mental illness.

Doctors need to recognise that they are just one source of information fighting for the patient's loyalty. Targeting other agencies which patients trust such as patients' rights groups and community groups has been shown to be effective.

The informed understanding of risk that people have depends on a complex mix of social context and general knowledge from everyday experience. Access to this Pandora's box is a prerequisite for effective risk communication.

How doctors discuss major interventions with high risk patients: an observational study
Corke CF, Stow PJ, Green DT et al.
BMJ, 2005; **330**: 182

We all love role play and this Australian study put 30 junior doctors (not vocationally trained GPs) in a staged no-win scenario (leaking abdominal aortic aneurysm in someone unlikely to survive surgery) to assess their consultation skills. They found that doctors were fine at discussing the medical bits but not so good at engaging with the patient's wishes and fears.

Research estimates at least 75% of patients want their doctor to offer a recommendation when faced with an end-of-life decision. In this study, only 36% of doctors gave advice even when it was directly requested. They suggest this approach is consistent with modern day medical school teaching but proclaim that a role limited to merely providing information is failing our patients. Those that suggested they go and discuss things with their family also came in for criticism, as it was felt such a patient would be too sick to relay all the arguments. Fortunately, they are starting a course to cure the problem.

Managing controversy through consultation: a qualitative study of communication and trust around MMR vaccination decisions
McMurray R, Cheater FM, Weighall A et al.
Br J Gen Pract, 2004; **54**: 520–525

This study in general practice illustrates the points above quite nicely using the MMR controversy. Interviews with parents in the Leeds area found that the medical evidence played little role in their decision to vaccinate their children. Even though doctors were usually trusted sources, too many concerns over the legitimacy of their role, financial impartiality and political bias got in the way.

A new collaborative approach to information exchange is needed to help people tackle decisions like this ready for when the next scandal happens.

Randomised controlled trial of effect of leaflets to empower patients in consultations in primary care
Little P, Dorward M, Warner G et al.
BMJ, 2004; **328**: 441

This randomised study of 635 patients in five UK general practices empowered patients ('patient activation') by giving them a leaflet before the consultation encouraging them to mention difficult issues. However, GPs worry about the clock and pressure to prescribe when activities like this go on.

Two leaflets were used – one general one which had an impact and one looking for depression which didn't.

The general leaflet increased patient satisfaction and communication and was more effective in shorter consultations. There was a small non-significant increase in consultation time and an increase in the number of investigations not thought to be strongly indicated by the doctor. There was no difference in prescribing or referral.

Effect of patient completed agenda forms and doctors' education about the agenda on the outcome of consultations: randomised controlled trial
Middleton JF, McKinley RK, Gillies CL
BMJ, 2006; **332**: 1238–1242

Two interventions were studied here: patients completing forms detailing their agenda for the consultation and doctors undergoing a one day workshop to help them recognise the layers of the patient's agenda (in terms of ideas, concerns, expectations and reasoning) and then negotiate a management plan.

In this randomised controlled trial of 46 UK practices and nearly 900 patients, using the forms added a minute to the consultation but more problems were identified and patients were more satisfied. Consultations were longer but still only took around five minutes per problem. However, the number of 'by the way, while I'm here' consultations were unchanged.

An accompanying editorial (*BMJ*, 2006; **332**: 1225–1226) comments that the form may be used to expand on the problem, select the desired outcome (prescription, explanation, investigation or certificate), or perhaps most usefully, allow all embarrassing problems to be voiced which may be the last item to be mentioned.

However, the efficiency gain is unclear from this study as we do not know if there was a successful reduction in future attendances. It is also possible that the extra problems are unnecessarily medicalised, as patients have been shown to have good judgement about whether or not to consult a doctor with their symptoms.

Importance of patient pressure and perceived pressure and perceived medical need for investigations, referral, and prescribing in primary care: nested observational study
Little P, Dorward M, Warner G et al.
BMJ, 2004; **328**: 444

This paper looked at the pressures on doctors in consultations.

They found that perceived medical need was the strongest predictor of behaviours of examination, prescribing and referral. However, after controlling for the actual preferences of patients, how doctors perceived pressure from patients also had an impact. Doctors felt there was little or no medical need for 15% of their examinations, 19% of their prescriptions, 22% of their referrals and nearly half their investigations.

Doctors need to work harder to elicit actual expectations from patients.

PERSONAL CARE

Qualitative study of the meaning of personal care in general practice
Tarrant C, Windridge K, Boulton M et al.
BMJ, 2003; **326**: 1310

NHS reorganisation may reduce continuity of care and therefore personal care but is this concept still valued?

Interviews with staff and patients were performed in six Leicestershire general practices.

They agreed that the three ingredients of personal care were human communication, tailored management and 'whole person' care.

- Good interpersonal skills, evidence of empathy and efforts to deal with someone as a person rather than as a patient went down well. This even enabled personal care to be provided by locum doctors in one-off consultations.
- Continuity of care was thought to be essential in long-term complex problems but busy people leading chaotic lives favoured quick access and were more likely to feel they could get personal care on a one-stop basis.
- Knowledge of the patients' social circumstances and family history was valued but this did not qualify as personal care unless opportunities were taken to refer back to this previous knowledge and build on it.
- Personal care was not always desirable particularly if the issue might cause embarrassment or damage the doctor–patient relationship.
- The wider practice team and receptionist in particular were very important in making care personal.

The authors conclude that practices should be able to provide continuity when patients desire it.

Personal knowledge

Sweeney K
BMJ, 2006; **332**: 129–130

Research has shown that doctors with personal experience of their warfarin patients undergoing a haemorrhage had lower odds of prescribing warfarin in the future. Yet adverse events associated with underusing warfarin do not exert the same influence.

This editorial expands the discussion that doctors are not simple conduits nor passive recipients for clinical evidence. They undergo an inner consultation where dramatic experiences which are easy to recall add a dimension of personal significance to more scientific evidence.

Two ways of 'knowing' – biomedical and biographical – compete for influence and personal judgements result in sometimes failing to follow through on that which is conventionally known.

The importance of patient preferences in treatment decisions – challenges for doctors

Say RE, Thomson R
BMJ, 2003; **327**: 542–545

Involving patients in treatment decisions poses several challenges looked into by this literature search and a set of interviews with doctors.

- Doctors may not have appropriate knowledge, ability to communicate risk or general interpersonal skills. Those with the right information to hand, however, were aware they could influence choices with their choice of language (and statistics).
- Patients for their part may get their information from websites but be unable to evaluate it. Doctors unskilled in debate may find it difficult to beat the persuasive but flawed evidence presented to them on the spot.
- Some patients see uncertainty in doctors as lack of confidence which undermines the relationship.
- Patient expectations may be unreasonable or may differ from guidelines or the doctor's opinion and this can create conflict. Such conflict between individual and societal needs is inevitable in a publicly funded NHS but an essential part of gatekeeping.
- Differences in education and experience may affect how a patient understands risk. Access to services is already known to be affected by sex, race and socioeconomic status and less successful articulation of preferences can further exacerbate inequality.
- Some patients do not even want to be involved in the process and we know that many doctors find difficulties eliciting such preferences.
- Add to this that most of the information dispensed is either forgotten or misremembered and it becomes obvious that new approaches are needed.

From research evidence to context: the challenge of individualising care
Weiner SJ
Evidence-Based Medicine, 2004; **9**: 132–133

This original article highlights the practical difficulties that may prevent implementation of evidence. Contextual issues include availability of transport, family support, drug interactions, ability to afford prescriptions, difficulty remembering to take tablets and a host of other factors that affect care.

A doctor can know how to apply evidence but assessment of cognitive abilities, emotional states, cultural and spiritual beliefs and social support may be much more crucial. Contextualising care in terms of so many variables is a challenge in the time available. The term 'categorisation' is used to describe the pairing of the label (diagnosis) with the best evidence (management). But clinical reasoning must extend to the next phase – 'discovery'. This examines the patient's life for elements relevant to the process and it is this that makes up the qualitative component of the clinical decision-making.

CHAPERONES

Chaperones: who needs them?
Richardson C
BMJ Career Focus, 2005; **330**:175–176

An accusation of inappropriate behaviour would be devastating for any doctor and would have far-reaching consequences for investigative proceedings and adverse publicity.

The Ayling report publicised in September 2004 provides recommendations on the back of an independent inquiry into a GP from Kent convicted of indecent assault and imprisoned for four years.

They recognise the patient's right to decline a chaperone as many find it intrusive and embarrassing. It recognised that a chaperone may not always be available and you may need to trust your instincts before performing an intimate examination (that is related to breast, genitalia or rectum). Defer examination if there are any concerns.

The report also stated that untrained administrative staff should not be expected to act as chaperones although to train them up would be acceptable. Similarly, family or friends should not be used in a formal chaperoning role. It may worsen embarrassment and lead to inadvertent breaches in confidentiality.

The chaperone should be introduced and the name documented in the notes.

Chaperones for intimate examinations: cross sectional survey of attitudes and practices of general practitioners
Rosenthal J, Rymer J, Jones R et al.
BMJ, 2005; **330**: 234–235

A questionnaire answered by over 1200 GPs in England revealed that for intimate examinations:
- only 37% of respondents had a policy on the use of chaperones

- two-thirds of males but only 5% of female GPs usually or always offered a chaperone
- over half the male doctors and only 2% of female doctors usually or always used one
- 8% of males and 70% of females never used one
- although practice nurses were most popular, family and friends were frequently used, as were administrative staff
- most never recorded the offer or the identity of the chaperone in the notes
- although use of chaperones has increased in the last decade, more flexible guidance is needed for GPs other than the universal recommendations from the royal colleges to always use chaperones for intimate examination

CONCORDANCE AND PRESCRIBING

What we know already:

- Half of all drugs are not taken as prescribed
- Most patients would prefer not to take any medicines and many try to minimise their doses
- As quickly as 10 days after prescription of a new medication, 30% of elderly chronic disease sufferers may not take it as prescribed. This was intentional in almost half of the cases
- There are massive consequences of this disparity in term of missed benefits and health economics
- Concordance describes an agreement which respects the beliefs and wishes of patients rather than the following of instructions
- Doctors mistakenly think they know what the patient's preferences are
- Many patients want to be involved in prescribing decisions but not all
- Patients for their part find it hard to adjust to their new role of drug-taker
- Doctors rarely discuss whether a patient will go along with a treatment plan
- Decision-making and concordance are dynamic concepts needing continual exploration and not are necessarily linked to a behavioural outcome
- Concordance is particularly challenging for preventative therapy in asymptomatic conditions and for those drugs with significant side effects, as increasing concordance increases side effects
- Low cost prescribers find it easier to refuse patients prescriptions and subscribe more strongly to the importance of a local consensus, a practice formulary and cost-consciousness
- Both high and low prescribers of new drugs considered themselves to have conservative prescribing behaviour
- Placebo comes from the Latin for 'I will please' and there has been little debate about their use

Recent Papers

CONCORDANCE

A meta-analysis of the association between adherence to drug therapy and mortality
Simpson SH, Eurich DT, Majumdar SR *et al.*
BMJ, 2006; **333**: 15–18

This meta-analysis of nearly 47 000 patients in 21 studies found that good adherence to medication was associated with lower mortality even if the tablets were placebos. This flies in the face of the theory that placebos do not influence health outcomes and supports the 'healthy adherer' theory that speculates that taking your tablets is an overall marker for generally healthy behaviour. This may manifest as better diet, exercise, follow-up, screening, immunisations and use of other drugs.

Mortality of good adherers was half that of patients with poor adherence.

Not to be taken as directed
Marinker M, Shaw J
BMJ, 2003; **326**: 348–349

Patients do not comply with medication for reasons which may be intentional or not. When drugs 'fail', doctors too often look to their own prescribing choices but it is time to recognise that it is the patients' agenda that determines whether medicine will be taken.

There can be conflict between being both patient-centred and evidence-based but we need to reconcile where the pharmacology meets the patient's desires and beliefs.

Doctors and patients needed to learn how to 'do concordance', but as yet there is no blueprint for this.

Analysis of polypharmacy in older patients in primary care using a multidisciplinary expert panel
Denneboom W, Dautzenberg M, Grol R *et al.*
Br J Gen Pract, 2006; **56**: 504–510

In this study an expert panel of pharmacists and physicians in the Netherlands looked at 102 older patients on multiple drug therapy. They found that:
- for almost all, improvement in pharmacotherapy could be made
- 30% of possible improvements were considered to be of 'direct clinical relevance'
- in 60% this involved adding another medicine to improve pharmacotherapy

The authors stress the need for regular medication reviews for older people in primary care.

Managing multiple morbidity in mid-life: a qualitative study of attitudes to drug use
Townsend A, Hunt K, Wyke S
BMJ, 2003; **327**: 837

Interviews with community-based middle-aged people in Scotland who had four or more chronic illnesses shed some light on the under-researched issue of how users view their use of medication.

Complex strategies were employed. Resourcefulness in stopping, varying or minimising doses was shown reflecting a widespread cultural belief that drugs should be used as little as possible. Self-regulation was common and might vary between the conditions the drugs were for.

All respondents expressed their dislike for drugs. Some feared dependency, side effects or interactions, but most acknowledged their need for drugs to improve their life or lifespan.

Insight into these tensions may help doctors to support the self-care of patients and optimise concordance.

Does a prescribed treatment match a patient's priorities?
Britten N
BMJ, 2003; **327**: 840

This commentary on the paper above describes several central notions:
- the futility of labelling patients as compliant or non-compliant when the same person may take one drug regularly while varying another
- the ambiguous yet powerful impact that taking medication has on people's identity
- patients organise drug taking around their own priorities which are often related to non-medical aspect of their lives
- clinicians need to use the consultation to engage with patients' priorities to find the real place of the proposed medication in the patients' life

Prescribing and taking medicines
Jones G
BMJ, 2003; **327**: 819

This editorial comments on our failure so far to execute a concordant strategy.

The problem may start with health professionals not having heard of the term or not understanding it.

Information pathways may be shared but does the internet with all its inaccuracies, irrelevancies, biases and contradictions really mean people are better informed?

Do we even sing from the same hymn sheet in the real world or is it possible that our advice on drug taking is contradicted 10 minutes later by a pharmacist?

Do doctors accept smaller benefits than patients in preventative health care?

Are we surprised that asymptomatic patients do not persist with preventative medication?

When the patient is a child, how can we communicate well enough to allow concordance with a third party – parents?

More questions than answers I am afraid.

Factors involved in deciding to start preventive treatment: qualitative study of clinicians' and lay people's attitudes
Lewis DK, Robinson J, Wilkinson E
BMJ, 2003; **327**: 841

This paper looks at the opinion of Liverpool GPs, nurses and lay people when given information on the benefits of starting a drug to treat an asymptomatic risk factor for heart attacks.

This is useful information as we have little understanding of the rationale behind patient's decisions. It found that:
- there is an enormous variation in what is considered a minimal acceptable benefit to patients regarding taking a drug long term. Some would only take a 'perfect' treatment.
- many dislike the idea of taking pills and preferred options of lifestyle change
- few doctors or lay people knew that increased length of treatment meant increased benefit (absolute benefit roughly doubles over double the time)

- 10 year estimates of risk inflate apparent benefits of treatment (assuming 30% risk reduction in patients with a 10 year coronary risk of 30% means 9 out of 10 patients take the drug for 10 years with no benefit)
- doctors accepted lower benefits from medication than lay people or nurses
- doctors made more confident decisions but not necessarily more logical or consistent ones
- high quality decision-sharing dialogue is required to bridge the gaps between guidelines and patients

INTERVENTIONS

Interventions to enhance medication adherence
Haynes R, Yao X, Degani A, *et al.*
Cochrane Database Syst Rev, Oct 2005

A Cochrane review of 49 RCTs confirmed that around half of the interventions used improved adherence to medication, but only one-third of interventions improved any of the outcomes.

Almost all of the effective interventions for long-term care were complex, including combinations of more convenience, better information, reminders and reinforcement, self-monitoring, counselling and psychological therapies, crisis intervention and telephone follow-up.

With such improvements still being fairly small, the full benefits of treatment are limited and new methods of achieving concordance are required.

PLACEBOS

Sham device v inert pill: randomised controlled trial of two placebo treatments
Kaptchuk TJ, Stason WB, Davis RB *et al.*
BMJ, 2006; **332**: 391–397

A study of 270 patients with arm pain compared two placebos treatments – acupuncture with a sham device and inert pills (pretending that they might be amitriptyline). In the long run, there was a larger improvement in reported (subjective) symptoms in those using the sham acupuncture device. The superiority of one placebo over another implies that the rituals involved may be of key importance.

Questionnaire survey on use of placebo
Nitzan U, Lichtenberg P
BMJ, 2004; **329**: 944–946

This study was performed in Israel and the questionnaire administered in Hebrew. Interview of 89 physicians and nurses revealed:
- 60% prescribed placebos such as saline infusions and vitamin C tablets for a wide-ranging array of conditions
- 68% of these prescribers told their patients they were receiving an actual medication

- 28% used them as a diagnostic tool to uncover 'real' pain or treat suspected pseudoseizures
- 94% found them effective
- only 5% thought placebos should be banned

The authors argue for the legitimacy of placebo use in therapeutics or at least for more debate in this ethical minefield. Should we have bans or guidelines for use?

Placebos in practice

Spiegel D
BMJ, 2004; **329**: 927–928

There is controversy about using biologically inert substances therapeutically. This editorial accompanies the paper above and follows up the claim that placebos are in widespread use. Those of us who assumed that the use of placebos had been all but stamped out by 20th century medicine and relegated to coffee-break anecdote seem hopelessly and slightly worryingly misguided. And yet only about half of all medical treatments are evidence-based.

The concept of placebo responders being healthy, histrionic dimwits is not supported by research. It even has its own industry which incorporates many holistic 'therapies' that harness and market the effect and that are increasingly capturing the public's 'imagination'. Its evil brother – the nocebo effect – describes negative expectations producing negative results. This, so far, has failed to find much of a market share except in a sadomasochistic minority.

A US body recently called for research to optimise use of the placebo phenomenon while attending to the ethical considerations.

Most easy to criticise was the claim that use of placebos helped to differentiate organic pain from psychogenic pain. This involves concepts of pain long since discredited.

New scientific domains such as psychoneuroimmunology and psychoneuroendocrinology are helping to explain the mechanisms of how the mind affects the body and explain associations between, for example, depression and cancer that have been recognised for years.

Deception is not necessary for the placebo effect but ethical considerations need looking at.

Can we afford to dispense with any interventions that work?

Why do doctors use treatments that do not work?

Doust J, Del Mar C
BMJ, 2004; **328**: 474–475

Why? Well, how about:
- the need to do something (and the difficulty of doing nothing) in the face of perceived expectation. Are errors of omission 'worse' than errors of commission?
- using our personal clinical experience (which is a poor judge of what works and what doesn't)

- being misled by the pathophysiological approach, e.g. the apparent contraindication of beta-blockers in heart failure, now dismissed by high quality trials
- harms are sometimes uncovered too late, e.g. HRT for cardiovascular protection
- nobody thinks to ask the question

TEAMWORK AND MORALE

What we know already:

- Working with other GPs in practices of increasing size has become *de rigueur* in the NHS
- Partnerships reduce professional isolation and provide the opportunity for a supportive environment
- A major reason for new GPs to express regret at joining a practice is the stress from the partnership where complex interactions as well as personal style influence morale
- Other grievances in doctors relate to pay, workload and ever-increasing patient demand
- Personal morale and ability to cope with workload depends on fairness in allocation of work and remuneration – a topic often too emotive to discuss
- A general lack of respect for the medical profession has been perceived by some and compounded by media reports
- GPs are at risk of high levels of stress and burnout. They have a tendency to deny personal illness, to self-prescribe and have a high suicide rate
- Managers are under increasing pressure to reach new targets and achieve major structural reform
- Doctors do not like to give up professional autonomy to managers. Management styles that make doctors unhappy may adversely affect quality of care

Recent Papers

JOB SATISFACTION

Selecting and supporting contented doctors
Peile E, Carter Y
BMJ, 2005; **330**: 269–270

Unhappy doctors underperform and can drag their colleagues down with them according to this editorial.

However, much of the perception of the stress in their lives can be directly attributed to their own personality, according to research on over 1600 medical graduates followed up 12 years after they had entered medical school. The trait of neuroticism, for example, predicts a disordered approach to work and perceptions of high workload and stress. Perhaps if we cannot socially engineer to fill medical schools with easy going contended candidates (after all where are we to get our supply of academics from?), we should use this psychological profiling to identify those in need of help. A process of mentoring and appraisal with the chief aim of supporting doctors and students can detect unhappiness early and do something to effect change.

National survey of job satisfaction and retirement intentions among general practitioners in England
Sibbald B, Bojke C, Gravelle H
BMJ, 2003; **326**: 22–24

This postal survey compared intentions to quit in UK GPs and was able to compare its results on two occasions. They noted an increase in those intending to quit in the next 5 years from 14% in 1998 to 22% in 2001.

Factors associated with a higher intention were older age (obviously) and ethnic minority status. The rise was mainly due to reduction in job satisfaction followed by a slight increase in the number of ethnic doctors and in the mean age.

Those with higher job satisfaction and children under 18 were less likely to throw in the towel.

The results also reflect societal change towards early retirement and more flexible patterns of work.

Threats are threats (and doctors may still stay in healthcare in some other capacity) but previous research has shown strong associations of intention to quit with actual action.

PRACTICE RELATIONSHIPS

General practitioners' perceptions of sharing workload in group practices: qualitative study
Branson R, Armstrong D
BMJ, 2004; **329**: 381

Hats off to the authors! This paper looks at a how GP partners get on with each other. Not generally without resentments and resignations of one kind or the other, it seems.

All the 18 GPs who agreed to be interviewed recognised the problems of inequitable distribution of workload. The most common cause of tension was between 'fast consulters', who felt they inherited extra visits, appointments and more repeat prescriptions, and 'slow consulters' who saw themselves as providing a higher quality service with more stress resulting from attending to psychosocial issues.

Doctors were irritated when covering a fast consulter's clinic made them realise they were bringing patients back for trivia.

Perceived inequality is a major source of resentment and stress in general practice but erosion of trust is shared with many areas of modern society. Interestingly, legitimate data fails to back up perceptions of being a harder worker with actual facts. The conclusion is that workload is not as misallocated as presumed.

Small practices needing more flexibility between colleagues in order to provide a full service relied on mutual trust to manage this hurdle. Larger practices had more rigid systems that allowed them to predict workload. Some even allocated points linked to financial rewards, but fairness still depended on who designed the system.

Practice meetings could be useful to air grievances but a lot of lengthy meetings became self-defeating and increased stress levels.

Ultimately, solutions to the problem depended on a cyclical acceptance of periods of contentment and resentment or, like any other marriage, divorce.

I like the comment in the rapid responses: "[In the complex work of general practice] if you don't think you are working harder than your partners then you're not working hard enough".

MANAGEMENT COLLEAGUES

Managing change in the culture of general practice: qualitative case studies in primary care trusts
Marshall MN, Mannion R, Nelson E *et al.*
BMJ, 2003; **327**: 599–602

This is an excellent look at management styles and how they apply to the NHS infrastructure. Interviews with 39 senior and middle managers in six primary care trusts identified two distinct and polarised styles.

A directive style:
- an authoritarian style characteristic of hierarchical organisations
- most of these were senior managers driven by political imperatives
- more likely to see doctors as obstacles to be overcome rather than relating problems to organisational or environmental factors
- may effectively achieve short-term measurable change at a cost of conflict with doctors and dysfunctional consequences

A facilitative style:
- more characteristic of a clan-type culture
- more likely to facilitate change from within rather than forcing it from outside
- keen to achieve a collaborative co-operation with attention to the values of those that deliver health services
- accepts this is a complex but important time-consuming task and dismisses quick fixes
- middle managers needed these skills, as they had to negotiate with those with the power to achieve their aims
- most of these were middle managers acting as 'buffers' between health professionals and senior managers
- more likely to see problems as environmental and organisational rather than relating them to attitudes of an individual
- they were more likely to be able to perceive an individual's ability to cope with change, but risked oversensitivity to the demands of conservative professionals

Opposing styles can lead to tensions between tiers of management. Facilitative middle managers were more likely to see seniors as being out of touch. Sound familiar? The authors conclude that primary care trusts should value versatile, high quality facilitative managers who can be partners in the complex reform of the culture of the NHS.

Doctors and managers: a problem without a solution?

Edwards N, Marshall M, McLellan A *et al.*
BMJ, 2003; **326**: 609–610

This editorial accompanied the BMJ theme issue on doctors and managers. The authors describe the paradox of a call for common values between doctors and managers and the need to recognise that each group thinks differently.

Badly managed organisations fail patients and are at least as lethal as bad clinical practice. Yet if doctors prioritise delivery of policy over the patient in front of them, then quality of care and public support would evaporate.

Traditional values differ. Doctors focus on patients, desire professional autonomy and work towards evidence-based practice, while yearning for a bygone age when managers knew their place. Managers look at allocating resources to populations and the need for public accountability.

Patients are best served by a tension between the doctors and managers.

To bridge the gap, everyone from educators to government need to work hard to improve dialogue, mutual respect and the ability to live with different points of view.

ACCESSING CARE

What we know already:

- Critics have worried about legitimising demand for minor illness and fragmenting care
- Walk-in centres were introduced in the NHS in 2000, partly to reduce demand on GPs and A&E
- Although popular with the public, a government report, 'Improving Emergency Care in England', confirms primary care demand is higher than ever and recent services such as NHS Walk-in centres have failed to relieve pressure
- NHS Direct is a direct access health advice line with nurse advisers using computerised decision support systems to advise callers. It is popular, safe and expensive
- Both walk-in centres and NHS Direct improved access for the white middle class but may have increased health inequalities
- Between 6% and 10% of patients in primary care are referred to a specialist
- Nearly two-thirds of general and acute hospital beds are occupied by people over 65. Average length of stay in the UK is more than twice that in the US where there is greater use of intermediate care facilities
- A shared care model with a GP liaising with specialists improves clinical skills, is a logical use of resources and can reduce investigation, referral and follow-up. It improves treatment strategies, patient satisfaction and concordance although cost-effectiveness is unclear
- Joint consultations between GPs and consultants can improve patient management with fewer investigations, referrals and follow up
- Requests for laboratory analysis in the UK went up by over 80% between 2000 and 2004, raising concerns that some primary care doctors are investigating inappropriately

Guidance

Advanced Access – This model from the National Primary Care Collaborative aims to reduce waiting times and allow greater control over how demand from patients is addressed. Appointment capacity is balanced with demand on a daily basis reducing non-attendance and home visits while increasing satisfaction all round.

Those practices implementing the model have shown, for example, that triaging requests for same-day appointments by telephone can reduce face-to-face consultations by up to half and follow-ups by 20%.

Recent Papers

ADVANCED ACCESS

Preferences for access to the GP: a discrete choice experiment
Rubin G, Bate A, George A *et al.*
Br J Gen Pract, 2006; **56**: 743–748

The NHS Plan states patients should be able to see a health professional within 24 hours and a GP within 48 hours. How this competes with patients who prefer flexibility in choosing their timing and doctor is unclear.

This study of six practices in Sunderland found that the waiting time until an available appointment was only important for children and new health problems. Others would happily wait longer to see their own choice of doctor or choose their own time. This was particularly important for those who worked – they valued it six times more important than the waiting time. It was also of particular importance for those with a chronic illness, women and the elderly.

Evaluation of advanced access in the national primary care collaborative
Pickin M, O'Cathain A, Sampson FC *et al.*
Br J Gen Pract, 2004; **54**: 334–340

Practices in this programme were more likely to be training practices and less likely to serve urban or deprived populations.

Data from about 400 practices implementing Advanced Access has shown:
- improved availability of GP appointments by showing times to the third available appointment shortened from 3.6 days to 1.9 days
- availability improved in 66% and worsened in 18% of practices
- increased sense of control over workload, benefits for staff morale and perceptions of increased patient satisfaction
- it was well-received by most GPs, although 39% thought it involved an excessive amount of work and 1 in 12 would not recommend it
- concerns were expressed about favouring immediate access over continuity and offering easier appointments for trivia at the expense of reviewing chronic patients
- some were concerned that the improvements were cosmetic as same day appointments may have been bookable on the day only

---

Open-access versus bookable appointment systems: survey of patients attending appointments with general practitioners
Pascoe SW, Neal RD, Allgar VL
Br J Gen Pract, 2004; **54**: 367–369

This study included over 800 patients and looked at preference for open-access (non-bookable) appointments compared with bookable appointments.

It was bookable appointments that were reported to be more convenient for patients and unsurprisingly more patients with these planned appointments saw their doctor of choice. One-fifth of patients felt they were not seen as soon as they should have been regardless of group.

The findings support use of a combined appointment system offering choice. Patients have been shown in other research to have a good sense of when they value continuity over speed of access.

Implementation of Advanced Access in general practice: postal survey of practices
Goodal S, Montgomery A, Banks J *et al.*
Br J Gen Pract, 2006; **56**: 918–923

This survey, to which 63% of 391 UK practices replied, found few differences between those claiming to be offering Advanced Access (two-thirds) and those who made no such claim. Both types of practice had made a wide range of measures to improve access to appointments. The Advanced Access group has more appointments available on the same day but less than half had used all four of the recommendations – measuring demand, matching capacity to demand, managing demand in different ways, and contingency planning.

WALK-IN CENTRES

Effect of NHS walk-in centre on local primary healthcare services: before and after observational study
Hsu RT, Lambert PC, Dixon-Woods M *et al.*
BMJ, 2003; **326**: 530–532

This observational study looked for changes in consultation rates in A&E, general practice and a minor injury unit when a walk-in centre was opened nearby. They compared results to a town without one.
- The centre was well-used but there was no luck for the GPs: their workload did not change.
- Neither did it affect the number of calls to NHS Direct or out of hours services. A&E attendances seemed to go up.
- The only clear difference was an increase in attendance at the local minor injury clinic which was in the same building.
- Fears of a major increase in demand or hopes of a decrease seem unjustified.

At best, walk-in centres may still have a role in uncovering certain types of demand for particular care needs. Our chances of spotting these needs and then showing that the approach is cost-effective are not looking good.

Walk-in centres in primary care: a review of the international literature
Salisbury C, Munro J
Br J Gen Pract, 2003; **53**: 53–59

Review of the international literature on walk-in centres shows that users tend to be a more affluent group of working age but are a different population from conventional users of general practice.

They used the service particularly when other options are closed and mainly for minor illness and injury. People like the convenience and the quality of care tends to be reasonable. But even in countries that have had walk-in centres for a long time, there is a dearth of research on important issues such as cost-effectiveness and how they could develop a clearer role in the future.

TELEPHONE TRIAGE

NHS Direct versus general practice based triage for same day appointments in primary care: cluster randomised controlled trial
Richards DA, Godfrey L, Tawfik J et al.
BMJ, 2004; **329**: 774

In-house telephone triage by practice nurses is effective but no cheaper than standard appointment systems for screening requests for same day appointments.

Delivering a truly comprehensive service would involve expanding this to an off-site service. That service is NHS Direct. But is it effective and is it worth the expense?

This trial from York randomised nearly 5000 callers to one service or the other and found that external management by NHS Direct was feasible but only at a higher cost.

Management options were to refer to a nurse or a GP for a phone call, appointment or home visit.

NHS Direct nurse advisers:
- were less likely to resolve the problem on the phone and more likely to recommend a GP appointment
- took around 7 minutes longer to triage a patient using complex algorithms. This was two and a half times longer than a practice nurse
- did not achieve equivalent outcomes to, and cost more than, practice-based triage

Practice nurses had the advantage of being able to access the medical record and provide a personal flexible service based on previous knowledge of the patient. They could also book a slot to see the caller themselves and use their own competences more efficiently knowing there was always a GP nearby. This seems like the closest thing we have to an ideal option.

NHS Direct on the other hand tended not to refer to nurses. Most NHS Direct nurses had never worked in general practice.

Survey of the impact of nurse telephone triage on general practitioner activity
Richards DA, Meakins J, Godfrey L et al.
Br J Gen Pract, 2004; **54**: 207–210

Delegation of management of minor illness to nurses may result in a change in patients' presenting problems and have consequences for the GP.

This paper from the same York-based team as above looked at the practice records before and after introduction of a nurse telephone triage system.

It found that patients seen by GPs after introduction of the triage system had a higher number of presenting complaints and received more consultations, prescriptions, and investigations. Numbers of referrals were unchanged.

Appointment systems may have to be adjusted to ensure this particular 'distillation' of patients receive the time they appear to need from their GP.

Evaluation of a general practitioner with special interest service for dermatology: randomised controlled trial
Salisbury C, Noble A, Horrocks S *et al.*
BMJ, 2005; **331**: 1441–1446

This study randomised non-urgent skin problems to a GP with special interest in dermatology (as introduced by the NHS Plan in 2000) or care from a hospital consultant dermatologist. There was no noticeable difference in quality of care or clinical outcome, but the GP service was considerably more accessible with appointments around 40 days earlier. Patients also expressed slightly greater satisfaction for the GP service after 9 months. Only 12% of the GP's patients needed to be referred on to the hospital but this affected the economic analysis which made the GP service more costly than hospital care.

JOINT CONSULTATIONS

Virtual outreach: economic evaluation of joint teleconsultations for patients referred by their general practitioner for a specialist opinion
Jacklin PB, Roberts JA, Wallace P *et al.*
BMJ, 2003; **327**: 84

Over 2000 people were randomised to 'virtual outreach' (videoconferencing between doctors and patients) or standard conventional outpatient care.
    After a 6 month period, there were:
  • greater total costs for virtual outreach by over £100 per patient due mainly to clinicians' time
  • fewer investigations in the virtual outreach group
  • significantly lower transport costs, childcare costs and loss of pay in the virtual outreach arm
  • no significant differences in prescription costs or number of clinical contacts
  • no differences in health outcomes
Widespread adoption of virtual outreach cannot yet be justified in the NHS on economic grounds. Improved selection of patients and clinical speciality may improve its value in the future.

INDEPENDENT FEEDBACK

Effect of enhanced feedback and brief educational reminder messages on laboratory test requesting in primary care: a cluster randomised trial
Thomas R, Croal B, Ramsay C *et al.*
Lancet, 2006; **367**: 1990–1996

Feedback from laboratory services can help to reduce the number of tests ordered. This study chose nine such tests. It directed feedback to the GPs in the form of helpful educational tips about the test and attached it to the test results. It also produced a quarterly report on the number of investigations ordered, enhanced with graphs comparing their practice's request rates with the region as a whole. It compared the impact of these measures alone and together with no intervention in 85 Scottish practices and 370 GPs. Both measures fared equally well and together reduced requests by around 20%.

EARLY DISCHARGE

Discharge destination and length of stay: differences between US and English hospitals for people aged 65 and over
Jarman B, Aylin P, Bottle A
BMJ, 2004; **328**: 605

In the US, 39% of patients are discharged from hospital to intermediate care compared with 10% in England. People are more likely to die out of hospital in the US with in-hospital death rates of 5% compared to 9% in England.

Using community facilities and other forms of non-inpatient care could allow earlier discharge and alleviate pressure on hospitals. Strong financial incentives exist in the US to facilitate this and as a result, mean length of hospital stay is more than halved compared to the UK.

Admission rates were similar in the two countries suggesting that the Americans are not admitting more trivial cases. These figures could have implications for the choice of environment in which we care for elderly people in the future and lead to a significant impact on primary care resources.

MISSED APPOINTMENTS

Missed appointments in primary care: questionnaire and focus group study of health professionals
Husain-Gambles M, Neal RD, Dempsey O, *et al.*
Br J Gen Pract, 2003; **54**: 108–113

It is a wonderful thing when a patient does not turn up and you have a chance for a breather. But far from being a stress-relieving gift from the heavens, it turns out that this is, in fact, a waste of resources.

The authors sent out a questionnaire to practice staff which showed that:
- GPs felt that patients usually missed their appointments because they forgot or couldn't be bothered
- waiting area notices with information on how many appointments were wasted were seen as effective
- there were prevalent negative attitudes towards the "offenders" and most felt some sort of punishment was in order
- receptionists felt strongly that doctors should sort the patients out by addressing the problem in the next consultation but doctors did not really fancy the idea.

Reasons for and consequences of missed appointments in general practice in the UK: questionnaire survey and prospective review of medical records
Neal RD, Hussain-Gambles M, Allgar VL, *et al.*
BMC Fam Pract, 2005; **6**: 47

A postal survey of nearly 400 patients who missed appointments achieved a return rate of around one-third.

Over 40% of these said they had forgotten the appointment and around one-quarter said that they had tried to cancel it. Over 90% went on to consult in the next three months. More than half came with the original problem. Measures such as reminders, greater freedom with appointments and making cancellations easier might help. Disengaged groups may be potentially vulnerable.

FUTURE OF GENERAL PRACTICE

What we know already:

- The evidence shows that patients value 'humaneness' in their doctors above all other qualities. They want GPs who engage, take time, explain and have up-to-date skills
- Although younger patients are willing to trade continuity for faster access, older ones particularly value continuity of care
- Patients want a service that will be there when they need it which is free at the point of delivery
- They tend to resist structural change that undermines the foundations of the NHS, but major structural review of the delivery of primary care is well under way
- Associations between practice size and quality of care have not been consistently demonstrated. Research has implied that size of practice does not itself impact on the quality of chronic disease management
- Marked improvements in quality of care of chronic disease in UK general practice has been shown between 1998 and 2003 after measuring a host of variables
- The new GMS contract of 2004 constitutes the biggest change in primary care for decades. Financial incentives are closely linked to improvements in quality

Guidance

The future of general practice. A Statement by the Royal College of General Practitioners. **London: RCGP, September 2004**
(www.rcgp.org.uk/PDF/Corp_future_of_general_practice.pdf)

Investing in general practice—the new general medical services contract
(www.nhsconfed.org/docs/contract.pdf)

Recent Papers

Who needs health care—the well or the sick?
Heath I
BMJ, 2005; **330**: 954–956

This beautifully poetic article is well worth a read.

Dr Heath suggests there is a paradox that the more we concentrate on health at the expense of some of the other joys of living, the unhealthier we become. Rich countries are swept along in the 'excessive self confidence of preventative medicine' which could be tipping them towards a 'foundation of fear' and misery. Self-reporting of illness can be too low in poorer nations but is extremely high in the United States despite their health care never having been more advanced.

The measure of health care in rich countries seems to have become the simple prolongation of life. Swarms of protocols seem to express certainties where they do not exist and this may be a form of bullying. Bullying by doctors, by politicians and by multinationals who may have a lot to gain from the medicalisation of populations into the 'worried well'. We live in a time where more money is invested into research into the prevention of disease than into treatments. Money that could make a huge difference to poorer nations contributes towards relabelling risk factors as the latest illness.

As each generation looks back on the ignorance of the last, are we really sure we are doing more good than harm? Are we really addressing our patients' concerns? Or just doing everyone a favour by saying we can deliver life from its inherent thrill – uncertainty?

Competition in general practice
Marshall M, Wilson T.
BMJ, 2005; **331**:1196–1199

This is one of the articles under the issue banner 'The NHS Revolution' and looks at how competition might affect general practice. Alternative models of primary care have already arrived in communities that have failed to replace retiring GPs and challenged the priority of continuity of care which has been so successful in minimising competitive forces at the expense of patient choice.

General practice performs well in term of equity (although some inequalities remain), efficiency (where it is one of the most cost-effective healthcare systems in the developed world, with its emphasis on dealing with uncertainty and rationing expensive services), and quality (where clinical governance is starting to bear fruit).

But other models could be used:
- Commercial takeover, e.g. by a high street retailer or pharmaceutical company
- Mergers of existing practices allowing a common executive team
- Hospital-based services with primary care clinics closely linked to hospitals
- Population-specific services in which a provider might deliver all services aimed at a specific age group, e.g. teenagers
- Condition-specific services – where independent providers might deliver hypertension clinics or investigative facilities

The trade off in personal care might suit those who want technically efficient, accessible care. But fragmentation might lead to exacerbation of inequalities and reduce care for the growing number of people with comorbidities. And if general practice has been as cost-effective as it is claimed, new entrants in the market may be unable to compete with current providers.

Either way, the monopoly is disappearing and the article opines that positive things will come of integrated measures such as takeovers and mergers. Negative effects are more likely with different packages of care coming from different directions such as population-specific and condition-specific approaches.

PRACTICE SIZE

The future of singlehanded general practices
Majeed A
BMJ, 2005; **330**: 1460–1461

This editorial is a good summary of the position regarding single-handed practices.

Between 2003 and 2004 the proportion of such practices in the UK fell to 6% with a larger fall over that one year than in the preceding nine years. Yet the value of such doctors in communities, especially rural and inner city practices, has been unquestionable. Although they have the shadow of Harold Shipman leering over them, the balance of evidence for general practices does not insist that bigger is better. Government recommendations to do something about the clinical isolation of single-handed practitioners flies in the face of a well-liked service that offers patients a choice (at a time when choice is quite a popular idea) and has been found by patients to be more accessible and deliver higher rates of satisfaction than larger practices.

Doctors may well like the flexibility of working in a large practice to allow time for family or other interests as well as the opportunity to work with more support staff. But for those that might choose single-handed practice, perhaps the market rather than the government should decide their fate. Good comparative information on measures of quality of care will identify those underperforming. Perhaps in the future these data will even be published so patients can vote with their feet. Single-handed practices can then die a fair and equitable death. But who would bet against them flourishing? Nearly half the family practitioners in the US are single-handed.

Determinants of primary medical care quality measured under the new UK contract: cross sectional study
Sutton M, McLean G
BMJ, 2006; **332**: 389–390

This study in 60 Scottish general practices found that higher quality scores were obtained in deprived areas (contrary to early concerns that the new contract would increase health inequalities) and where the teams of doctors and practice nurses were larger. Practices with fewer than four full time clinicians had lower recorded quality.

Factors not statistically associated with quality were accreditation, training status and age of the GP. This implies that the size and the composition of the clinical team are the most important determinants of the quality of primary medical care. We should focus on this structure when looking to the future.

CHILDREN

Primary care for children in the 21st century
Hall D, Sowden D
BMJ, 2005; **330**: 430–431

This editorial opens with a pat on the back for the model of general practice and then goes on to say how inadequate it will be in treating the children of the 21st century. It proposes that the lack of 24 hour care will mean more and more concerned parents will bypass primary care in favour of a trip to the hospital.

It suggests that GPs do not have a major role in managing chronic disorders in children and while the preventative care may be fine, this can easily be taken over by health visitors and other non-medical staff.

Teenagers need special attention and, despite some practices making an effort to make things more accessible in sensitive areas such as sexual health, clinics not attached to 'the doctor's' seem to be more popular with adolescents.

We are told that tomorrow's parents will expect their doctor to have 'confirmed competencies in acute and non-urgent children's care particularly psychological disorders and chronic disease'. It proposes the abandoning of the concept of the whole family doctor in favour of a new generation of general paediatricians who can work in the community as well as in hospitals.

It is written by a professor of community paediatrics.

VISIONS OF PRIMARY CARE IN 2015

The following articles appear as part of a themed *BMJ* discussing possible futures for general practice.

Good general practitioners will continue to be essential
Lakhani M, Baker M
BMJ, 2006; **332**: 41–43

These authors argue there will still be a need for care from a doctor with whom they have a relationship. Care will flow from a relationship-based model which commits to interpersonal care and becomes more necessary as health care becomes more complex. Patients will take part in planning health services and assessing quality as well as self-management of chronic illness.

The unique skills of GPs are dealing with uncertainty and managing comorbidity. Cost-effective management of undifferentiated problems will be more important than ever. There will be more mediation with specialists and GPs will work within communities to develop partnerships to promote an agenda for health in schools and workplaces.

A broader range of professionals will be based in primary care and providing a range of skills in an integrated fashion at a convenient location close to home will be crucial to match what the public requires. Virtually all problems including mental health will be dealt with in primary care, with short term referral to specialists as needed. Interfaces of care are dangerous for patients and primary care clinicians. Good clinicians will help prevent fragmentation of care using intelligent systems which ensure quality and accountability.

The magic roundabout
Lapsley P
BMJ, 2006; **332**: 43–44

In 2015, unreasonable targets to be seen by a doctor within 2 days have been dropped due to effectively penalising working patients. Working out of hours has been made more attractive to GPs. Patients have finally been recognised to have responsibilities as well as rights in terms of leading healthy lifestyles, turning up for appointments and conforming with care plans. This seems to have started with the ban on smoking in public places.

Health promotion messages have started to hit home and alternative health practices have been coordinated into NHS new age clinics which are well placed to provide practical advice on diet and fitness, as well as offering services such as acupuncture and chiropractic. Doctors and nurses are free to spend more time with patients who really are partners in their own health care.

General practice under pressure
Meldrum H
BMJ, 2006; **332**: 46–47

A darker vision is that of GPs feeling undervalued due to eroded incomes and ongoing political interference.

Charges have been introduced for many non-essential items including sickness certificates. Mobile video phones allow consultations with healthcare professionals in their practice and, if investigations are needed, patients visit a mobile resource centre which feeds results back to the practice.

The clutches of the private sector are extending as Tesco Health takes over a failing NHS Direct. NHS facilities have found it difficult to compete with an aggressive cherry-picking private sector but a few larger practices (with many more salaried doctors) have succeeded in radically improving the number and quality of services offered.

INFORMATION TECHNOLOGY

What we know already:

- Evidence is awaited on how best to translate the potential of technology into daily care
- Over 90% of doctors use computers in clinical care and over 90% of prescriptions are now issued on computers
- Computers have already increased safe prescribing by as much as 60% with legible, complete prescriptions
- The NHS Plan, NSFs and NHS information strategy all promote use of electronic patient records
- Work is in progress for an integrated care record service for the use of all NHS staff
- Health information is some of the most retrieved information on the internet. Patients use it to check the experiences of others, identify questions to ask the doctors and check their advice and treatment
- Online discussion groups for 'e-patients' can be highly organised and complex
- Electronic medical records in general practice contain inaccuracies in 40% of their summaries
- The internet comes with the appealing characteristics of 24 hour availability and privacy and the unappealing ones of poor quality sites and unscrupulous marketing
- Online learning for patients can produce objectively measured changes in behaviour as well as knowledge that are at least as good as learning 'live'

Recent Papers

What next for electronic communication and health care?
Jadad AR, Delamothe T
BMJ, 2004; **328**: 1143–1144

This editorial for the technology theme issue of the *BMJ* glances over several points raised by the papers that were submitted.
- Most papers focus on measures far removed from health outcomes.
- Assessment of clinical gains from use of decision software and hardware is seriously lacking.
- New tools for old tricks may be 'acceptable' for doctors but that is hardly a measure of a revolution in clinical care.
- Technologies may move too rapidly to make randomised controlled trials as useful as we need them to be, outpacing our ability to judge them.
- When things go wrong, people blame the technology. Focus on gadgets needs to shift to focus on people.
- To use these advances, we need to change behaviour and incorporate the human element.
- Impact on doctors' workload, income, liability and quality of life are under-addressed.
- Elderly and disabled people are most disenfranchised by new online communication tools.

Soft paternalism and the ethics of shared electronic patient records
Norheim OF
BMJ, 2006; **333**: 2–3

> This paper discusses the ethics relating to the proposed network of integrated databases regarding patients records.
>
> Rapid access to a single resource may improve quality of care but also makes patients vulnerable when records contain sensitive private information.
>
> They note that the Royal College of General Practitioners strongly recommends an 'opt in' policy for citizens whereas Connecting For Health, the agency building the new electronic records service, wants an 'opt-out' policy.
>
> Standard medical ethics suggests that where the path is unclear the public should be fully informed and only be included if they give explicit consent. This preserves freedom of choice, but as people are not always rational and may be too lazy to make a well-informed opinion, their health and welfare may suffer. On the other hand, automatic opt-in without the possibility to opt out promotes health and welfare at the cost of liberty
>
> This article puts the case for 'soft paternalism', automatically opting people in unless they strongly disagree. This preserves freedom of choice and promotes health.
>
> However, there are some caveats. The NHS must convincingly show that technical and legal safeguards are bulletproof and that the control of access is strict and transparent.

The electronic patient record in primary care – regression or progression?
A cross sectional study
Hippisley-Cox J, Pringle M, Cater R *et al.*
BMJ, 2003; **326**: 1439–1443

> This review examined the use of electronic records by 53 GPs in 25 practices in the UK to see if concerns over briefer note-taking and lesser engagement with the consultation were valid. They were not.
>
> In fact, paperless records compared very favourably with paper-based systems.
>
> They were more understandable and fully legible. They contained more information in terms of diagnoses, advice, referral details and drug doses. They contained significantly more words, abbreviations and symbols.
>
> Written records might stimulate memories of consultations through pattern recognition but this was not shown to be so. Paperless doctors could recall more of the advice they gave to patients.
>
> Generally GPs remembered fewer than 1 in 5 patients and 1 in 20 specific consultations implying that the doctor–patient relationship may not be as personal as many think.

Patients' experiences when accessing their on-line electronic patient records in primary care
Pyper C, Amery J, Watson M et al.
Br J Gen Pract, 2004; **54**: 38–43

This study gave 100 patients private access to their electronic records in a secure facility to see how they felt about it.

Most found viewing their record useful and understood most of the content after medical terms and abbreviations were explained. They expressed worries about security, confidentiality and potential exploitation of the information.

Many expected more detail, wanted to add their own information and identified errors most of which were not medically significant.

ELECTRONIC PRESCRIBING

Prescribing safety features of general practice computer systems: evaluation using simulated test cases
Fernando B, Savelyich BSP, Avery AJ et al.
BMJ, 2004; **328**: 1171–1172

This study tested four different general practice computer systems with 18 scenarios which highlighted the use of alerts. Unfortunately they kept quiet which system was which. No one system detected all the important potential prescribing errors. They conclude that these systems, which serve three-quarters of UK general practices, have important deficiencies.

Better system design that matches the patient record with external sources of data is needed to improve safety features.

Warnings need to be relevant and prioritised in order to be useful on an everyday basis.

Electronic transfer of prescription-related information: comparing views of patients, general practitioners, and pharmacists
Porteous T, Bond C, Robertson R et al.
Br J Gen Pract, 2003; **53**: 204–209

This Scottish study questioned 800 lay people, 200 GPs and 200 community pharmacists with a response rate of around 70%. They wanted opinions on electronic transfer of prescription-related information between GPs and community pharmacists as advised in the NHS Plan. All three groups were in favour of it. Patients liked the potential for convenience, GPs thought it would improve repeat prescribing and pharmacists liked the enhanced professional role. The problem was security and confidentiality. Wider access for community pharmacists to parts of the patient record not related to medication was frowned upon by GPs and needs further research.

Automated quality checks on repeat prescribing
Rogers JE, Wroe CJ, Roberts A *et al.*
Br J Gen Pract, 2003; **53**: 838–844

Repeat prescriptions have usually been checked manually but this study looked at a how a software application fared at the job in three practices in Manchester.

In 15% of the alerts raised, there was no apparent rationale for prescribing the drug documented in the electronic patient record. Almost two-thirds of alerts were wrong due to errors in the drug information resource used in the software or idiosyncrasies of local coding and doctors' documentation. Tightening up on these should improve the process.

EHEALTH

Email consultations in health care: 1 – scope and effectiveness. 2 – acceptability and safe application
Car J, Sheikh A
BMJ, 2004; **329**: 435–438, 439–442

Electronic communication has revolutionised the industries of banking and retail but what can it do for healthcare? Although little evidence currently exists on electronic models of care, patients want email access to doctors and this pair of papers considers its potential.

Advantages are:
- user-friendly, efficient and versatile in facilitating asynchronous communication
- increases patient choice and many would be prepared to pay for this service
- may be cost-effective, time-efficient and reduce need for face-to-face contacts
- addresses unmet need and delivers care to those who would not normally present
- plenty of scope for preventative health care and managing non-urgent conditions
- role in receiving straightforward test results or doing follow up checks
- useful for improving non-attendance rates with cheap reminders
- certain responses can be automated
- avoids face to face embarrassment of rescheduling appointments
- written record of important points to remember or clarify
- increased reporting of adverse events
- delivering information to many people simultaneously
- feedback from patient selfcare assignments particularly in chronic care
- surveys report greater honesty in electronic questionnaires that in person by an interviewer

Disadvantages are:
- potential for overwhelm due to increased communication burden

- satisfaction decreases markedly if replies take longer than 48 hours
- may widen social disparities of care
- loss of subtle emotive clues and patient-centredness
- inability to examine and risk of diagnostic errors
- lack of data security measures results in threats to confidentiality
- system must seamlessly integrate e-contacts with the usual medical record
- not currently recommended outside existing doctor–patient relationships

Guidance will be needed on organising the service with suitable standards and strategies that mitigate risk at all stages. Patients and doctors will need to understand the limitations and risks involved. Ideally, informed consent should be obtained.

Remote working: survey of attitudes to eHealth of doctors and nurses in rural general practices in the United Kingdom
Richards H, King G, Reid M, *et al.*
Fam Pract, 2005; **22**: 2–7

This survey of remote Scottish regions showed that more than two-thirds of responders had at least an ISDN line but only around a third had a digital camera and the ability to videoconference.

The most important barriers expressed from the 1112 respondents were 'lack of suitable training' (55%), 'high cost of buying telemedicine equipment' (54%), and 'increase in GP/nurse workload' (43%). Concern was also expressed about the impact of videoconferencing on patient privacy and on the quality of the consultation itself.

More than half used eHealth mainly for obtaining laboratory results using the internet, 20% were most familiar with videoconferencing for education or clinical purposes, and 27% used it mainly for a 'variety of other applications'.

So it is underused as we stand but there is a lot to be gained in terms of levelling out health inequalities in remote areas, and technology will be an essential part of that.

THE INTERNET

Googling for a diagnosis – use of Google as a diagnostic aid: internet based study
Tang H, Ng JHK
BMJ, 2006; **333**: 1143–1145

Using one year's worth of case histories from one journal (*New Engl J Med*), this study looked at the accuracy of Google in coming up with the correct diagnosis.

Doctors chose the search words and opted for distinctive combinations of three to five terms. The three most prominent diagnoses that seemed to fit the signs and symptoms were selected and compared to the case record. If one of these was the right answer, the search was deemed a success. Google got it in 58% of cases.

Physicians have been estimated to carry 2 million facts in their heads in order to be a diagnostician. Google already accesses 3 billion articles.

Searches by patients may be less efficient than this figure but, at the very least, search engines can clearly be an additional tool to help doctors diagnose difficult cases with unique symptoms.

Diagnosis using search engines
Gardner M
BMJ, 2006; **333**: 1131

Although thousands of computer systems have been developed, most have made little impact. That said, they have not had the same speed, accessibility, simplicity and lack of cost as Google. No special equipment is required and no maintenance bills will come your way.

This editorial asks clinicians not to feel too discouraged. Although the press loved this story, we are reminded that doctors chose the search terms in the study above and that inferring a diagnosis also depended on the assessment of doctors.

However, developments in years to come will herald a much more powerful 'semantic web'. When future search engines can access data and resources that reside in databases other than HTML code, they will be increasingly important assets.

Patients' experience with a diabetes support programme based on an interactive electronic medical record: qualitative study
Ralston JD, Revere D, Robins LS *et al.*
BMJ, 2004; **328**: 1159

Clinic visits alone do not meet the needs of patients with chronic conditions.

This pilot study of a web-based disease management programme involved interactive diabetic disease management tools and electronic records which were accessible to patients and providers. It had the following effects:
* patients valued the unique environment to voice their worries
* they felt an enhanced sense of security about their health
* they were very disappointed at times when the programme did not meet their expectations and this is hard to resolve in web-based care

Web-based care will have an important role in collaborative health care if everyone understands what can actually be delivered.

Advertising campaign on a major internet search engine to promote colorectal cancer screening
Purvis Cooper C, Williams KN, Carey KA *et al.*
BMJ, 2004; **328**: 1179–1180

Advertising a colorectal screening campaign on Yahoo! over 6 weeks generated 26 000 visits to the website at a cost of £1.33 per visit. Compared to television advertising this is fairly cheap and showed that online advertising is a viable strategy to attract internet users to health promotion websites.

PHARMACISTS

What we know already:

- Calls have been made for greater collaboration between GPs and community pharmacists in primary care
- Reviewing elderly patients' medication is a requirement of the National Service Framework for Older People but difficult for GPs to prioritise given current pressures
- A pharmacist could manage an estimated 8% of adult attendances at A&E according to one study from St Thomas' Hospital
- Community pharmacists given a little training in asthma management can successfully self-manage plans and basic follow up care
- In 2006 the Department of Health extended considerable prescribing power to pharmacists

Recent Papers

BARRIERS

Perceived interprofessional barriers between community pharmacists and general practitioners: a qualitative assessment
Hughes CM, McCann S
Br J Gen Pract, 2003; **53**: 600–606

This qualitative study looked at how GPs and pharmacists see each other in the light of possible shifts in roles in the future.

GPs expressed themes related to the 'shopkeeper' image of community pharmacy and lack of knowledge about their training and activities. They expressed concern over giving pharmacists prescribing rights. They were also concerned about the marriage of profit-making and healthcare and felt that the limited opening hours of the local chemist imparied their ability to provide a service.

Community pharmacists considered themselves to be healthcare professionals and felt that GPs had no appreciation of their role in health care.

Identifying these barriers is the first stage to challenging them if there is to be a useful liaison between the profession of medicine and the role of the community pharmacist.

Patients' views of a pharmacist-run medication review clinic in general practice
Petty DR, Knapp P, Raynor DK *et al.*
Br J Gen Pract, 2003; **53**: 607–613

Another qualitative study looked at what elderly patients thought of sitting down with a pharmacist to review their use of medication. The aim was to provide more information about the medicines, review repeat prescriptions and inquire about side-effects and efficacy.

A range of opinions about these medication review clinics revealed some suspicion about the purpose of the clinic and some disappointment about unfulfilled expectations. However, there was also appreciation of the in-depth review and further explanation of their treatment. More research is needed to inform the development of the service.

EXTENDED ROLES

Effectiveness of telephone counselling by a pharmacist in reducing mortality in patients receiving polypharmacy: randomised controlled trial
Wu JYF, Leung WYS, Chang S et al.
BMJ, 2006; **333**: 522

Telephone follow-up from a pharmacist to non-compliant patients saves lives according to this Hong Kong study. The patients were on five or more drugs and received periodic telephone counselling to reinforce the benefits of the medication, clarify treatment regimes and clear up any misconceptions.

Over the two years of this intervention there was a 40% reduction in death with the NNT being 16. Use of health resources was also reduced in this group showing the value and necessity of continuous support in order to change behaviour.

Pharmacist led, primary care based disease management reduced risk factors and improved glycaemic control in diabetes. *Evidence-Based Medicine,*
2005; **10**: 154
The following paper is reviewed
A randomised trial of a primary care-based disease management program to improve cardiovascular risk factors and glycated haemoglobin levels in patients with diabetes
Rothman RL, Malone R, Bryant B, et al.
Am J Med, 2005; **118**: 276–84

Pharmacists have show that they can be as useful as nurses in chronic disease management programmes, in this case for poorly controlled diabetics. After some additional training, clinical pharmacists used evidence-based algorithms to help them give intensive teaching sessions and succeeded in showing improvement in the usual diabetic parameters and risk factors. The pharmacists could track, co-ordinate and implement individualised care which, assuming these non-physicians stick to their remit, should be as good as the protocols they are working from.

Does home based medication review keep older people out of hospital? The HOMER randomised controlled trial
Holland R, Lenaghan E, Harvey I et al.
BMJ, 2005; **330**: 293

This interesting study looked at sending in pharmacists to the homes of 872 patients over 80 years old who were on at least two medications and who had been recruited during a recent emergency admission to hospital. The pharmacists visited twice around two and eight weeks after discharge to educate about medication, look for drug interactions and assess adherence to medication.

The NHS advocates such medication review for older patients but this approach resulted in significantly more admission to hospitals, more GP home visits and a worse quality of life while failing to reduce mortality.

This counterintuitive finding might be explained by better help-seeking behaviour or just by creating more dependence through anxiety and confusion, but also may be due to an increase in side-effects with improved compliance causing more iatrogenic illness.

Either way, more research is needed before we go down this line too far.

OTC MEDICATION

Switching prescription drugs to over the counter
Cohen JP, Paquette C, Cairns C
BMJ, 2005; **330**: 39–41

Prescription drugs are usually considered for over the counter availability when they ease a non-chronic condition that is fairly easy to self-diagnose and has low potential for harm. But recent switches, such as simvastatin in May 2004, break this pattern. What are the motives? This article suggests three possibilities, pharmaceutical firms' desire to extend their market, attempts to reduce NHS costs, and the self-care movement. Cost has caused omeprazole to jump over the counter in Switzerland but that is unlikely to be the main motive for simvastatin in the UK as those at moderate risk of heart disease will still receive it on the NHS.

The number of drugs available this way will undoubtedly grow as pharmaceutical companies whose patents are expiring explore new markets.

NURSE PRACTITIONERS

What we know already:

- Rising demand and expectations have led to a shift of care to different health professionals, notably nurses
- Nurses can successfully undertake much of the health promotion work of general practices and they have a leading role in chronic disease follow up
- The term 'nurse practitioner' is often used vaguely
- The role of nurse practitioner involves responsibility for assessment and treatment decisions. They work as co-practitioners in the primary care team.
- The different abilities, training and degree of autonomy of nurse practitioners makes the role difficult to recommend with evidence
- Research in the area is homogenised and draws conclusions not necessarily relevant to general practice
- Generalisations regarding the value of the role sometimes extend beyond the conditions actually studied which are often trivial illness and minor injury

Guidance

Consultation on options for the future of independent prescribing by extended formulary nurse prescribers. Dept of Health, Medicines and Healthcare Products Regulatory Agency (www.dh.gov.uk).

Recent Papers

Systematic review of whether nurse practitioners working in primary care can provide equal care to doctors
Horrocks S, Anderson E, Salisbury C et al.
BMJ, 2002; **324**: 819–823

There has not been much written in this area recently so I have included this review which seems to be the 'biggest' paper around on the subject. It succumbs to some of the generalisations mentioned above but taking it in context with the letters that it provoked allows us some understanding of where current thinking lies.

The review includes 34 studies from both sides of the Atlantic dating back as far as 1975 and included minor injury work in emergency rooms as well as baby-checks in paediatrics. This makes the generalisations of their conclusions questionable.

- Nurse practitioners spent around 4 minutes longer consulting.
- Patients were more satisfied with care from a nurse practitioner than from a doctor.

- Health outcomes were the same.
- Nurses ordered more investigations than doctors
- There were no differences in prescriptions, return consultations or referrals.

The authors conclude that in some ways nurse practitioners provided higher quality of care than doctors and boosting their numbers is a good idea.

In the letters, a nurse practitioner voices her opinion that nurses communicate better than doctors and that therefore nurses are the 'professional with the right skill' that the patient should see. Expression of patient confidence in the nurses' clinical ability is identified as a surrogate equivalent of medical experience.

There are replies from doctors too who draw comparison with GP registrars with their 4 years of post-graduate experience and who still need to pass assessment in video-taped consultation technique. They express discomfort that these are standards that do not apply to nurse practitioners. They also suggest that responsibility for indemnity should lay with the nurse themselves rather than their practice and note that demonstration of basic pathology and pharmacology does not seem to be on the agenda.

They note that the oft-quoted 'patient satisfaction' correlates with adherence to treatment but not with standards of care. It plays no part in ability to diagnose and provide medical care. Spending more time ordering more tests may suggest a lack of ability to diagnose or provide time-efficient care.

We need to focus more carefully on improving delivery of care within the limited scope of nurse practitioner training.

This is the one paper in this book where I have concerns that the conclusions and abstract have the genuine potential to mislead but I think the varied opinions in the *BMJ* letters round out the discussion.

Comparing the cost of nurse practitioners and GPs in primary care: modelling economic data from randomised trials
Hollinghurst S, Horrocks S, Anderson E *et al.*
Br J Gen Pract, 2006; **56**: 530–535

This cost analysis of two randomised controlled trials included costs of training and estimated the cost of nurse practitioner consultation (£30.35) as costing much the same as a salaried GP (£28.14). Confidence intervals overlapped. The costs were higher because of the time spent by GPs contributing to the nurses consultations and doing return visits.

They point out that proven abilities of nurse practitioners are very mixed and employment should depend more on the actual role fulfilled than a cost analysis like this.

Impact of nurse practitioners on workload of general practitioners: randomised controlled trial
Laurant MGH, Hermens RPMG, Braspenning JCC *et al.*
BMJ, 2004; **328**: 927

This study does relate directly to general practice.

It was a randomised trial that looked at the impact of allocating a nurse practitioner to a Dutch general practice to look after specified elements of care in COPD, asthma, dementia and cancer.

Adding a nurse practitioner failed to reduce workload for GPs in this study compared to the control group.

Consultations by doctors actually increased during surgery hours by around five per week. This implies that nurse practitioners may supplement or extend GP care rather than substitute for aspects for it. It is possible they were uncovering previously unrecognised problems which would diminish with time.

Nurse practitioner and practice nurses' use of research information in clinical decision making: findings from an exploratory study
McCaughan D, Thompson C, Cullum C et al.
Fam Pract, 2005; **22**: 490–497

How do nurses deal with uncertainty? They ask a doctor. This qualitative study of information-seeking behaviour on a sample of 29 practice nurses and 4 nurse practitioners in the North of England showed that human sources of information were overwhelmingly preferred to books or the internet. The nurses involved, including the more independent role of nurse practitioner, rarely used evidence-based resources to seek answers to questions regarding diagnosis and treatment.

NURSE PRESCRIBERS

Extended prescribing by UK nurses and pharmacists
Avery AJ, Pringle M
BMJ, 2005; **331**: 1154–1155

In 2005, the Department of Health announced that nurse and pharmacist prescribers will be able to independently prescribe any licensed drug except controlled drugs. This is the most radical and far reaching development of its type anywhere in the world and stunned more than a few.

With a relative absence of evidence of either safety or benefit, the BMA has suggested that diagnostic skills just might be a valid part of safe prescribing, but this diplomatic article seems to get behind the propositions, reassuring itself that nurses will always act within their own areas of competence. There is no mention of the unknown incompetence that haunts some of us on a day-to-day basis. The authors admit it 'is impossible to draw clear conclusions on the safety and appropriateness of extended prescribing' and want to rely on clinical computer systems (as yet poorly developed) to provide the safety net. By the end of the article they seem to change their tune with the phrase 'thorough risk assessments should be done nationally and locally before prescribing is extended to new clinical areas'.

Epilepsy and supplementary nurse prescribing
Hosking PG
BMJ, 2006; **332**: 2

This editorial written by an epilepsy nurse specialist points out that we can do a lot more to prevent epilepsy-related deaths. Incentives can encourage GPs to conduct annual reviews and nurse specialists are known to improve patient management, reducing the need for contact with doctors.

However, she tells us that less than half of all epilepsy nurse specialists have postgraduate qualifications relevant to the responsibility of case management, casting doubt on titles such as 'specialist nurse'.

They propose that the correct level of education is a generic masters degree which can be adapted for epilepsy. This will provide the necessary familiarity with classification, differential diagnosis, pharmacology, neurophysiology, neuro-imaging, and psychosocial aspects of care. They would be able to advise GPs directly and be responsible for a caseload of around 1000 epileptics each.

TRAINING

What we know already:

- Twelve months' training may not adequately prepare doctors for general practice
- Many feel the year is too pressured and too focused on examinations
- Concerns about entering into partnership centre on balancing life with work
- The GMC views general practice as an appropriate setting to learn the duties of a doctor in advance of full registration
- Schemes throughout the country have given junior doctors the opportunity to rotate through general practice
- In April 2004 'Modernising Medical Careers – The Next Steps' was published and the new 2 year Foundation Programme for all medical school graduates went 'live' in August 2005, effectively replacing the PRHO year and the first SHO year

Recent Papers

Evaluation of extended training for general practice in Northern Ireland: qualitative study

Sibbett CH, Thompson WT, Crawford M *et al.*
BMJ, 2003; **327**: 971–973

The length of GP training is currently 1 year out of a 3 year vocational scheme. This pilot scheme increased the time spent in general practice to 18 months and interviewed GP registrars and trainers about this.

After a busy exam-orientated year, many grievances were expressed in the interviews.

- Registrars were left feeling averse to further continuing education and did not feel prepared for GP life.
- Registrars covered for practices who said they were providing training when they were not. Some were frightened of their trainer and were worried their report would not be signed.
- Several areas of training were not covered at all.
- Confidence was reduced by not being treated as a team member and being 'just the trainee'.

Neither the 12 or 18 month courses were thought to provide the necessary competencies and confidence to enter independent practice or know enough about practice management.

The 6 months' extension appeared to go some way towards developing confidence, restimulating desire to learn and promoting teamwork but this would be only a part of the solution as extended training may be unlikely to fill all these gaps.

Preregistration house officers in general practice: review of evidence
Illing J, van Zwanenberg T, Cunningham WF et al.
BMJ, 2003; **326**: 1019–1022

This literature review looked at the strengths and weaknesses of schemes where house officers spend four months of their year in general practice. It encompassed the views of 180 preregistration house officers, 45 GP trainers and 105 consultants.

- All 19 studies valued the educational benefits of the placements.
- Most doctors, even those not considering a career in general practice, were generally positive about the experience and would recommend it.
- Concerns about spending the first four months of the year (before experience in medicine or surgery) in the post did not appear to be upheld although confidence grew after these conventional placements.
- Participants reported enhanced communication skills, patient-centred consulting, learning to deal with diagnostic uncertainty and developing understanding of doctor-patient relationships in the community.
- However, doctors were likely to feel isolated, most jobs required a car and their inability to sign a prescription did not help.
- Tutorials were held more often in general practice than in hospitals.
- GP trainers reported a 10% increase in workload and wanted paying for it. As a result, the schemes will not be expanding.

The authors suggest an improved model may be to have SHOs rather than house officers attached to general practice. This would overcome difficulties of supervision, prescription and independence.

Indeed in March 2005 the Department of Health announced that from August 2006 there would be funding made available for 55% of all doctors on the Foundation Programme to undertake part of their training in general practice (it has been announced that this will be increased to 80% from August 2007). The experience is to be fundamentally different from the training of a GP Registrar within the VTS but allows early exposure to general practice.

THE PHARMACEUTICAL INDUSTRY

What we know already:

- Doctors need to use the products the pharmaceutical industry comes up with and it is reasonable that the industry should promote these products
- Drug companies are allowed to advertise to doctors but not patients
- Contact with pharmaceutical representatives increases prescribing costs
- Requests from patients for specific medications increases their prescribing
- Most medical journals have a substantial income from drug companies who crave favourable editorial coverage in credible journals above all things
- Doctors like to get journals for free even if they have lots of adverts in. Free publications work hard to increase their attractiveness to readers and therefore advertising revenue
- Advertising is often misleading. Caution should be exercised even with claims that appear to be supported by referenced evidence
- The pharmaceutical industry funds an increasing number of trials at all stages of a product's life cycle
- There is potential for huge conflicts of interest and corruption charges have been brought in high profile cases in Italy

Recent Papers

The influence of big pharma
Ferner RE
BMJ, 2005; **330**: 855–856

A government report on '*The influence of the pharmaceutical industry*' from April 2005 paints a picture of an industry that buys influence over doctors, charities, patient groups, journalists and politicians, and whose regulation is at worst weak and at best ambiguous. Half of all postgraduate medical education, and a great deal of nurse education, is funded by the pharmaceutical companies. They finance 90% of drug trials but come up with few innovative products while publishing positive results in a variety of guises and dismissing negatives results as flawed.

Advertising associates their brands with emotional attributes to appeal to doctors as they push their promotions as powerfully as they can.

The report suggests new limits on marketing and prescribing during 'probationary periods' for new drugs, with formal trials of efficacy performed within the NHS to improve pharmacovigilance.

Medical journals and pharmaceutical companies: uneasy bedfellows
Smith R
BMJ, 2003; **326**: 1202–1205

This article takes a closer look at the complex relationship between drug companies and medical journals.

Studies have shown that references cited in drug advertising can be impossible to track down and independent review of the evidence quoted often leads to different conclusions than those claimed.

The BMJ itself does not censor adverts (and the revenue they produce) but relies on readers and competing drug companies to follow up on overbloated claims while it focuses its resources on its own content.

This article offers a 'quick guide to corrupting science'. It suggests for example that a little healthy bribery to doctors funds 'postmarketing surveillance' into adverse effects. And if they have to push the drug in question a little harder, well ... who's to know? The answer is a delighted pharmaceutical industry, of course.

Other trials will be carefully designed to show 'equivalence' or 'non-inferiority'. Trials powered to detect superiority would be a disaster if the new drug did not win the head-to-head race. If in doubt, use your competitor's drug in the wrong dose. Keep the dose nice and high so you can show your drug has fewer toxic effects or nice and low so you can say yours is more effective. If it all goes wrong of course, you can bury the results in a drawer labelled 'unpublished'.

Add in a hideously complex economic evaluation paper and the brain of the average journal editor could be spinning, never mind the poor pressured GP trying to divine the truth.

Characteristics of general practitioners who frequently see drug industry representatives: national cross sectional study
Watkins C, Moore L, Harvey I *et al.*
BMJ, 2003; **326**: 1178–1179

This questionnaire survey of the behaviour of over 1000 UK GPs found that frequent contact with a drug rep was associated with:

- a greater willingness to prescribe new drugs
- increased likelihood of agreeing to a request for a drug not clinically indicated
- reluctance to end consultations with advice only and no prescription
- isolation from colleagues (single-handedness or non-training practice)
- working in deprived areas

Increases in reattendance and future workload could be substantial if these results are repeated. This study could not identify the direction of causality. Drug reps may well target 'responsive' GPs and those who like a bit of company behind the wooden door from time to time.

Who pays for the pizza? Redefining the relationships between doctors and drug companies. 1. Entanglement 2. Disentanglement
Moynihan R
BMJ, 2003; **326**: 1189–1192, 1193–1196

This pair of papers is based on the American system but looks at how doctors and drug companies are 'twisted together like the snake and the staff'. There is a new urgency to address this area in the face of rising pharmaceutical costs.

- In the US about 90% of doctors see drug reps. They receive gifts and attend events which highlight the sponsor's drug.
- Most deny their influence despite evidence to the contrary.
- Entanglement is widespread and undermines rational prescribing strategies.
- Medical journals rely on drug company-funded trials, advertisements, company-purchased reprints and ad-laden supplements.
- The impact is to fundamentally distort the evidence base of healthcare.
- 'Food, flattery and friendship are all powerful tools of persuasion'.
- Increasing access to young medics means that a culture of gift-giving could breed a long-term sense of entitlement and indebtedness.
- Young doctors unrealistically believe they are immune to promotional influences.
- Calls for disentanglement are being made by medical reform groups (such as www.nofreelunch.org).
- The 'systematic bias' in sponsored research comes not from bad science but the fact that the questions asked in the first place are in the interests of the sponsors not the patients.
- Reporting all trials rather than burying important negative findings should be job number one.
- The analogy that we would not tolerate judges taking money from those they judge may be a realistic one.

The debate seems to have started now that the American healthcare system is at a crisis point. There may still be some valid points for the UK system.

Relationships between the pharmaceutical industry and patients' organisations
Herxheimer A
BMJ, 2003; **326**: 1208–1210

Even patients' organisations are at it!

Pharmaceutical companies are rich and patients' organisations are poor. The inequality of the partners in this relationship raises serious questions.

The need to recover money quickly on newly developed products mean that persuading patients to lobby for them against restrictive health service policies has massive potential since the companies cannot market directly to patients.

Patients' organisations welcome cash for project funding and publicity to enable growth of the group. Drug companies have exploited this in various sneaky ways in the US and may be able to misrepresent real agendas.

Guidelines from the Long Term Medical Conditions Alliance offer advice to voluntary health organisations on keeping the relationship in the patients' best interests and not selling out their credibility.

Direct to consumer advertising
Mansfield PR, Mintzes B, Richards D, et al.
BMJ, 2005; **330**: 5–6

With New Zealand introducing a ban in 2005, the United States is left as the only industrialised country allowing full direct-to-consumer advertising of prescription medicines.

Generally, nations feel that there is no net benefit for their communities from minimising risk information and exaggerating benefits with advertising gloss. It increases prescriber workloads and expenditure for the larger employers that provide healthcare benefits.

Advertising is most profitable for new drugs where long-term health effects are unknown. It may increase knowledge but not in a balanced way as the idea is to persuade rather than inform. It also provides a potential conflict for doctors striving to be both patient-centred and evidence-based.

Pharmaceutical industry sponsorship and research outcome and quality: systematic review
Lexchin J, Bero LA, Djulbegovic B et al.
BMJ, 2003; **326**: 1167–1170

This review of 30 studies showed that research funded by pharmaceutical companies was more likely to have favourable outcomes for the sponsor's drug than that funded by other sources. The high quality of the work, however, was not in question. The bias must have slipped in in other ways, perhaps by use of inappropriate comparators in the trials or publication bias.

One suggestion for the future is that all clinical trials are registered prospectively to avoid admitting to only the favourable ones when the results are out.

How conducting a clinical trial affects physicians' guideline adherence and drug preferences
Andersen M, Kragstrup J, Søndergaard J et al.
JAMA, 2006; **295**: 2759–2764

This Danish study in 10 general practices shows how a pharmaceutical company-sponsored clinical trial can influence doctors to prescribe their drugs. Over 5000 asthma patients were compared to 60 000 control patients from 165 practices.

There was no influence on adherence to guidelines but the sponsor's share of the asthma drugs prescribed rose by a healthy 6.7% over the 2 years of the trial. This could be attributed to a higher preference for the company's drugs but we know pharmaceutical companies use various means to influence doctors. GPs in this trial were paid around £440 for each recruit. The trial compared two different dosage regimens and was never published. 'Seeding trials' were first described in 1994 and pay doctors for trials of dubious virtue while the hidden agenda is really to influence physician and patient behaviour.

How to dance with porcupines: rules and guidelines on doctors' relations with drug companies
Wager E
BMJ, 2003; **326**: 1196–1198

Many guidelines are now in existence to guide on the ethics involved in pharmaceutical medicine. They involve standards for clinical trials and calls for disclosure of all results.

Codes of conduct for drug companies tend to be voluntary but are backed up by procedures which can look into complaints from rival companies.

The Association of the British Pharmaceutical Industry (ABPI) has a national Code of Practice that prohibits all but the most modest hospitality towards doctors. The going rate is £6 per present and it has to be relevant to the doctor's work. Venues for clinical meetings must not be chosen for their leisure and recreational facilities and the temperature must be turned down to 'uncomfortably cold'. Anyone who cracks a joke is removed from the building.

CLINICAL GOVERNANCE

What we know already:

- Many clinicians feel that the 'cookbook' approach to practice promoted by prescriptive guidelines can undervalue clinical experience
- Successful implementation of evidence requires a profound understanding of how decisions are made
- GPs prefer punchy guidelines but brevity alone may not be enough to make them more likely to be implemented
- Guidelines are more likely to be followed by GPs if they are clear, applicable to daily practice, avoid complex decision trees, require no new skills and are supported by evidence
- Society acknowledges the importance of the views of users of health services and increased participation of patients is seen as desirable
- The National Institute for Clinical Excellence was introduced in the NHS Plan of 1998
- It aims to promote evidence-based medicine, improve standards of care and reduce inequalities in access to innovative treatments
- Government guidelines in the form of national service frameworks have aimed to increase quality through concepts of clinical governance

Recent Papers

INPUT FROM PATIENTS

Can patients assess the quality of health care?
Coulter A
***BMJ**, 2006; **333**: 1–2*

Coulter reflects on a paper in the same issue (Rao *et al. BMJ*, 2006; **333**: 19) that showed no correlation between patients' evaluations of the quality of technical care by a GP, compared with evidence-based indicators. The authors conclude that patients cannot reliably assess technical aspects of care but this editorial says this is a generalisation too far.

The public tends to value excellent communication skills and sound up to date technical skills as equally important, and together these are the two most importance factors in having confidence in their doctor.

Questionnaires continue to be popular tools for practice accreditation and clinical governance, appraisal and revalidation. The General Practice Assessment Survey used in Rao's paper has now been replaced with the General Practice Assessment Questionnaire which has no such assessment of technical skill (www.gpaq.info).

The authors comment that it is difficult enough for doctors to rate the technical skills of other doctors, so it is nigh on impossible for patients with no training.

However, asking the right question can still be a useful ingredient of the assessment. Recall of an individual's experience of a consultation in terms of specific events and information shared really is valuable information.

BIAS IN EVIDENCE

Evidence b(i)ased medicine – selective reporting from studies sponsored by pharmaceutical industry: review of studies in new drug applications
Melander H, Ahlqvist-Rastad J, Meijer G, *et al.*
BMJ, 2003; **326**: 1171–1173

This review illustrated that published data alone could not be relied upon to recommend a specific drug. Although this review looks at serotonin reuptake inhibitors, the conclusion can probably be extended to research on other drugs.

They discovered multiple publications of results, selective publication (with positive effects more likely to make it into print) and selective reporting by, for example, failing to report intention to treat. All these efforts bias the claims made.

All 42 studies in the investigation were initiated by the sponsors of the drug and the investigators were not primarily researchers. The accusation is that the sponsor would then have free reign over whether or not to publish.

USE OF GUIDELINES

Evidence based guidelines or collectively constructed 'mindlines?' Ethnographic study of knowledge management in primary care
Gabbay J, le May A
BMJ, 2004; **329**: 1013

This paper studies in depth how primary care clinicians formulate their healthcare decisions. They coin the term 'mindlines' which nicely describes the tacit internal guidelines which are 'knowledge in practice' or perhaps 'evidence-informed' rather than 'evidence-based' practice.

The doctors involved rarely accessed explicit guidelines or used sources of research directly. They would not, for example, take a clinical case, find a relevant guideline whether on a computer or on paper and prescribe their care package.

Shortcuts to evidence were employed. Their daily practice was informed more by brief reading of trusted sources, for example, free GP magazines, topped up with their own experience and that of colleagues. They listened to input from patients and valued interactions with respected opinion leaders. Pharmaceutical representatives rounded out the mix.

The information gleaned adapted their internalised mindline while leaving room for individual flexibility. It they were stumped by a new problem, they would read up or ask around and develop a mindline for the future. The end result was a formula for day-to-day practice which buffered against rigid thinking.

The authors conclude that it is unreasonable to expect even the best clinicians to rely on the full process of evidence-based healthcare. Recognition that such information networks power general practice may allow their exploitation when it comes to conveying important information to clinicians.

NICE

What's the evidence that NICE guidance has been implemented? Results from a national evaluation using time series analysis, audit of patients' notes, and interviews
Sheldon TA, Cullum N, Dawson D, *et al.*
BMJ, 2004; **329**: 999

The pattern of implementation of NICE guidelines has been mixed. Prescribing, such as use of orlistat for example, was more amenable to change than surgical recommendations such as promotion of laparoscopic hernia repair.

The extent to which trusts have put in place a structure for implementation of the guidelines was variable. The study recognises that NICE advice is just one factor influencing professional practice and that it is not capable on its own of stimulating rapid universal implementation of evidence.

Guidance is more likely to be adopted where it is properly funded, clear, relevant to clinical realities and where the evidence base is strong and stable. Add in a bit of professional endorsement from opinion leaders such as professional bodies and changes can pick up speed.

National Institute for Clinical Excellence and its value judgments
Rawlins MD, Culyer AJ
BMJ, 2004; **329**: 224–227

This paper from the originators of NICE tells us how they dovetail scientific evidence with what is good for society (social value judgements) in order to create guidelines for the NHS.

NICE aims for the highest attainable standards based on evidence which may not be very good and is rarely complete.

Cost as well as clinical effectiveness must be taken into account. NICE prefers the QALY – the cost per quality adjusted life year – but if quality of life data are not available, alternatives such as the cost per life year gained are used.

They avoid an absolute threshold as there may be circumstances where they wish to ignore it but they would need a good reason to adopt a treatment over £25 000–£35 000 per QALY.

NICE claims not to consider affordability. If it decides something is cost-effective then deeming it unaffordable is a matter for the government.

To facilitate social value judgements, NICE has formed a Citizen's Council to ensure these values resonate broadly with the public. They aim to achieve equity with no disadvantages for age, productivity, sex, perceived deservedness or how many QALYs have already been enjoyed. Lack of equity in location (postcode prescribing) was one of the reasons it was set up in the first place.

Challenges for the National Institute for Clinical Excellence
Maynard A, Bloor K, Freemantle N
BMJ, 2004; **329**: 227–229

Although Rawlins (see above) has stated there is 'no role for NICE in the rationing of treatments to NHS patients', these authors disagree.

They argue that NICE must expand into fully informed rationing in the NHS. The issue is 'not whether but how to ration'.

They argue that the government should make it impossible to adopt expensive new technologies until they are approved by NICE.

Different values systems compete and overemphasis on new technologies means relatively little attention is paid to old technologies that may be redundant and could be withdrawn.

Approval of expensive marginal therapies such as some cancer treatments cause NHS provider organisations financial headaches.

They have several suggestions. Tightening the threshold to less than £15 000 per QALY would lead to rejection of many more technologies. Giving NICE a notional budget to fund its recommendations would mean they would have to stay within it or find services to withdraw.

The NHS cannot afford to be 'nice'. Although funding is up, so are demands from the national service framework targets and the economic climate will only get more difficult.

Going the whole hog and giving NICE a real budget to fund all its advice is what the authors recommend as the most efficient path.

They claim that the political consequences would require 'careful management'. The phrase 'political suicide' springs a little easier to mind.

HEALTH INEQUALITIES

What we know already:

- New socioeconomic classification is based on current occupation and employment. The seven main classes are based on responsibility within the job and an eighth class is for long-term unemployed
- Reducing inequalities between socioeconomic groups is a government priority but the new general medical services contract takes no account of deprivation or ethnicity on target levels
- Measurement of population health has largely depended on mortality data
- Research has shown reduced access to angiography for lower social class groups
- Lower socioeconomic groups are under-represented in medical schools
- Over the past decade, the UK ethnic minority population has grown by 53% and now comprises 8% of the total population, with South Asians, the largest group, now accounting for 50% of ethnic minority groups
- Homelessness poses serious health risks and high mortality rates
- Inhibited access to general practice mean homeless people often access healthcare inappropriately through A&E

Guidance

Tackling health inequalities: a programme for action. *Dept of Health,* 2003.
An updated status report was published in August 2005 showing narrowing of the gaps in some indicators (see also www.dh.gov.uk/healthinequalities).

Recent Papers

DEPRIVATION

Is there a north–south divide in social class inequalities in health in Great Britain? Cross sectional study using data from the 2001 census
Doran T, Drever F, Whitehead M
BMJ, 2004; **328**: 1043–1045

The north–south divide in social class inequalities is real but it is more of a north-west–southeast divide.

Questions from the 2001 UK census on self-rated general health were used to explore these patterns:
- within each social class, there were considerable inequalities depending on region (with the South East coming off best)
- within each region of Britain, there were large inequalities of health related to social class

- those in class 7 had rates of poor self-rated health more than double those of class 1
- scores were also worse in women than in men in each region and class
- Wales, the North-East and North West fared badly in all classes. Women in class 1 in Wales, for example, fared worse than women in class 4 in the South West
- Scotland and London had the widest health divides, adding to the debate on how to allocate resources to tackle the divide

Some questions remain:

- What aspect of population health is represented by this type of self-assessment?
- How does this outcome measure compare to mortality figures from earlier studies?

Influence of socioeconomic deprivation on the primary care burden and treatment of patients with a diagnosis of heart failure in general practice in Scotland: population based study

McAlister FA, Murphy NF, Simpson CR *et al.*
BMJ, 2004; **328**: 1110

Previous research has shown that deprivation is associated with more hospital admissions and mortality from heart failure independent of age, sex or co-morbidity.

This study in 53 practices and over 2000 heart failure patients showed that:

- incidence of heart failure increased by 44% between the most affluent and most deprived socioeconomic strata
- the most deprived patients were 23% less likely to see their GP for follow up
- there was no bias in prescribing patterns, eliminating this as an explanation of the inequalities

Perhaps deprived groups behave in a more fatalistic way towards illness or they seek out care through A&E more often.

We know that closer follow up leads to better outcomes so these patients might have be worse off as a result of less ongoing contact with their GP.

Area deprivation predicts lung function independently of education and social class.

Shohaimi S, Welch A, Bingham S *et al.*
Eur Respir J, 2004; **24**: 157–161

Being in a manual occupational social class, having no educational qualifications and living in a deprived area all separately predict reduced lung function, even after controlling for smoking. Lung function is an important indicator of general health. These factors may exert their influence through poor diet, lack of exercise, poor housing that increases respiratory infections, or environmental tobacco smoke.

Association of deprivation, ethnicity, and sex with quality indicators for diabetes: population based survey of 53 000 patients in primary care

Hippisley-Cox J, O'Hanlon S, Coupland C
BMJ, 2004; **329**: 1267–1269

This study used data from 237 general practices to look at the effect of deprivation and ethnicity on the standard of care in diabetes.

They found that people living in areas of high deprivation or with large ethnic minorities are less likely to have their diabetes care recorded thoroughly.

The less affluent areas had fewer recorded assessments of BMI, BP, urinalysis, cholesterol levels and smoking status.

Diabetic women were also less likely to have these assessments recorded than men. This mirrors the less adequate care for women shown elsewhere for heart disease.

Practices in deprived areas will need to work harder to achieve recommended standards.

Perceptions and experiences of taking oral hypoglycaemic agents among people of Pakistani and Indian origin: qualitative study

Lawton J, Ahmad N , Hallowell N, *et al.*
BMJ, 2005; **330**: 1247

Interviews with British Pakistani and Indian diabetics illustrated that ambivalent attitudes towards oral hypoglycaemics exist. Many perceive such medication as necessary but also harmful which backs up the particularly poor adherence to medication and poor glycaemic control noticed in this group.

Most trusted their doctors' expertise, appreciating the NHS delivery of prescriptions free of financial incentive for the doctor, and considered the medicines available in Britain to be better than those available in the Indian subcontinent. Their beliefs about Western medicines, however, may lead them to self-regulate their doses in ways that seem rational to them but go against medical advice.

The authors make recommendations to tackle these observations by having a high index of suspicion that patients will self-regulate, asking about it in a non-judgmental way, asking the patient what they think each medication is doing for them and, in particular, if they make dietary changes (which may be counter to their diabetes recommendations) as a result of taking the medications.

Influence of practices' ethnicity and deprivation on access to angiography: an ecological study

Jones M, Ramsay J, Feder G *et al.*
Br J Gen Pract, 2004; **54**: 423–428

This paper looked at data from 143 general practices and used nitrate prescriptions and admission data as measures of need. Practices with more South Asian patients had higher rates of angiography after allowing for age, deprivation, admission rates and nitrate prescribing. This challenges suggestions of inequality related to ethnicity in treatment of coronary heart disease. In addition, there was no association between deprivation and angiography.

Excess coronary heart disease in South Asians in the United Kingdom
Kuppuswamy VC, Gupta S
BMJ, 2005; **330**: 1223–1224

This editorial, however, suggests that inequalities are indeed widening with death rates in South Asians from Bangladesh, Pakistan and India (in order of how badly they fare in coronary mortality statistics) declining at a slower rate than the 'indigenous' population.

They theorise that the increased prevalence of the metabolic syndrome and diabetes in second and third generation Asians is the most compelling aetiology. Lack of exercise, unhealthy diets and a reduced likelihood to receive statins as well as drop out of cardiac rehabilitation all add to the mix.

The authors argue that the usual methods for risk stratification, such as Framingham data, underestimate risk in this ethnic group and that treatment ranges may need to be redefined. They also point to possible linguistic and cultural barriers and the need for more patient education, a higher index of suspicion among doctors and perhaps 'well Asian' clinics to provide some intensive primary care.

Religious beliefs about causes and treatment of epilepsy
Ismail H, Wright J, Rhodes P, *et al.*
Br J Gen Pract, 2005; **55**: 26–31

A study of the use of healers and complementary therapies by South Asian epileptics in Yorkshire revealed that over half of responders attributed their illness to fate, the will of God, or as punishment for the sins of a previous life. There was a network of healers who were seen as providing a parallel and complementary system of care.

Although families of Asians encouraged them to turn to these traditional religiospiritual treatments in desperation for a cure, many were sceptical about their effectiveness. It is important doctors are aware of these belief systems and consider if there are conflicts with Western health care.

EDUCATION

'Not a university type': focus group study of social class, ethnic, and sex differences in school pupils' perceptions about medical school
Greenhalgh T, Seyan K, Boynton P
BMJ, 2004; **328**: 1541–1544

Academically able 14–16 year olds from lower socioeconomic backgrounds are markedly less likely to want to be a doctor. They underestimate their chances of succeeding and stereotype medical school as 'culturally alien' and geared towards 'posh' students.

They liked the idea of the financial rewards but were not so keen on what they perceived as prohibitive personal sacrifice. Pupils from less deprived backgrounds were more attracted by the challenge of medicine and potential for achievement and fulfillment.

There were no such differences between backgrounds on the basis of sex or ethnicity.

All pupils had concerns about the costs of going to medical school, but only those from poor backgrounds allowed cost to affect choices.

Policies to broaden entry to medical school must address these complex social and cultural perceptions.

HOMELESSNESS

10 year follow up study of mortality among users of hostels for homeless people in Copenhagen
Nordentoft M, Wandall-Holm N
BMJ, 2003; **327**: 81

This Danish study found that homeless people staying in hostels are four times more likely to die early than the general population. This applied particularly to young women, those in the 15–43 year age group, and in a transient population that stayed only a short time in the hostel. Other predictors of early death included drug and alcohol misuse and bad experiences in childhood such as death of a parent.

ETHICS

What we know already:

- Decisions to withhold or withdraw treatment are among the most difficult that health professionals face
- Advance directives are written statements made by patients concerning future treatment preferences in the event that they become incapable of expressing them
- In the UK, advance directives should be given consideration and respect but are not bound by statutory law
- Guidance exists in case law but an obligation to follow advance directives has not been tested in the courts
- It is not known to what extent patient's perspectives are integrated into clinical decisions
- Euthanasia has been pioneered in Holland and debate on legalisation is growing in many countries
- Supporters claim euthanasia is a continuation of palliative care and that doctors must respect patients' autonomy
- Evidence suggests we may lack sufficient training in palliative care at the end of life. Tackling this might be a good place to start before clarifying a place for euthanasia
- The RCGP withdrew opposition to legalisation of assisted dying in October 2004 and the BMA followed in June 2005

Guidance

Advance statements about medical treatment – code of practice. *BMA*, April 1995.

Withholding and withdrawing life-prolonging treatments: good practice in decision-making. *GMC*, August 2002.

Recent Papers

ADVANCE DIRECTIVES

Adherence to advance directives in critical care decision making: vignette study
Thompson T, Barbour R, Schwartz L
BMJ, 2003; **327**: 1011

This study looked at how doctors differed in their interpretation of an advance directive in a fictional clinical vignette.

The scenario was designed to create dissonance and many of the 12 participants demonstrated an 'it depends' response. They took individual judgements on 'what the patient really meant' and what was a reasonable quality of life worth preserving.

Ambiguities of terminology explained some of the variation. Some decided, for example, that antibiotic treatment was palliative and therefore allowable and those who overruled the directive did what they felt was in the patient's best interests. There was difficulty in balancing these subjective impressions with the patient's expressed desire for autonomy and the right to have treatment withdrawn.

The authors concluded that anyone creating an advance directive cannot assume that any particular outcome will result from its implementation.

EUTHANASIA

GPs' views on changing the law on physician-assisted suicide and euthanasia, and willingness to prescribe or inject lethal drugs: a survey from Wales
Pasterfield D, Wilkinson C, Finlay IG *et al.*
Br J Gen Pract, 2006; **56**: 450–452

There is little information on how GPs feel about legislation and possibly taking part in euthanasia. This survey of over 1200 Welsh GPs that responded found that:
- 62% said they did not favour a change in the law to allow physician-assisted suicide
- 56% said they did not favour legal backing for voluntary euthanasia

Time for change
Branthwaite MA
BMJ, 2005; **331**: 681–683

In physician-assisted suicide, a doctor provides a patient with the means to end life. In voluntary euthanasia, the doctor ends that life if the patient is physically unable to do so.

In this paper from a cluster in the same issue of the *BMJ*, a barrister argues that assisted suicide is an extension of an individual's right to withdraw consent to life-sustaining interventions.

Unfortunate cases have been highlighted where determined patients have acted alone to visit countries such as Switzerland where euthanasia is legal.

Assisted dying is legal in Holland, Belgium and the US state of Oregon where all but one death in 2004 took place at home and those choosing it tended to be younger and more highly educated.

Public support seems to be growing and even the BMA has revised its position in favour of a neutral stance allowing parliament to decide.

A proposed UK parliamentary bill incorporates safeguards for patients and physicians for whom the requirement for 'unbearable suffering' is still subjective.

Legalised euthanasia will violate the rights of vulnerable patients
George RJD, Finlay IG, Jeffrey D
BMJ, 2005; **331**: 684–685

This paper fails to see a distinction between legalised euthanasia and therapeutic killing. This 'insoluble ethical conflict' may mean that the voice of the vulnerable and incapable is drowned out, making coercion and the inference of a 'duty to die' a real risk. In Oregon requests for physician-assisted suicide because of 'being a burden' have increased as people shop around for compliant doctors. Can we afford the moral cost to society?

And this at a time when research consistently shows that GPs, each dealing with fewer than five dying patients per year, could do a lot better with the palliative care they deliver.

CONSENT

Gillick or Fraser? A plea for consistency over competence in children
Wheeler R
BMJ, 2006; **332**: 807

This article emphasises the difference between the terms 'Gillick competence' and 'Fraser guidelines'. Synonymy has been encouraged following an urban myth that Mrs Gillick did not want to associate her name with the ruling.

Adulthood is reached at 18 years in the UK and, to a limited extent, 16 and 17 year old children can make medical decisions independent of their parents.

The Gillick test for competence in those under 18 dates from 1983 and requires the child to demonstrate sufficient maturity and intelligence to understand and appraise the nature and implications of the proposed treatment (age alone is recognised as an unreliable predictor of this capacity).

Lord Fraser was one of the Law Lords in the Gillick judgement and specifically addresses the dilemma of contraceptive advice without parental knowledge. To protect the welfare of these girls he emphasised the desirability of parental involvement and understanding the risks for unprotected sex. So Gillick is a general assessment of competence. Fraser fuses this with the specific provision of contraceptive advice.

Remembering this will protect the concept of Gillick competence as the central doctrine with which to judge capacity in children.

ALCOHOL

What we know already:

- The 'U-shaped curve' describes non-drinkers and heavy drinkers having higher mortality rates than light/moderate drinkers
- Rising alcohol consumption costs the British economy an estimated £30 billion a year
- The benefits of light to moderate drinking on cardiovascular outcomes have been proven even after MI
- Men drinking over 35 units a week double their risk of stroke
- Alcohol use is increasing in teenagers
- There is a high prevalence of alcohol problems in those who commit suicide
- Most problem drinkers are unknown to their GPs
- GPs are strongly encouraged to identify cases of alcohol excess and intervene. They need simple screening instruments high in specificity and sensitivity to accomplish this
- Delving using screening questionnaires is seen by doctors as creating serious problems with rapport and hijacking the consultation. One has likened it to having to do a rectal examination on everyone who walked in
- Brief advice interventions undertaken in ideal conditions in primary care have shown it is possible and cost-effective to reduce excessive drinking
- Real effectiveness of these measures in everyday practice is unproven
- Laboratory tests such as GGT and MCV are poor at identifying problem drinkers
- Non-drinkers are at greater health risks but should not be encouraged to start drinking alcohol
- The BMA is calling on the government to legislate to compel manufacturers of alcoholic drinks to clearly label their products with the number of units of alcohol
- Preventing alcohol-related morbidity and mortality is a key priority of the UK's government health strategy

Guidelines

A report from the RCGP and the Royal Colleges of Physicians and Psychiatrists recommends no more than 21 units per week and 14 units per week for men and women respectively.

The UK Government Guidelines define 'a drink' as 8 g (1 cl of pure alcohol) and define moderation as 3–4 drinks a day (28 units a week) for men and 2–3 drinks a day (21 units a week) for women.

LIFESTYLE

Recent Papers

Screening in brief intervention trials targeting excessive drinkers in general practice: systematic review and meta-analysis
Beich A, Thorsen T, Rollnick S
BMJ, 2003; **327**: 536–542

Screening for excessive alcohol use and providing brief interventions is not effective in general practice according to this meta-analysis of eight eligible studies that focused on alcohol use rather than dependency.

For every 1000 patients screened, 90 (9%) screened positive, 25 qualified for brief interventions and after a year, only two to three drank less than the maximum recommended level.

The authors claim that due to methodological difficulties such as lack of blinding and short follow-up, previous reports have overestimated the impact of brief interventions.

The competition for GPs' time means this model of universal screening is questionable as a case finding approach. Alcohol problems might be better approached through the rapport of a good consultation.

Opportunistic screening for alcohol use disorders in primary care: comparative study
Coulton S, Drummond C, James D *et al.*
BMJ, 2006; **332**: 511–517

In this study of nearly 200 males, the Alcohol Use Disorders Identification Test (AUDIT) – a 10 item questionnaire – proved more efficient than levels of GGT, MCV and AST at correlating with alcohol consumption when used for opportunistic screening in six Welsh primary care practices. It had a higher sensitivity, specificity and positive predictive value than the biochemical markers for hazardous consumption, including binging as well as alcohol dependence. It was also cost-efficient at around £1.70 per patient.

Some 25% of attendees screened positive, showing the scale of the hidden problem.

Sensitivity of the CAGE questionnaire for the DSM diagnosis of alcohol abuse and dependence in general clinical populations was 71% at cut points ≥2. Evidence-Based Medicine 2005; **10**: 26
The following paper is reviewed
The value of the CAGE in screening for alcohol abuse and alcohol dependence in general clinical populations: a diagnostic meta-analysis
Aertgeerts B, Buntinx F, Kester, A
J Clin Epidemiol, 2004; **57**: 30–39

Scoring 2 or more on the CAGE questionnaire has a sensitivity of 71% and specificity was 90% for diagnosis of alcohol abuse and dependence according to this meta-analysis. This limits its value using its recommended cut-off point but, as the commentary says, likelihood ratios increase with higher scores, particularly in ambulatory patients. So the kind of patients we get in general practice can be

LIFESTYLE

screened by the tool with the legitimacy of treating the score like a graded measure rather than simply positive or negative.

British drinking: a suitable case for treatment?
Hall W
BMJ, 2005; **331**: 527–528

Britain has one of the highest rates of alcohol dependence in the European Union and the usual remedies of public education and improved policing do not seem to be making much headway.

Australians, on the other hand, have imposed lower taxes on weaker beer and low alcohol beer now accounts for 40% of beer consumed. Random breath testing on a large scale (and lower driving limits for alcohol) have gained public support following reductions in deaths and serious injuries.

Regarding treatment, the time may now be right for investment in two relatively brief psychosocial interventions – motivational enhancement treatment and social network therapy – allowing the UK government to make headway on their targets for alcohol related disease.

Effectiveness of treatment for alcohol problems: findings of the randomised UK alcohol treatment trial (UKATT)
and
Cost effectiveness of treatment for alcohol problems: findings of the randomised UK alcohol treatment trial (UKATT)
UKATT Research Team
BMJ, 2005; **331**: 541–544, 544–548

These two papers compared the effectiveness of social behaviour and network therapy (up to eight 50-minute sessions) – a new treatment for alcohol problems aimed at building social networks to support changes in behaviour – with the proven track record of motivational enhancement therapy (three 50-minute sessions).

No previous British randomised trial of non-pharmacological treatments for alcohol problems had had the statistical power to reliably detect effectiveness.

This randomised trial followed over 600 outpatients for a year and showed that both interventions showed similar and substantial reductions in alcohol consumption and dependence as well as improvements in mental health. Both therapies saved about five times as much in term of GP/hospital resources, social consequences and legal services as they cost.

The two therapies were equally cost-effective despite the average cost of social behaviour and network therapy being £221 and that of motivational enhancement therapy being £129.

Alcohol dependence and driving: a survey of patients' knowledge of DVLA regulations and possible clinical implications
Culshaw M
Psychiatric Bulletin, 2005: **29**: 90–93

A Glasgow survey of 58 patients with alcohol dependence showed that most

LIFESTYLE

heavy drinkers with a licence continue to drive, unaware that there are any restrictions from the DVLA. Only 14% said that a health professional had discussed the regulations with them – of these, four were GPs, one was a nurse, and one a psychiatrist. Doctors have a duty to inform the DVLA if they are aware such a patient continues to drive but are either unaware of this, avoid the issue, or worry about breaches of confidentiality and the effect on the doctor–patient relationship.

Further Research

CARDIOVASCULAR EFFECTS

- A large US study in 14 000 hypertensive men with 76 000 person-years of follow-up, supported the many reports that link alcohol consumption with lower cardiovascular risk. Those who had some alcohol every day came off best with a 40% reduction in cardiovascular mortality. Total mortality also reduced significantly as frequency of consumption increased. No cancer link with moderate alcohol consumption was spotted. *Arch Intern Med*, 2004; **164**: 623–628.

- Coronary calcification was detected by CT and used as a measure of coronary atherosclerosis in this cross-sectional study. The risk of extensive calcification was 50% lower in individuals who consumed 1 to 2 alcoholic drinks per day compared to nondrinkers. *Arch Intern Med*, 2004; **164**: 2355–2360.

EFFECTS ON STROKE

- Meta-analysis results indicate that heavy alcohol consumption around 50 units a week markedly increases the relative risk of stroke, both ischaemic and haemorrhagic. One unit a day seemed to protect against total stroke but two daily drinks only protected against ischaemic stoke. The relationship between alcohol intake and total and ischaemic stroke was nonlinear whereas the relationship with haemorrhagic stroke was linear. *JAMA*, 2003; **289**: 579–588.

- This prospective study followed nearly 20 000 middle-aged Japanese men for an average of 11 years. Heavy drinking (around 50 units per week), more than doubled the risk of stroke after controlling for hypertension and other cardiovascular risk factors. Strokes were mainly haemorrhagic. For those who drank two drinks a day or less, the increase in haemorrhagic stroke was balanced by a decrease in ischaemic stroke and total stroke was not affected. *Stroke*, 2004; **35**: 1124–1129.

LIFESTYLE

EFFECTS ON CANCER

- Pooled data from eight large prospective studies involving nearly half a million people in five countries indicate that, as suspected, alcohol moderately increases the risk of cancer of the colon and rectum. The increased risk only applied if consumption was two or more drinks a day as it was in 4% of women and 13% of men. Over five drinks per day led to a 40% increased risk. Type of drink and gender were irrelevant. *Ann Intern Med*, 2004; **140**: 603–613.

DRUG MISUSE

What we know already:

- Some 3.2 million people in Britain smoke cannabis
- The number of cannabis smokers is increasing with large rises in adolescents
- One-quarter of boys and girls age 14–15 years have tried cannabis
- Cannabis use appears to be associated with onset of schizophrenia
- Between 1993 and 1998 psychotic illness related to drug misuse increased by 50%. The average age of these cases decreased from 38 years to 34 years
- Most users of cannabis also smoke tobacco
- Cannabis was reclassified from a Class B to a Class C drug across the UK in January 2004. As a controlled drug, production, supply and possession remains illegal, only the penalties have changed
- Despite pressure and fears over psychosis, the Home Secretary refused in January 2006 to reclassify cannabis as a Class B drug
- Amongst drug misusers, heroin is the most used drug followed by methadone then cannabis and amphetamines
- Most users are in their twenties and males outweigh females by 3:1
- All doctors will see drug users for a variety of medical and social problems
- Methadone maintenance in a primary care setting can be effective in reducing crime and HIV risk-taking behaviour while improving physical and psychological well-being

Guidance

The BMA are trying to highlight the driving risks related to drugs including cannabis. Between the mid-eighties and mid-nineties there was a four-fold increase in those testing positive for cannabis after fatal collisions. It is an offence involving the same penalties as for alcohol but legal limits are not defined, public awareness is low and good testing devices are needed.

Cannabis and the lungs. A smoking gun? *British Lung Foundation,* London 2002.
This document serves as a useful summary of current evidence. It recommends a public health education campaign aimed at young people and further research on consequences of cannabis smoking.

Drug Misuse and Dependence – Guidelines on Clinical Management. *Dept of Health,* 1999/2007.
This is a comprehensive document of the growth of drug use and measures aiming to tackle it. Updated guidelines incorporating NICE guidance on detoxification, maintenance therapy and psychosocial interventions for opiate users are expected by Summer 2007.

Guidance for working with cocaine and crack users in primary care. *RCGP,* Sept 2004.
This is a detailed document looking at issues related to primary and shared care for different types of user communities.

LIFESTYLE

Recent Papers

CANNABIS

Comparing cannabis with tobacco
Henry JA, Oldfield WL, Kon OM
BMJ, 2003; **326**: 942–943

This editorial explains that both cannabis and tobacco smoking lead to inhalation of 4000 largely identical chemicals. Smoking cannabis is known to entail a two-thirds larger puff volume, a one-third larger inhaled volume, a four-fold longer time holding the breath and a five-fold increase in carboxyhaemaglobin. In addition, the amount of the main active constituent, tetrahydrocannabinol (THC), in cannabis has increased ten-fold in the last 20 years in Britain and is still only half the strength of that smoked in Holland. Cannabis cigarettes deposits four times as much tar on the respiratory tract as an unfiltered cigarette of the same weight.

As well as triggering mental illness, other effects on the heart and respiratory system are inevitable. But solace for the users may be taken in the dearth of evidence against it, much as for smoking a few decades ago. There will undoubtedly be a latent period for the damage to be seen and evidence to mount up. All the indications are that the effects of smoking cannabis will be at least as bad as those of smoking tobacco, except at a younger age where it also notably starts causing bullous lung disease. Sudden death and myocardial infarction have been attributed to acute effects of smoking cannabis but not yet linked to progressive CAD.

The article concludes there is no momentum for attacking the problem and no clear public health message.

Prospective cohort study of cannabis use, predisposition for psychosis, and psychotic symptoms in young people
Henquet C, Krabbendam L, Spauwen J et al.
BMJ, 2005; **330**: 11

This study of nearly 2500 young people aged 14–24 years found that use of cannabis moderately increased psychotic symptoms at follow up 4 years later. The effect was not exclusive to but was more pronounced in those with a predisposition for psychosis (such as paranoid ideation), but independent of use of other drugs, tobacco or alcohol.

This supports the accumulation and converging evidence of a pro-psychotic effect of cannabis which followed a dose–response pattern. The study was able to establish the association as causal.

A 25-year prospective study in New Zealand found rates of psychotic symptoms more than 60% higher in users than non-users. *Addiction,* 2005; **100**: 354–366.

Another from the same country found that cannabis users had a 10-fold increased risk of serious car crashes. *Addiction,* 2005; **100**: 605–611.

LIFESTYLE

The effectiveness of community maintenance with methadone or buprenorphine for treating opiate dependence

Simoens S, Matheson C, Bond C, *et al.*
Br J Gen Pract, 2005; **55**: 139–146

This systematic review of maintenance therapy in primary care found that methadone and the lesser used buprenorphine were both effective and that higher doses were associated with better treatment outcomes.

This is important as a recent survey showed that almost half the GPs surveyed were prescribing substitute medication – three times as many as 16 years previously. However, most doses were too low to constitute optimal methadone maintenance risking adverse patient behaviours and poor outcomes (*Br J Gen Pract,* 2005; **55**: 444–451). Primary care could truly be an effective setting to expand high quality substitute prescribing in treatment of opiate dependence.

Incidence of hepatitis C virus and HIV among new injecting drug users in London: prospective cohort study

Judd A, Hickman M, Jones S *et al.*
BMJ, 2005; **330**: 24–25

This recent reassessment of prevalence rates of HIV and hepatitis C infection in injecting drug users shows that our harm reduction strategies have not been as successful as first thought. Testing users mostly from London who had started their habit within the previous 6 years showed baseline prevalence to be 44% for hepatitis C and 4.2% for HIV.

Over the year of study, the incidence of new cases of hepatitis C virus among new injecting drug users was 42 per 100 person years and of HIV was 3.4 cases per 100 person years. The suggestion is that transmission may have recently increased perhaps due to greater injection of crack and riskier behaviour in the new recruits.

LIFESTYLE

DIET

What we know already:

- The burden of food-related ill health mainly due to unhealthy diets has been estimated as similar to that attributable to smoking in terms of mortality and morbidity
- The Mediterranean diet relying on plant foods and unsaturated lipids has been shown to reduce cardiovascular end-points, cancers and overall mortality
- It is characterised by a high vegetable intake, legumes, fruits, and cereals, a moderate to high intake of fish, a low intake of saturated fats but high intake of unsaturated fats, particularly olive oil, a low intake of dairy products and meat, and a modest intake of alcohol, mostly as wine
- An Indo-Mediterranean diet in which green leafy vegetables, mustard or soybean oils, certain nuts and whole grains replace fish, rapeseed and olive oils, also reduces risk of cardiac death by up to half – at least in Indian men
- Total fruit and vegetable intake is inversely associated with risk of cardiovascular disease – at least five 'servings' a day are recommended. A once-daily serving of a green leafy vegetable has been shown to claim most of this benefit by cutting cardiovascular disease by over 10%
- Research has concentrated on dietary patterns in order to accommodate a complex interplay between nutrients
- The Atkins diet books have sold more than 45 million copies over 40 years
- Omega 3 fatty acids can protect against coronary heart disease
- Dietary magnesium (from whole grains, nuts, and green leafy vegetables) appears to protect against diabetes and heart disease

Recent Papers

GENERAL

Health claims for functional foods
Katan, MB
BMJ, 2004; **328**: 180–181

This editorial looks at functional foods that claim to improve well-being or health and examines who safeguards the truth in an area full of dubious claims.

Some ingredients certainly promote health – the value of folic acid for example is well established. But some are questionable – anyone for a zinc lozenge?

Non-nutritive ingredients in functional foods include sorbitol in chewing gum (which reduces dental caries), plant stanols and sterols (which lower LDL) and probiotic bacteria which may diminish rotavirus in infants. There are also unproven candidates such as phytoestrogens for breast cancer and many herbal remedies are under review for benefit and more importantly for potential harm.

Functional foods are marketed directly to consumers who cannot assess these claims. If doctors are not there to do it, the government needs to. Current regulations allow an articulate commercial enterprise to dance round them. Soft claims compellingly imply health benefits without naming a disease and 'quackery' is rife.

Little research is being done to identify the ingredients with the positive therapeutic effects as regulation does not require it.

While safety is well regulated, health claims are not. Even the US which used to require 'significant scientific agreement' for food claims has seemingly thrown in the towel to allow 'qualified health claims' as long as a disclaimer is included. The EU regulations are such that a claim (e.g. for folic acid preventing neural tube defect) cannot be made even when it is true!

Fruit and vegetable consumption and stroke: meta-analysis of cohort studies
He F, Nowson C, MacGregor G
Lancet, 2006; **367**: 320–326

This meta-analysis totalled 250 000 subjects with nearly 5000 stroke events and showed that eating more than five servings of fruit and vegetables per day can cut the risk of stroke by as much as 26%. Three to five servings managed a reduction of 11%.

It is probably the combination of nutrients that does the trick. A portion might be a medium-sized apple, a cup of raw salad greens, half a cup of cut-up vegetables, half a cup of cooked beans or peas, or three-quarters of a cup of 100% fruit or vegetable juice.

DIET REGIMES

Comparison of the Atkins, Ornish, Weight Watchers, and Zone diets for weight loss and heart disease risk reduction. A randomized trial
Dansinger ML, Gleason JA, Griffith JL, et al.
JAMA, 2005; **293**: 43–53

So which is the best diet, doctor?

A total of 160 participants in the US were randomly assigned to Atkins (carbohydrate restriction), Zone (macronutrient balance), Weight Watchers (calorie restriction), or Ornish (fat restriction) diet groups. After 2 months of maximum effort, participants selected their own levels of dietary adherence.

All the diets performed equally. At one year, about 25% of each group had a more than 5% loss and 10% had a more than 10% loss.

Adherence to the diets was not good so patients should choose the diet they will find the easiest to stick to.

LIFESTYLE

The BBC diet trials
Arterburn D
BMJ, 2006; **332**: 1284–1285
and
Randomised controlled trial of four commercial weight loss programmes in the UK: initial findings from the BBC 'diet trials'
Truby H, Baic S, deLooy A *et al.*
BMJ, 2006; **332**: 1309–1314

The BBC diet trials were an attempt to compare the effects of four commercially available diets – Dr Atkins' new diet revolution ('the Atkins' – a low carbohydrate diet), Slim-Fast plan (meal substitution), Weight Watchers pure points programme (energy control), and Rosemary Conley's Eat Yourself Slim diet and fitness plan.

- Compared to a control group, there was little to choose between them – all produced weight loss of around 6% (6 kg) at 6 months
- Atkins produced faster weight loss in the first four weeks but was no more effective by the end. It did not adversely affect cholesterol and was the cheapest option. The Atkins book costs £8, 24 weeks of Rosemary Conley classes were £140, Weight Watchers classes cost £170, and twice daily Slim-Fast meal replacements cost £240
- Dropout rates were slightly higher for Slim-Fast and Atkins – the programmes which had less ongoing support

The BBC picked up the tab for the first 6 months but after that persistence with the diets was low and long-term inferences become impossible.

MEDITERRANEAN DIETS

Modified Mediterranean diet and survival: EPIC-elderly prospective cohort study
Trichopoulou A, Orfanos P, Norat T, *et al.*
BMJ, 2005; **330**: 991

EPIC – the European Prospective Investigation into Cancer and Nutrition study – is a very large prospective study reaching 9 European countries and 478 000 men and women from many European countries. It investigates the role of biological, dietary, lifestyle and environmental factors in cancer and other chronic diseases. It is coordinated by the International Agency for Research on Cancer and is the largest available database for investigating the role of diet in health.

This part of EPIC studied 75 000 men and women from 9 countries, aged over 60 and free of serious disease at enrolment. They aimed to see if the advantages for cardiovascular end points with the Mediterranean diet translated into years of longer life. They did better than they expected.

The diet was modified to make it more Euro-friendly by including polyunsaturates (much commoner in non-Mediterranean countries) in with the measure of the monounsaturated lipids so common in the olive oils of Greece and Spain.

A scoring system out of 10 was invented to measure adherence to the diet which may be a little arbitrary and discriminatory. However, the results were still impressive.

LIFESTYLE

- There was significantly longer life expectancy in the healthy elderly cohort
- A 2 point increase in the score corresponded to an 8% reduction in mortality and a 4% increase led to a 14% reduction
- A healthy 60 year old adhering to the diet can expect to live a year longer than one who does not adhere well
- They conclude polyunsaturates are an acceptable substitute for monounsaturates
- The benefits were strongest in Greece and Spain where they have the true Mediterranean diet.

Effects of a Mediterranean-style diet on cardiovascular risk factors

Estruch R, Martínez-González MA, Corella D *et al.*
Ann Intern Med, 2006; **145**: 1–11

This Spanish study is finding that the impact of the Mediterranean diet can be quick. They randomised 772 patients with a high risk of cardiovascular disease to a low fat diet or one of two Mediterranean diets – one provided free virgin olive oil and one provided free nuts.

Short term benefit on surrogate markers of cardiac disease were illustrated within 3 months. The Mediterranean diet improved plasma lipid profiles and CRP more than a low fat diet, reduced systolic blood pressure by 6 mmHg (oil) and 7 mmHg (nuts) and reduced serum glucose by 0.4 mmol/l and 0.3 mmol/l, respectively.

OMEGA 3

Omega 3 fatty acids and cardiovascular disease – fishing for a natural treatment

Din JN, Newby DE, Flapan AD
BMJ, 2004; **328**: 30–35

This review looks at the evidence for omega 3 fatty acids derived from fish oils, namely eicosapentanoic acid and docosahexanoic acid. (A further one – α-linolenic acid – is available from certain plants.) Oily fish such as mackerel, herring, tuna, salmon, sardines and trout are rich sources of the two fish oils. Although optimal intake remains to be established, the often-quoted two to three servings per week should provide approximately 1 g/day omega 3 fatty acids. Cod and haddock are leaner and have less oil and frozen / fast food products have very little.

A coronary benefit has been shown following observations that Greenland Inuits who largely consume fish, seal and whale, have a low mortality from CHD.

Most studies have confirmed an inverse association between fish consumption and CHD. The DART trial involved over 2000 men with recent MI and showed that advice to eat more fish reduced mortality in the following 2 years by 29%.

Fish oil capsule supplementation in a large Italian study showed a 15% reduction in total mortality over 3.5 years.

Most of the rest of the studies (that showed no such association) were in populations with an already moderate fish intake who perhaps already had reached a ceiling of benefit.

Various mechanisms have been suggested, originally dwelling on antithrombotic effects, but recent evidence showing substantial reductions in sudden death

LIFESTYLE

indicate the predominant effect may be antiarrythmic. Improvements in atherosclerosis on angiography have also been shown after omega 3 supplementation. This may be due to effects on inflammation, lipids, production of growth factor or endothelial vasomotor function.

A meta-analysis has also shown a benefit on blood pressure by 2.1 / 1.6 mmHg. But contaminants, including lead, that accumulate in particularly larger fish may attenuate the cardioprotective benefit.

The Americans recommend supplementation of fish oil for those with 'documented' CHD but high quality trials are awaited before routine recommendations can be validated.

Further Research

Fish

- In an American trial of nearly 5000 elderly adults followed for 12 years, weekly consumption of broiled or baked fish – not fried fish or fish sandwiches – was associated with a 30% lower incidence of atrial fibrillation. *Circulation*, 2004; **110**: 368–373.

- A meta-analysis of eight studies showed a 13% reduction in stroke for those who ate fish once a week (compared to those who ate it less than once a month), and a 31% reduction for those who ate it more than four times per week. The benefit is principally for ischaemic stroke. *Stroke*, 2004; **35**: 1538–1542.

Meat

- EPIC found that eating more than 160g of red meat per day means a 35% higher chance of developing bowel cancer than those who eat less than 20g per day after adjusting for other variables. The risk also increased in those on a low-fibre diet. These findings were consistent through all the European populations in the EPIC study. *J Natl Cancer Inst*, 2005; **97**: 906–916.

- In another large study of 25 000 people followed up for 9 years, researchers found that people who ate the most red meat in the study were twice as likely to develop rheumatoid arthritis as people who ate half as much red meat or less. *Arthritis Rheumatism*, 2004; **50**: 3804–3812.

Calcium

- Consumption of milk and calcium is inversely associated with the risk of cancers of the distal colon and rectum. Dietary information gathered by food questionnaires showed a benefit threshold at around 1000 mg per day of calcium. Unfortunately some studies point to a higher risk of fatal prostate cancer when calcium intake is high. *J Natl Cancer Inst*, 2004; **96**: 1015–1022.

LIFESTYLE

- A meta-analysis of 19 studies regarding calcium supplements in children showed only a slight increase in bone density in the upper limb but none at the hip or lumbar spine. The authors tell us that supplements are unlikely to make a significant difference to the risk of fracture in childhood or later adult life. An editorial suggests we might have to change assumptions and revise guidelines for calcium intake. *BMJ*, 2006; **333**: 763–764, 775.

Probiotics

- Influencing the gut microflora by administration of probiotic bacteria – live, non-pathogenic, micro-organisms – is a new idea. This study indicated that treatment with *Lactobacillus GG* helped reduce symptoms of atopic eczema/dermatitis but only in IgE-sensitised infants. *Allergy*, 2005; **60**: 494–500.

- A probiotic preparation containing *Bifidobacterium infantis* relieves symptoms of IBS while reducing inflammatory cytokine levels suggesting an immune-modulating effect. It was head to head with a *Lactobacillus* which was ineffective. The effect was similar in magnitude to that shown for the recently approved tegaserod and alosetron. *Gastroenterology*, 2005; **128**: 541–551.

- The first placebo-controlled randomised trial of co-treatment with *Saccharomyces boulardii* in children showed an impressive 80% reduction in the risk of antibiotic-associated diarrhoea. *Aliment Pharmacol Ther*, 2005; **21**: 583–590.

Fibre

- A high quality meta-analysis has found no evidence that higher fibre intake reduces the risk of colorectal cancer. It seemed protective until the intake of dietary folate was adjusted for. A diet high in whole plant foods is still a good idea, however. *Gut*, 2006; **55**: 1461–1466.

LIFESTYLE

VITAMINS

What we know already:

- Folate, vitamin B6, and B12 deficiency are related to elevated blood homocysteine level
- Raised homocysteine is thought to be an independent risk factor for cerebral and coronary vascular disease and is usually due to deficiency of folate and B vitamins
- However, higher concentrations of vitamins in the blood have not been shown to reverse the disease process, so the role of supplementation is far from clear
- Folate intake, at least as part of the diet, appears to have a protective effect on stroke and there is an ongoing debate regarding mandatory folate fortification of foods
- There is a lot of controversy about the role of vitamin supplements for prevention of vascular disease and cancer. There is much research to be done but they are not as harmless as many would like to believe
- Reports suggest that use of multivitamin supplements in early life could lead to a higher risk of asthma and food allergies
- The largest randomised trials we have conclude that antioxidant supplementation with vitamin E, vitamin C and beta-carotene cannot be recommended for CHD prevention. Wasting more time on them may reduce compliance with proven medications such as aspirin, ACE inhibitors and statins
- Beta carotene (even in over-the-counter formulations) leads to a small but significant increase in all-cause mortality and cardiovascular death
- Promotion direct to consumer by health food outlets has been widespread
- At least 25% of older people in the UK take nutritional supplements

Recent Papers

FOLIC ACID

Lowering homocysteine with folic acid and B vitamins did not prevent vascular events in vascular disease or after myocardial infarction. *Evidence-Based Medicine,* 2006; **11**: 104–105
The following papers are reviewed
Homocysteine lowering with folic acid and B vitamins in vascular disease
Lonn E, Yusuf S, Arnold MJ *et al.*
N Engl J Med, 2006; **354**: 1567–1577
and
Homocysteine lowering and cardiovascular events after acute myocardial infarction
Bønaa KH, Njølstad I, Ueland PM *et al.*
N Engl J Med, 2006; **354**: 1578–1588

Does folate really help to reduce cardiovascular disease by lowering homocysteine?

Good observational evidence and some small trials said yes. These two large randomised trials provide a clear 'no'. Confidence intervals were tight enough to rule out an important effect.

The first study – HOPE-2 – randomised 5522 patients over 55 with cardiovascular disease in 145 centres in 13 countries. A combined pill with folic acid, vitamin B6 and B12 did increase the blood concentrations of these vitamins and lowered plasma homocysteine by around 22%. But it failed to have a positive effect on cardiovascular death, MI or stroke.

Similarly, the NORVIT (Norwegian Vitamin) trial of 3749 patients with recent MI were randomised to various combinations of the same vitamins or to placebo. Again they lowered homocysteine to a similar degree but after 3 years there was no evidence of improvement in end-points. The combination tablets that contained all three ingredients even showed a trend towards an increase in fatal or non-fatal MI in stroke and sudden cardiac death.

It seems the one untested element of the 'polypill' can now be dropped.

The commentator espouses how similar the pattern is to the fallen arguments for vitamin E and HRT. It seems that in CVD prevention there is 'simply no substitute for large randomised controlled trials that measure clinical, not surrogate, end-points'. We end up 'chasing rainbows' when we should be focussing on ensuring that all patients are receiving the therapies that we know work.

Effect of folic acid supplementation on risk of cardiovascular diseases: a meta-analysis of randomized controlled trials
Bazzano LA, Reynolds K, Holder KN et al.
JAMA, 2006; **296**: 2720–2726

Meta-analysis of 12 RCTs found that folic acid supplementation does not reduce the risk of cardiovascular events or reduce all-cause mortality in those with a history of vascular disease. Nearly 17 000 such patients were included and secondary prevention with folate was not shown to have any value.

Low folate levels may protect against colorectal cancer
Van Guelpen B, Hultdin J, Johansson I et al.
Gut, 2006; **55**: 1461–1466

It is widely thought that folate protects against colorectal cancer. Most of the studies claiming this have estimated dietary intake. However, this study took the trouble to actually measure circulating folate. It found a decreased risk of colorectal cancer in subjects with low folate status. In addition, subjects with the highest folate seemed much likelier to develop colorectal cancer than those with the lowest.

It remains to be seen how this study fits in with the balance of evidence in the long run. Mandatory folic acid fortification in foods is a hot debate and would be an enormous public heath intervention. Research such as this must give pause to the notion of folate fortification for all.

International retrospective cohort study of neural tube defects in relation to folic acid recommendations: are the recommendations working?
Botto LD, Lisi A, Robert-Gnansia E, et al.
BMJ, 2005; **330**: 571.

Folic acid supplements consumed before conception can reduce spina bifida and other neural tube defects by over 80%. This retrospective study in

LIFESTYLE

13 countries that issued advice to take folic acid in this way found no detectable improvement in incidence of neural tube defects up to 6 years after the recommendation.

Preventable new cases of neural tube defects are still appearing. The time may be right to join the US and Canada who ensure their citizens get at least some folate by fortifying their flour with it.

ANTIOXIDANTS

Meta-analysis: high-dosage vitamin E supplementation may increase all-cause mortality
Miller ER , Pastor-Barriuso R, Dalal D, *et al.*
Ann Intern Med, 2005; **142**: 37–46

A meta-analysis of 1 135 000 subjects in 19 trials indicated increased mortality with increasing doses of vitamin E, further refuting suggestions of a benefit for heart disease or cancer.

About 11% of adult Americans consume at least 400 IU of vitamin E daily, more if they are older and take other antioxidants. Doses above this can kill and those who choose to take vitamin E for the reasons above should be aware of the risk to their health or better still, just stop (*Ann Intern Med*, 2005; **143**: 116–20). It probably leads to heart failure in the long run and it may be time to finish with this discredited supplement. (*JAMA*, 2005; **293**: 1338–1347).

Antioxidant supplements for prevention of gastrointestinal cancers: a systematic review and meta-analysis
Bjelakovic G, Nikolova DMA, Simonetti RG, *et al.*
Lancet, 2004; **364**: 1219–1228

A meta-analysis of 14 randomised trials (*n*=170 525) looked at effects of supplementation with vitamins A, C and E on oesophageal, gastric, colorectal, pancreatic, and liver cancer incidences. None was shown to be protective and a combination of beta carotene with vitamin A was even associated with a 30% increased risk of death. Combination of beta carotene with vitamin E led to a 10% increase.

MULTIVITAMINS

Effect of multivitamin and multimineral supplements on morbidity from infections in older people (MAVIS trial): pragmatic, randomised, double blind, placebo controlled trial
Avenell A, Campbell MK, Cook JA, *et al.*
BMJ, 2005; **331**: 324–329

This placebo-controlled trial of the effect of multivitamin and multimineral supplementations was done in Scotland over a period of a year.

There was no effect on self-reported infections, prescriptions, admission, quality of life or contacts with primary care. The study was of good quality and largely

LIFESTYLE

confirms previous research but biases can creep in. The doses used were low and the populations were relatively fit.

Role of multivitamins and mineral supplements in preventing infections in elderly people: systematic review and meta-analysis of randomised controlled trials
El-Kadiki A, Sutton AJ
BMJ, 2005; **330**: 871

Older people are susceptible to infection and vitamin supplements have been used on an *ad hoc* basis. This review looked at the available evidence for and against and found little evidence to suggest that multivitamin and mineral supplements actually prevent infections in elderly people,

Overall, a lot of the evidence was weak, flawed and conflicting. It does not support a policy of routine supplementation in all elderly people as things stand.

LIFESTYLE

EXERCISE

What we know already:

- Physical inactivity is an independent risk factor for cardiovascular and other diseases
- It is difficult to change longstanding and complex patterns of physical inertia
- General practice is ideally placed to identify sedentary adults and deliver brief interventions
- Young adults assessed by treadmill test as having low fitness were twice as likely to develop diabetes, high blood pressure, and the metabolic syndrome than participants with high fitness levels, even after accounting for body mass index
- Early interventions could create massive health benefits for the population
- Interventions promoting physical activity can help to reduce cardiovascular risk factors, diabetes, obesity, osteoporosis, and symptoms of depression
- Exercise training lowers CRP levels linked to high risks of diabetes and cardiovascular disease
- Measuring CRP levels could help to identify the high-risk people that will benefit from the anti-inflammatory and anti-atherosclerotic effect of exercise
- Research has shown that for both sexes, moderate physical activity delays cardiovascular disease and extends life in the over fifties by 1.3 years. High physical activity extends life by 3.7 years
- Physical functioning and quality of life can also benefit from such interventions making physical activity 'today's best buy in public health'

Guidelines

At least five a week: Evidence on the impact of physical activity and its relationship to health (April 2004). This report from the Chief Medical Officer recommends that adults do at least 30 minutes a day of moderately intense activity on five or more days a week. It also advises that children and young people do at least 60 minutes every day. Walking, golf, mowing the lawn, decorating and cycling are considered examples of moderate physical activity.

Recent Papers

THE VALUE OF EXERCISE

Exercise is associated with reduced risk for incident dementia among persons 65 years of age and older
Larson EB, Wang L, Bowen JD *et al.*
Ann Intern Med, 2006; **144**: 73–81

This study followed 1740 subjects over the age of 65 years who were clear of cognitive impairment at baseline. Those who exercised regularly over a mean follow-up period of 6 years reduced their risk of developing dementia by 38%.

The elderly have particularly low exercise levels and the most benefit in this large robust study went to those who were the least fit. Walking 15 minutes three times a week was enough to delay dementia.

What level of physical activity protects against premature cardiovascular death? The Caerphilly study
Yu S, Yarnell JWG, Sweetnam PM, *et al.*
Heart, 2003; **89**: 502–506

This interesting study involved 1975 men aged 49–64 years in Caerphilly – 90% of the 'middle-aged' male population in this part of Wales.

They were free of evidence of CHD and were followed up over 11 years with the intention of identifying how hard we need to exercise to get cardiovascular benefits.

Heavy intensity exercise such as swimming and jogging reduced the risk of premature death in this otherwise fit cohort after adjustment for age and other risk factors. Light and moderate intensity exercise, such as walking, golf and dancing, had inconsistent and non-significant effects on all cause, cerebrovascular and cardiovascular mortality. The conclusion? Habitual leisure exercise of vigorous intensity extends life.

Relative intensity of physical activity and risk of coronary heart disease
Lee IM, Sesso HD, Oguma Y, *et al.*
Circulation, 2003; **107**: 1110–1116

This paper followed 7337 men, mean age 66 years, for 7 years and adds another piece of information to the mix when deciding what levels of exercise to recommend.

Rather than prescribing a certain intensity, which may not be appropriate, this paper shows that benefits are gained relative to the individual's perceived level of their own exertion. This inverse association of exercise intensity and cardiovascular disease extended to men not fulfilling current activity recommendations.

This is good news and the authors caution that it is important that we are not over-prescriptive of exercise regimes that have not considered individual fitness.

It was previously unknown whether moderate intensity exercise, relative to an individual's capacity, was associated with reduced CHD rates.

INTERVENTIONS

Promoting walking and cycling as an alternative to using cars: systematic review
Ogilvie D, Egan M, Hamilton V, *et al.*
BMJ, 2004; **329**: 763

Promoting physical activity as leisure is one thing but changing the public's approach to transport is another option.

This review of 22 studies looked at the impact of promotion campaigns to use 'healthier' modes of transport. Campaigns with buzzy names such as 'Walk In to Work Out', 'TravelSmart', 'Curb Your Car' and 'Bikebusters' were assessed.

LIFESTYLE

They found some evidence that motivated subgroups could be influenced on around 5% of all trips. But the evidence in favour of many interventions and campaigns seems to suggest they are generally not very effective. Short-term improvements in cycling or walking to work were evident but no population strategy was shown to be effective. Raising awareness is not enough. Interventions that engage people and address personal relevance are likely to be more effective.

Effectiveness of counselling patients on physical activity in general practice: cluster randomised controlled trial
Elley CR, Kerse N, Arroll B, et al.
BMJ, 2003; **326**: 793–796

This study from New Zealand showed that when GPs (from 42 practices) gave written and oral advice to patients to get moving, it seemed to be beneficial. Previously no health benefits have been shown from the increases in physical activity that such advice leads to.

Attending patients age 40–79 years were screened by giving them a form which asked them about their physical activity or lack of it.

This study used something they called a 'green prescription' which outlined basic medical details and personal exercise goals. This was faxed to a local sports foundation and exercise specialists followed up the good word with telephone calls.

Motivational interview techniques were used throughout (the GPs had been trained in this) and the staff of the practice provided feedback on subsequent visits.

The proportion of people taking 2.5 hours of exercise a week increased by 10% with corresponding improvements in 'general health', vitality and bodily pain over 12 months.

Exercise training meta-analysis of trials in patients with chronic heart failure (ExTraMATCH)
Piepoli MF, Davos C, Francis DP, et al.
BMJ, 2004; **328**: 189–192

Randomised trials have focused mainly on symptomatic benefits and we know that exercise training reduces the debilitative effects of CHD.

This meta-analysis by the ExTraMATCH Collaborative of nine trials that included 801 stable patients found that exercise training improved survival in patients with chronic heart failure (risk reduction 32%). It also increased the median time to hospital admissions.

The paper was reviewed by Massie (*Evidence-Based Medicine*, 2004; **9**: 137) and the authors are praised for nailing down an answer to the question of mortality improvements as a result of exercise. He compares the size of benefit to the best pharmacological agents. The caveats he mentions refer to the necessary lack of blinding of the exercise groups and the widespread variation in conclusions of the included studies. In addition, the nature of the exercise varied in terms of nature, intensity, duration and supervision. He concludes that although this may

LIFESTYLE

not be definitive evidence for a beneficial effect of exercise training on mortality and morbidity, there is good reason for additional enthusiasm for further research and confidence in the safety of exercise recommendations.

A randomised controlled trial of three pragmatic approaches to initiate increased physical activity in sedentary patients with risk factors for cardiovascular disease
Little P, Dorward M, Gralton S, *et al.*
Br J Gen Pract, 2004; **54**: 189–195

What approaches work best to persuade people to get out of their chairs?

This randomised controlled trial looked at 151 sedentary patients with at least one documented cardiovascular risk factor.

These three interventions were applied in a $2 \times 2 \times 2$ factorial design:
- prescription by GPs for regular brisk exercise not requiring a leisure facility
- counselling by practice nurses to modify intentions and implement new behaviours
- use of the Health Education Authority information booklet 'Getting active, feeling fit'

Only the most intensive programme (combined counselling plus exercise prescription) showed clear improvements in activity and fitness. Single interventions had modest effects. The approach was shown to be feasible in general practice.

LIFESTYLE

SMOKING

What we know already:

- Smoking is the leading preventable cause of death in the UK
- Existing evidence implicates passive smoking as a cause of lung cancer and coronary heart disease
- Deaths from passive smoking from exposure at work are estimated at more than 600 each year in the UK, with exposure at home accounting for 2700 deaths in those aged 20–64 and 8000 in those aged ≥65
- As randomised controlled trials are not going to happen, various data used to examine the effects of environmental smoke have been subject to problems with confounding and precision
- We are still unsure about which of the 4000 ingredients in cigarette smoke lead to the harm
- Secondhand smoke is known to cause rapid changes in platelet and vascular endothelial function and rapid reductions in heart attacks have been observed in areas with smoking bans
- Cardiac patients get more benefit from quitting than using beta blockers or ACE inhibitors
- This shows the potential for the enforcement of smoke-free workplaces and public spaces and eliminating exposure to secondhand smoke is a public health priority throughout the world
- Nicotine is extremely addictive but two-thirds of smokers want to quit
- About 27% of the UK population smokes; about 25% of 15 year olds smoke regularly. One-third of smokers try to quit each year
- Smoking is a chronic condition requiring long-term management plans
- Brief advice to stop smoking is successful in 1 in 40 cases making it one of the most cost-effective interventions in medicine
- Nicotine replacement and bupropion, an atypical antidepressant, both double cessation rates. Nortiptyline has also been shown to be effective
- Combining drugs with counselling using a cognitive behavioural therapy approach yields the best results, but the style and depth of counselling in studies varies greatly
- Increased intensity of counselling including messages which invoke fear, self-help material and additional follow-up sessions or phone calls all increase the success rates
- Most smokers who are trying to stop need several attempts (typically up to seven) to quit but half quit eventually
- Positive predictive indicators for success in quitting smoking were a low nicotine dependence score and those with previous attempts to stop (80% more likely to quit). Each ten years of age increased the chances of success by 32%

Recent Papers

GENERAL

Mortality in relation to smoking: 50 years' observations on male British doctors
Doll R, Peto R, Boreham J et al.
BMJ, 2004; **328**:1519–1528

The fifty year results of this most famous of all papers are in. Sir Richard Doll's analysis of smoking habits in nearly 35 000 male British doctors since 1951 has concluded that:

- long-term cigarette smokers die on average 10 years earlier than non-smokers
- the full mortal effects of smoking can take 50 years to mature
- about half of all persistent smokers are killed by their habit (this figure has even reached two-thirds for this particular cohort)
- stopping smoking at age 60, 50, 40, or 30 years gains, respectively, about 3, 6, 9, or 10 years of life expectancy
- stopping at age 50 halves associated risks. Stopping at 30 avoids almost all of the elevated risk
- medical progress has reduced mortality rates in the last fifty years but persistent smokers do not qualify for these improvements
- on current patterns of uptake and in the absence of widespread cessation, there will be about one billion deaths from smoking this century

---

Prevalence of hardcore smoking in England, and associated attitudes and beliefs: cross sectional study
Jarvis MJ, Wardle J, Waller J et al.
BMJ, 2003; **326**: 1061

There is an especially resistant group of 'hardcore smokers'. Although there is no consensus of definition, this study targeted those who had not attempted to quit, had no desire or intention to quit in the future, and had had less than a day without cigarettes in the past five years. A Californian study used a slightly different definition which included consumption of at least 15 cigarettes per day but these authors preferred to use a definition which solely reflects motivation. Some 16% of all smokers fell into this category – much higher than previously estimated.

Hardcore smoking was associated with increased nicotine dependence and socioeconomic deprivation but the strongest association was with age, rising from 5% in those under 24 years to 30% in those aged $\geq$65 years. They were more likely to be recalcitrant in their attitudes and deny the possibility of consequences on their health despite actually being able to benefit more from giving up. Doing so at age 65 years can extend life by two years.

Interventions that are targeted to the particular needs and perceptions of hardcore smokers are needed.

LIFESTYLE

PASSIVE SMOKING

Passive smoking and risk of coronary heart disease and stroke: prospective study with cotinine measurement
Whincup PH, Gilg J A, Emberson JR *et al.*
BMJ, 2004; **329**: 200–205

An excess mortality from domestic sources alone in never-smokers who live with a smoker has been estimated previously at 15%.

This fascinating research in nearly 5000 men in the British Regional Heart Study concluded that using smoking in partners as a measure of exposure underestimates the risks of passive smoking.

A biomarker, serum cotinine (a nicotine metabolite), was measured, meaning that all sources of smoke could be assessed. Only half the amounts found were explained by domestic exposure, the rest presumably coming from pubs, restaurants and the workplace.

They showed that passive smoking (in non-smokers) led to an excess risk of coronary heart disease of 50–60%. The risk of stroke was not increased.

Environmental tobacco smoke and risk of respiratory cancer and chronic obstructive pulmonary disease in former smokers and never smokers in the EPIC prospective study
Vineis P, Airoldi L, Veglia F, *et al.*
BMJ, 2005; **330**: 277

A large prospective case-control study of 123 479 subjects within the enormous EPIC cohort provided information about exposure to secondhand smoke. Analysis was limited to people who had not smoked for more than 10 years. The results showed that:

- exposure to passive smoking raises the risk of all respiratory diseases including lung cancer
- the risks of secondhand smoke exposure are greater for ex-smokers than for never smokers perhaps due to susceptibility of already existing mutations
- frequent exposure to environmental tobacco smoke during childhood was associated with a threefold risk of lung cancer in adulthood
- cotinine concentrations were not associated with the risk of lung cancer. (Cotinine relects the past 24 hours of exposure. It can be useful for rapid feedback as a point of care test rather than estimating long-term risks.)

LEGISLATION

Legislation for smoke-free workplaces and health of bar workers in Ireland: before and after study
Allwright S, Paul G, Greiner B *et al.*
BMJ, 2005; **331**: 1117

In March 2004 the Republic of Ireland banned smoking in all indoor workplaces, including bars and restaurants. This study looked at changes in exposure in bar staff and restricted analyses to the 158 who were still non-smokers at follow-up a year after the legislation.

The non-smoking bar staff (who were the majority) had salivary cotinine concentrations which dropped by 80%, consistent with their estimates of their reduction in exposure. Respiratory symptoms also declined in non-smoking bar staff.

A recent survey has confirmed overwhelming and growing support for the new law. Over 80% of Irish smokers said the law was a 'good' or 'very good' thing. Nearly half the smokers said it made them more likely to quit, and 60% said it made them cut down on their smoking. Of the quitters, 80% said the law helped them to quit and nearly 90% said it helped them to stay off the cigarettes.

SMOKING CESSATION

Systematic review of the effectiveness of stage based interventions to promote smoking cessation
Riemsma RP, Pattenden J, Bridle, C et al.
BMJ, 2003; 326: 1175–1177

This is a review of 23 randomised controlled trials using the stage-based approach to positive change in smoking behaviour.

Behavioural approaches using a transtheoretical model identify a sequence of stages:
- precontemplation – where an antismoking seed may be planted for the future
- contemplation – an opportunity to build on the patients' dissatisfaction with his habit
- preparation – where the smoker is making plans to break the habit
- action – the time of the attempt when as much support as possible is required
- maintenance – to keep the ex-smoker motivated and try to avoid ...
- relapse – which is all too common and starts the cycle off again

It is important with this model to identify accurately the stage the smoker is at in order to tailor an approach. Frequent reassessments should be done to reflect when a smoker is ready to change and interventions are adapted and repeated until a change is maintained. This is a popular model for smoking cessation courses and may be more efficient than a 'one size fits all' treatment.

Results seem to indicate a trend in favour of stage-based interventions but the review found difficulties with weighing up the value of the approach definitively as data were limited on what interventions were used and how if at all they were tailored to the patients involved.

'Catastrophic' pathways to smoking cessation: findings from national survey
West R, Sohal T
BMJ, 2006; **332**: 458–460

The prevailing model for smoking cessation is the stages mentioned above, but many feel this is too arbitrary. This study of nearly 2000 smokers found that

LIFESTYLE

almost half had made no organised plan to do so and the group that kicked the habit abruptly were more likely to succeed for 6 months than those who planned ahead regardless of age, sex or socioeconomic group.

The authors offer us a catastrophe theory whereby a tiny trigger leads to a sweeping change when the proper tensions are right. They describe the 3Ts – tension (personal dissatisfaction creating motivation), trigger (to activate the change when the smoker is 'on the cusp') and treatments (nicotine patches and counselling immediately available to support the attempts).

Self help interventions for smoking cessation are not effective unless tailored to the individual. *Evidence-Based Medicine* 2006; **11**: 48
The following paper is presented
Self-help interventions for smoking cessation
Lancaster T, Stead LF
Cochrane Database Syst Rev, 2005

This systematic review of 60 trials found that unless interventions for stopping smoking were personally tailored they were not much good. Handing out generic standardised materials whether written, audio or video gives very low levels of positive results. There may be a few who get the message and the interventions are at least cheap, but where at all possible, approaches that use healthcare professionals in face-to-face encounters yield the best results and must be emphasised.

The NNT for tailored materials compared to standard materials was 53 reflecting a 2% increase in smoking cessation.

Further Research

- Light smokers are not safe. The Norwegian tobacco industry has previously suggested there is probably a safe threshold for smoking. Not so. Recent follow-up of over 42 000 Norwegian men and women found that smoking 1–4 cigarettes per day was associated with triple the risk of dying from ischaemic heart disease and lung cancer. *Tobacco Control,* 2005; **14**: 315–320.

- Smoking is associated with lower body mass index but new research in nearly 22 000 men and women aged 45–79 from Norfolk shows it relatively increases abdominal girth (and this is a better measure of health risk). Current smokers had higher waist to hip ratios and bigger waists than former smokers and non-smokers. They conclude the metabolic consequences of smoking include an adverse fat distribution profile. *Obesity Research,* 2005; 13: 1466–1475.

- You can't win. In one large study, benefits of quitting on lung function (FEV_1) were lessened significantly due to weight gain but gains still outweighed losses. Quitting is good for your lungs but weight control should be part of the programme. *Lancet,* 2005; **365**: 1629–1635.

- A Cochrane review of six trials found that clonidine joins NRT, bupropion and nortriptyline as an effective option in smoking cessation but its side

LIFESTYLE

effects – drowsiness, dry mouth, and postural hypotension – mean it is not first choice. *Evidence-Based Medicine,* 2005; **10**: 19.

- Experts from the United States have given a cautious welcome to a new drug designed to help people quit smoking. Varenicline is a partial nicotinic agonist and is the first new smoking cessation agent in nearly a decade that does not contain nicotine. Trials in the US suggest it may be more effective than bupropion, although it probably will not work for everyone. Sleep disturbance and nausea were relatively common and relapse rates were high even in those motivated enough to volunteer for a randomised trial of a new treatment. *JAMA,* 2006; **296**: 94–95.

LIFESTYLE

OBESITY AND THE METABOLIC SYNDROME

What we know already:

- Worldwide over one billion adults and children are overweight
- More than half of British adults are overweight
- Nearly one-third of 11-year-olds are overweight and 17% are obese
- Obesity in pre-school children has increased by over 70% in the last generation
- It has been predicted that obesity will soon overtake smoking as the leading UK health problem
- Abdominal obesity probably reflects both visceral and subcutaneous fat and therefore total fatness, so is a better predictor of coronary risk than BMI which gives no indication of fat distribution
- Central fatness may be related more to physical activity which has decreased in spite of fairly static energy intake particularly recently in females
- Obesity shortens lifespan and the role of primary care in managing obesity is linked to the aims of the national service framework for CHD
- A large primary care study estimates that obesity more than doubles prescribing in most categories
- Small changes in energy intake and output can have a major impact on the risk of obesity. Two hours spent watching TV can raise the risk of obesity by 23% and of diabetes by 14%. Two hours of sitting at work is associated with increases of 5% and 7% respectively. But two hours of standing or walking around at home reduced obesity by 9% and diabetes by 12%
- The Department of Health requires primary care to deliver obesity management services but attempts so far have proved to be labour intensive and with modest results at best. There are serious questions of feasibility and new models may be needed
- Dedicated obesity specialists at primary care trust level, use of local leisure services and employment of the commercial weight loss sector may all play a role in the future

Guidelines

Obesity: the prevention, identification, assessment and management of overweight and obesity in adults and children. *NICE*, **Dec 2006.**

The first NICE clinical guideline to outline strategies to prevent and tackle obesity in adults and children was released in December 2006.
- Coordinated efforts are needed to maximise the effectiveness of interventions. Primary care trusts will be required to implement recommendations with audit criteria.
- BMI should be used to classify the degree of obesity bearing in mind it is less reliable in Asians, the elderly and highly muscular people.
- Waist circumference should be used to assess health risks but is unreliable when BMI exceeds 35 kg/m^2.
- Weight management programmes should include behavioural change strategies to increase activity and reduce energy intake with ongoing support and realistic targets. Guidance is also given on the role of drugs and bariatric surgery.

The National Audit Office (www.nao.org.uk) has issued a report 'Tackling Obesity in England'. This is a detailed account of the costs of the problem, management strategies in the NHS and population initiatives to address all aspects of obesity.

Recent Papers

THE SCALE OF THE PROBLEM

Fighting obesity
Jain A
BMJ, 2004; **328**: 1327–1328

Obesity is a growing problem with increases of 10–50% in the past decade throughout Europe and up to 75% in the developing world.

The consensus is that the cause is environmental – easy access for the modern human to food and little need for exercise.

Interventions to date have focused on dietary behaviour and exercise but as a whole have had little or no impact on the growing epidemic.

The UK House of Commons Health Committee report on obesity (May 2004) recommends simpler labelling of food, categorising healthfulness, the banning of vending machines and school sponsorship by fast food chains, whereas the WHO calls for immediate bans of advertising junk food to children and restriction of sugar content.

The UK report calls for more access to treatments but unfortunately only a few treatments have been shown to work. They include drug treatment, complex multicomponent weight-loss programmes and surgery in extreme cases. Apart from surgical intervention, weight loss tends to be modest. The best cost-effective evidence-based strategy to tackle obesity is awaited.

Association of bodyweight with total mortality and with cardiovascular events in coronary artery disease: a systematic review of cohort studies
Romero-Corral A, Montori V, Somers V *et al.*
Lancet, 2006; **368**: 666–678

A systematic review of 40 studies with 250152 patients and 4 years of follow up, looked at the association between obesity, and total mortality and cardiovascular events in cardiac patients (following angioplasty, bypass or MI).
- Morbidly obese people (BMI ≥35) had the highest risk for cardiovascular mortality but did not have increased total mortality.
- Obese patients (BMI 30–35) did best of all and had no increased risk for cardiovascular or total mortality.
- Overweight people (BMI 25–30) had the lowest risk for total mortality and cardiovascular mortality compared with those for people with a normal BMI.
- Patients with a low BMI <20 had an increased risk for total and cardiovascular mortality.

This all appears bizarre and paradoxical. It is unlikely weight protects against car-

CLINICAL ISSUES

LIFESTYLE

diac disease. The authors tell us that using BMI as an indicator of cardiovascular risk should stop. It may not distinguish between fat and lean mass.

A previous *Lancet* study of over 27 000 people covered a wide ethnic variation in 52 countries. They found that waist and hip circumferences (adjusted for BMI) and waist-to-hip ratio were closely and independently associated with risk of MI even after adjustment for other risk factors. Waist-to-hip ratio had the strongest association worldwide so in most ethnic groups it might be more clinically valuable to redefine obesity in this way. BMI was the worst and the authors suggested it should perhaps become obsolete as a measure of risk for heart attack (*Lancet*, 2005; **366**: 1640–1649).

Obesity and the risk of new-onset atrial fibrillation
Wang TJ, Parise H, Levy D *et al.*
JAMA, 2004; **292**: 2471–2477

This study showed an association of obesity with new-onset AF. It was based on over 5000 participants in the Framingham Heart Study who were free from AF at baseline and who were followed up for 13 years. There was a 4% increase in risk of AF per single unit increase in BMI in men and women. Compared with normal weight individuals, that amounts to around a 50% increase in the risk of AF in the obese. The excess risk of AF associated with obesity appears to be mediated by left atrial dilatation. Control for this factor and the association disappears.

Obesity is an important, potentially modifiable risk factor for AF, which means that targeting obesity may reduce the mortality burden associated with AF.

CHILDHOOD OBESITY

Parents' awareness of overweight in themselves and their children: cross sectional study within a cohort (EarlyBird 21)
Jeffery AN, Voss LD, Metcalf BS *et al.*
BMJ, 2005; **330**: 23–24

This study of the parents of 277 children found that:
- only one-quarter recognised when their child was overweight
- even when the children were obese, one-third of mothers and over one-half of fathers saw their child's weight as about right
- nearly half the overweight parents judged their own weight to be about right
- the apparent lack of parental concern probably stems from a lack of awareness
- this gap must be addressed as parents are crucial partners in the fight against childhood obesity
- the adults' obesity and perception of their children's weight was independent of socioeconomic grouping

LIFESTYLE

Early life risk factors for obesity in childhood: cohort study
Reilly JJ, Armstrong J, Dorosty AR, *et al.*
BMJ, 2005; **330**: 1357

This study of 9000 children in Avon, UK, was set up to identify risk factors in the early life environment for childhood obesity at age seven. It found associations with birth weight and weight gain in the first year, adiposity rebound by age 43 months, parental obesity, more than 4 hours a week watching the television at age 3 years and short (<10.5 hours) periods of sleep at age 3.

There was a relationship with maternal smoking *in utero* but no protective effect of breast-feeding.

Preventing childhood obesity by reducing consumption of carbonated drinks: cluster randomised controlled trial
James J, Thomas P, Cavan D *et al.*
BMJ, 2004; **328**: 1237

Few school-based or family-based programmes promoting activity and dietary change have had much impact. This study of 644 children aged 7–11 years in six English primary schools employed a focused educational programme called 'Ditch the Fizz' to discourage a single important factor – the consumption of carbonated drinks. A one-hour session each term was used to illustrate benefits on tooth decay and promote a healthy diet. After a year the intervention group drank fewer fizzy drinks and the control group drank more.

A small decrease in the percentage of overweight children in the intervention group occurred over the same twelve months that the control group had a 7.6% increase. Schools can have an important role in preventing childhood obesity.

METABOLIC SYNDROME

The metabolic syndrome
Meigs JB
BMJ, 2003; **327**: 61–62

The metabolic syndrome is proposed as the common antecedent of cardiovascular disease and type 2 diabetes. Diagnosing such a syndrome might hold promise for enhanced preventative measures. The syndrome is characterised by the co-existence of obesity (especially central), dyslipidaemia (especially high triglycerides and low levels of HDL), hyperglycaemia and hypertension. Specific thresholds are currently elusive.

Insulin resistance has been put forward as the unifying pathophysiology as has obesity but the argument still seems incomplete.

Does the metabolic syndrome predict adverse outcomes greater than the sum of its parts? Evidence is unclear. Inactivity fuels obesity fuels diabetes fuels cardiovascular disease. Prevention of obesity could break the vicious circle. More research on the metabolic syndrome is needed before targets can be located and effective interventions tailored.

Conflicting research persists in 2006 but there is a growth of feeling that the

LIFESTYLE

concept of the metabolic syndrome should be viewed as handy clinical summary of metabolic risk factors, rather than a real entity which predicts a cardiovascular endpoint independent of its constituents.

Metabolic syndrome
Khunti K, Davies M
BMJ, 2005; **331**: 1153–1154

Insulin resistance seems still to be the main underlying factor that leads to the metabolic syndrome, type 2 diabetes and cardiovascular disease. But different definitions now exist for metabolic syndrome with one body proposing a simpler definition – raised BP, low HDL-cholesterol, high serum triglycerides, high FPG and abdominal obesity – with no direct mention of insulin resistance.

In a recent joint statement, the American Diabetes Association and European Association for the Study of Diabetes questioned the diagnosis of metabolic syndrome and argued that too much emphasis has been given to this so-called 'syndrome' when there is so much uncertainty about its definition, pathogenesis, and known risk factors without regard for whether they can be clustered into a definition of 'metabolic syndrome' (*Diabetes Care,* 2005; **28**: 2289–2304).

This editorial finds the label a practical and useful one though. Definitions that omit the likes of a glucose tolerance test allow us to consider metabolic syndrome without too much increased workload.

Metabolic syndrome in normal-weight Americans: new definition of the metabolically obese, normal-weight individual
St-Onge MP, Janssen I, Heymsfield SB
Diabetes Care, 2004; **27**: 2222–2228

Data from the Third National Health and Nutrition Examination Survey (NHANES III) including 7602 adult participants demonstrated that the metabolic syndrome as described above is relatively common even in normal weight and slightly overweight men. Risk increased with weight and rose from 1–3% at BMI < 21 kg/m² to 10–22% at BMI 25.0–27 kg/m². Risk increases were even higher for women pound for pound.

There may be opportunities for a screening programme, but cost and the newness of this research make that seem a long time off. In the meantime an ever-lowering threshold to give good old fashioned advice to 'take up thy bed and walk' should bring the belt sizes down and save lives.

INTERVENTIONS

A primary care intervention programme for obesity and coronary heart disease risk factor reduction
Read A, Ramwell H, Storer H et al.
Br J Gen Pract, 2004; **54**: 272–278

This Nottingham study recruited 216 adults with BMI greater than 30 kg/m² and coronary risk factors. They were referred opportunistically by GPs or nurses or self-referred. Patients were invited to fortnightly sessions with a dietician who provided group education and support and concluded each session with a set of personal aims for each patient.

Periodic assessments showed that for the 60% still attending at 3 months, there were modest improvements in diabetic control, systolic blood pressure and lipid profiles as well as waist circumference. The average weight loss of around 3 kg was not earth-shattering but was at least maintained in the 34% that stuck it out for the whole year.

This intervention can seemingly change long-term habits in some, but effects are modest and the process is rather labour intensive.

An internet behavioural counselling weight loss programme reduced weight and BMI in patients at risk of type 2 diabetes. *Evidence-Based Medicine,* 2003; **8**: 181
The following paper is reviewed
Effects of internet behavioural counselling on weight loss in adults at risk for type 2 diabetes: a randomised trial.
Tate DF, Jackvony EH, Wing RR
JAMA, 2003; **289**: 1833–1836

In this study, 92 overweight or obese patients with at least one other risk factor for diabetes, received a 1-hour internet tutorial and written advice on diet and exercise. Some were randomised to a more detailed programme which provided personal e-counselling with feedback on their self-monitoring record, answers to questions and general support.

The intervention group lost twice as much weight as the basic internet weight loss programme.

The approach was innovative and popular, with 84% follow up at 12 months and showed that a patient-centred method was feasible. Barriers to its widespread implementation will include lack of reimbursement strategies for e-encounters and a lack of appropriate staff to support general practices.

Counselling, pharmacotherapy, and surgery help obese adults lose weight.
Evidence-Based Medicine, 2004; **9**: 110
The following paper is reviewed
Screening and interventions for obesity in adults: summary of the evidence for the U S Preventive Services Task Force
McTigue KM, Harris R, Hemphill B *et al.*
Ann Intern Med, 2003; **139**: 933–949

This review of approaches for obesity management highlights several points:
- no randomised controlled trials have evaluated the efficacy of screening for obesity
- counselling and behavioural interventions promoting exercise and dietary change achieve small weight reductions of 2–3 kg
- in the short term, sibutramine and orlistat were moderately effective with losses of 3–4 kg at one year
- drug treatments have not been evaluated in the long-term. Such use is contrary to NICE guidance
- evidence for metformin was inconclusive

LIFESTYLE

- surgical techniques reported considerable weight loss up to 40 kg with the main adverse effects being reoperation and wound infection
- long-term results are sparse. Most studies do not last anywhere near the 4 or 5 years required for a treatment trial in a chronic disease
- no study showed the desired end-point of a reduction in cardiovascular disease which is likely to depend on sustained weight loss
- the modest effects of a structured diet and exercise programme can lower BP, improve glycaemic control, lipid profiles and reduce the need for medication
- ultimately as weight loss is so hard to achieve and even harder to sustain, public and personal approaches should head rapidly towards prevention rather than treatment

Further Research

- GPs primarily believe that obesity is the responsibility of the patient, rather than a problem requiring a medical solution, according to a small qualitative study in London. They felt that obese patients wanted to hand them responsibility, creating possible friction. *Br J Gen Pract,* 2005; **55**: 750–754.

- Obesity in middle age independently increases the risk of future dementia. A Californian study found a 74% increased risk of dementia in obese people, and a 35% greater risk of dementia in overweight people (BMI 25–30) compared with those of normal weight. *BMJ,* 2005; **330**: 1360.

- A study in 10 000 British civil servants between 35 and 55, over a 14 year period, found that employees with chronic work stress had more than twice the odds of the metabolic syndrome than those without work stress. The effect was dose-related and persisted even after other risk factors such as smoking, alcohol and physical inactivity were taken into account. The study provides evidence that stress mechanisms may nudge us towards heart disease in neurophysiological ways. *BMJ,* 2006; **332**: 521–525.

ANTITHROMBOTICS

What we know already:

- Low doses of aspirin seem to be as effective as high doses for primary and secondary prevention of vascular events
- British Hypertension Society guidelines recommend low dose aspirin in high risk controlled hypertensives over 50 years old at a 10 year risk of cardiovascular disease of 20%
- In low risk patients there is no proven mortality benefit. Any advantages in numbers of coronary disease events are offset by the increased risk of major gastrointestinal bleeding
- Warfarin does not add additional benefit to aspirin alone after MI
- Nearly a million people in the UK are on warfarin and this is predicted to rise five fold in the next decade
- Atrial fibrillation (AF) is the most common cardiac dysrhythmia and has a risk of thromboembolic stroke of 5% per year – about five times the normal risk, accounting for 15% of all strokes
- Long-term anticoagulation reduces stroke in high-risk individuals but warfarin is massively underprescribed, with decisions being poorly based on evidence and fuelled by exaggerated fears
- Common reasons for not anticoagulating include non-compliance, fear of bleeding risk, dementia, risk of falls, and patient refusal. Prior GI bleeding and old age are not contraindications in themselves
- Over 100 000 Europeans monitor their own oral anticoagulation but studies sometimes show a lack of interest or confidence in doing this and high dropout rates
- After more than 50 years, a new oral anticoagulant – the first oral thrombin inhibitor, ximelagatran, has been developed. In a fixed dose, it may be as effective as adjusted-dose warfarin without the need for close monitoring and the fears of drug interactions

Recent Papers

ASPIRIN

Aspirin for the primary prevention of cardiovascular events in women and men: a sex-specific meta-analysis of randomized controlled trials
Berger JS, Roncaglioni MC, Avanzini F, et al.
JAMA, 2006; **295**: 306–313

> To determine if the benefits and risks of aspirin treatment in the primary prevention of cardiovascular disease vary by sex, this meta-analysis of randomized controlled trials included almost 95 000 people.
> In the women, aspirin:
> - reduced cardiovascular events by 12%
> - reduced ischaemic stroke by 24%
> - had no significant effect on MI

In the men, aspirin:
- reduced cardiovascular events by 14% and MI by 32%
- had no significant effect on ischaemic stroke

In both men and women in this low risk group (who did not have pre-existing cardiovascular disease):
- there was no apparent effect on cardiovascular mortality or all-cause mortality
- aspirin treatment increased the risk of major bleeding equally (by around 70%)

So, if aspirin reduces myocardial infarction in men and not women, and reduces ischaemic stroke in women and not men, we need to refer to sex-specific sets of data to help us discuss the risk and merits of taking aspirin as primary prevention.

Aspirin for everyone older than 50? "FOR"
Elwood P, Morgan G , Brown G, *et al.*
BMJ, 2005; **330**: 1440–1441

Whether or not to take aspirin for primary prevention of cardiovascular disease is still a thorny question. A pair of "FOR" and "AGAINST" articles appears in this *BMJ.*

The FOR article supports its use but covers the information void by suggesting the public should be given the evidence we have and should make their own decision on whether or not to take it. They consider that the crucial question is 'at what age does benefit outweigh risk?' But is it clear that even this question is valid?

They also consider side effects of aspirin to be 'unusual and seldom serious' and that for '[asymptomatic] people to consult a doctor before starting aspirin prophylaxis is unreasonable and places the doctor in an impossible position'. Everybody should evaluate the risks and benefits for themselves.

This reads as an extraordinary argument. They use the fact that many high-risk people are still undetected and therefore not on aspirin as a reason to consider a single low dose pill for larger populations.

Aspirin for everyone older than 50? "AGAINST"
Baigent C
BMJ, 2005; **330**: 1442–1443

High-risk patients with occlusive arterial disease can expect a benefit of about a quarter of their baseline risk for a vascular event. But in those without disease it is not so clear.

This "AGAINST" argument is much more scientifically rooted.

The balance of benefits for aspirin in people over 70 has not been clearly defined. Neither do the benefits clearly exceed risk of a major GI bleed in people younger than 60 without vascular disease. Age thresholds therefore seem illogical at present.

Meta-analysis of five of the six primary prevention trials performed show that aspirin reduces myocardial infarction by about one-third but, crucially, has little or no effect on stroke or death from vascular causes.

In 2005, data from the Women's Heath Study suggested low-dose aspirin protects against stroke in healthy women but has no effect on myocardial infarction.

Aspirin plus dipyridamole versus aspirin alone after cerebral ischaemia of arterial origin
The ESPRIT Study Group
Lancet, 2006; **367**: 1665–1673

Patients who have a stroke do better on aspirin and dipyridamole than on aspirin alone according to ESPRIT – the European/Australasian Stroke Prevention in Reversible Ischemia Trial.

In this vulnerable group, combined treatment reduced the combined mortality from vascular death, further stroke, heart attack and serious bleeding by 3 percentage points from 16% to 13%, with an NNT of 104 per year. Age, gender, race, and type of vessel involved did not seem to matter, but in the first week following the primary event, aspirin alone seemed preferable.

Adding the result to an existing meta-analysis gave a risk ratio for the combination of 0.82.

Results are about as clear as we can hope for and show that combination treatment (75 mg of aspirin and 200 mg b.d. of dipyridamole) is an effective option for ischaemic stroke or TIA. It caused no more serious bleeding than aspirin alone.

Giving aspirin and ibuprofen after myocardial infarction
Kimmel SE, Strom BL
BMJ, 2003; **327**: 1298–1299

Aspirin and NSAIDs bind to the same place on the COX-1 enzyme but NSAIDs take priority. Ibuprofen may therefore reduce or negate the antiplatelet cardioprotective effects of aspirin in people who take it before the aspirin or take it regularly. This is a problem as they are two of the world's most commonly used drugs.

- Increased cardiovascular and all-cause mortality in those on aspirin and ibuprofen has been found. There was no problem with diclofenac or other NSAIDs. The sample size was small and other confounders such as higher use of ibuprofen in high-risk obese, physically inactive people might have been an issue (*Lancet*, 2003; **361**: 573–574).
- Use of NSAIDs (not just ibuprofen) in The Physician's Health Survey was associated with a higher rate of MI (*Circulation*, 2003; **108**: 1191).
- A retrospective cohort study found no such increase. The study was larger but did not assess casual use of medication (*BMJ*, 2003; **327**: 1322–1323).

There is currently insufficient evidence for or against concomitant used of ibuprofen in patients needing prophylactic aspirin. But of the two, only aspirin should be used to specifically prevent MI. Further studies are awaited for a definitive answer but there are difficulties in doing this well:

- prescription records do not record drugs bought over the counter
- use of ibuprofen may be sporadic
- compliance with taking aspirin is suboptimal
- ibuprofen may also have good antiplatelet properties

CARDIOVASCULAR

WARFARIN

Self monitoring increases the efficacy and safety of anticoagulant therapy.
Evidence-Based Medicine, 2006; **11**: 103
The following paper is reviewed
Self-monitoring of oral anticoagulation: a systematic review and meta-analysis
Heneghan C, Alonso-Coello P, Garcia-Alamino JM, *et al.*
Lancet, 2006; **367**: 404–411

This meta-analysis of 14 randomised trials involving 3000 adults shows how successful the approach can be.

If patients are able to monitor their own INR, they spend more time in the therapeutic range and benefit from fewer thromboembolic events, fewer major bleeding episodes and a longer life. If they are capable enough to adjust their dose, they are likely to be better at it than their physician and benefit even more.

Not everyone can however. Some would not or could not. You need good manual dexterity, adequate vision and strong motivation as well as extensive education, a suitable device and lots of expensive test strips.

Impact of adverse events on prescribing warfarin in patients with atrial fibrillation: matched pair analysis
Choudhry NK, Anderson GM, Laupacis A, *et al.*
BMJ, 2006; **332**: 141–145

A doctor who has prescribed warfarin to a patient who goes on to have a major haemorrhage is less likely to prescribe appropriate anticoagulants for atrial fibrillation in the future. Patients treated in the 90 days following such an experience had reduced odds of receiving warfarin compared with prescribing before the event occurred. The odds reduced further in the following 90 days. The result was equivalent to a 12% absolute reduction in the likelihood that they would receive warfarin.

However, if patients suffered a thromboembolic stroke when they were not on warfarin, this did not instigate a change in the doctor's prescribing patterns for future patients.

Dramatic events are easily remembered and regretted. When those are acts of commission rather than acts of omission, physicians receive a harsh reminder of their 'do no harm' ethic. Future strategies should address physicians' perceptions of risk.

Further Research

- The CAPRIE trial – Clopidogrel versus Aspirin in Patients at Risk of Ischaemic Events – showed clopidogrel is more effective than aspirin at preventing ischaemic events particularly in high-risk patients with a history of atherosclerotic disease. *Stroke*, 2004; **35**: 528–532.

- The MATCH trial – Management of ATherothrombosis with Clopidogrel in High-risk patients – showed that giving additional aspirin to people already on clopidogrel (in high-risk patients with recent stroke/TIA) gave no advantage but did increase bleeding. *Lancet*, 2004; **364:** 331–337.

- The Warfarin/Aspirin Study in Heart Failure (WASH) showed no evidence that aspirin is effective or safe in patients with heart failure. This group had higher risk of adverse events due mainly to increased hospitalisation. Warfarin was not shown to benefit heart failure patients in sinus rhythm. Antithrombotics contribute to polypharmacy in these patients. *Am Heart J*, 2004; **148**: 157–164.

- Aspirin should be discontinued five full days before surgery according to this study. Platelet function in all the volunteers normalised 96 hours after stopping aspirin regardless of the dose they were taking. *J Am Coll Surg*, 2005; **200**: 564–573.

- High-risk patients who discontinued aspirin more than tripled their risk of ischaemic stroke or TIA in this study. This illustrates the importance of compliance and suggests we may need alternatives when patients discontinue aspirin. *Arch Neurol*, 2005; **62**: 1217–1220.

CARDIOVASCULAR

HYPERTENSION

What we know already:

- Hypertension is the most common treatable risk factor for cardiovascular disease in patients over 50 years
- The relationship with vascular mortality persists to pressure as low as 115/75 mmHg and is relevant for any incremental increase in systolic or diastolic pressure throughout ages from 40–89 years in adults with no history of vascular disease
- It affects about a billion people worldwide and in the UK fills 8% of total bed capacity of the NHS. It accounts for 30% of all UK deaths
- Cost to the NHS of antihypertensives in 2001 was around £840 million – 15% of total annual cost of all primary care drugs
- Surveys still show massive underdiagnosis, undertreatment (with predominant use of monotherapy), and poor rates of blood pressure control in the UK where it is controlled in only 10% of the hypertensive population
- Pulse pressure and systolic BP are better predictors of eventual development of congestive heart failure than diastolic BP, independent of age. Measures of night-time BP and morning surges have been similarly proposed as possible useful parameters to measure
- The PREMIER study showed that lifestyle interventions including advice on weight loss, reducing sodium intake, increasing physical activity, and limiting alcohol intake, can benefit BP and prevent progression to overt hypertension
- Effective implementation of these lifestyle measures requires time, effort, patience and reinforcement. It is best supported by well-trained health professionals such as practice nurses
- Getting blood pressure down is overwhelmingly more important than the drug cocktail used
- Lowering blood pressure by 10/5 mmHg reduces stroke by about a third and that of ischaemic heart disease events by about 25% at age 65 across all BP levels in Western populations
- False positives and false negatives are realities for all screening tests but low positive predictive values for BP measurement means that routine measurement of BP in those under 35 without other risk factors is more likely to misdiagnose than to diagnose hypertension correctly
- 'Masked' hypertension is the reverse of 'white coat' hypertension – BP is lower in clinical measurements than during ambulatory monitoring
- Prehypertension (120/80 to 139/89 mmHg) is an independent risk factor for major cardiovascular events and an early warning light according to analysis of the Framingham data

Key trials

***HOT – The Hypertension Optimal Treatment Trial** (**Lancet**, 1998; **351**: 1755–1762)*
This large trial of nearly 19 000 people provides our best evidence for blood pressure targets. Although it was underpowered, it reports an optimal blood pressure for reduction

of major cardiovascular events as 139/83 mmHg. However a target of 150/90 was not disadvantageous and the British Hypertension Society still uses this as an 'audit standard' target blood pressure.

ALLHAT – The Antihypertensive and Lipid-Lowering Treatment to Prevent Heart Attack Trial (*JAMA*, 2002; **288:** 2981–2997)

When it comes to deciding health policy, there is no substitute for a high quality randomised trial and ALLHAT was excellent. It was the largest anti-hypertensive trial to date and included 33 357 people including large numbers of women, black people, Hispanics and diabetics. Its conclusions are valid irrespective of sex, ethnicity or diabetes. It compared the calcium channel blocker amlodipine, the ACE inhibitor lisinopril, the thiazide diuretic chlorthalidone and the alpha blocker doxazosin. The alpha blocker arm was stopped early due to excessive mortality particularly due to heart failure.

ALLHAT looked at fatal coronary heart disease and non-fatal MI in patients over 55 with hypertension and at least one other risk factor.

It is well recognised that ACE inhibitors are less effective in lowering blood pressure in the elderly or black people as the renin-angiotensin system is more suppressed.

The thiazide was the best performer, reducing blood pressure more effectively and preventing cardiovascular end-points better than amlodipine or lisinopril with no evidence of impaired glycaemic control even in diabetics. It beat the ACE inhibitor group in terms of prevention of stroke and cardiovascular disease. Thiazides stake their claim to be the first line medication but there is an increasing lobby to start patients on combination therapy.

Further analysis of the ALLHAT data shows that diuretics may be more effective at reducing the incidence of heart failure than ACE inhibitors or calcium blockers, particularly during the first year of treatment (*Circulation*, 2006; **113:** 2201–2210).

LIFE – Losartan Intervention for Endpoint Reduction (*Lancet*, 2002; **359:** 995–1003)

This study looked at patients with hypertension and LVH and showed advantages in cardiovascular morbidity and stroke over atenolol despite similar drops in blood pressure. Recent work has indicated this is due to a lack of performance from atenolol due to its specific properties (*Lancet*, 2004; **364:** 1684–1689). We should no longer have to use beta blockers for hypertension as liberally as we should after MI.

SCOPE – The Study on Cognition and Prognosis in the Elderly (*J Am Coll Cardiol*, 2004; **44:** 1175)

This study supported LIFE's results. As part of antihypertensive therapy, it used candesartan or placebo in 1500 patients over 70 years old who had isolated systolic hypertension. There was 42% relative risk reduction in stroke with a candesartan-based regime compared with a mostly thiazide approach. Blood pressure reduction was the same but the ARB appeared to show specific vascular protective effects of AT1-receptor blockade in this age group.

STOP-2 – Swedish Trial in Old Patients with Hypertension-2 (*Lancet*, 1999; **354:** 1751–1756)

This trial randomised elderly hypertensives aged over 70 years to older drugs (thiazide or beta blocker) or to the newer drugs (ACE inhibitor or calcium channel blocker). It found no differences between older antihypertensives and newer more expensive drugs in terms of blood pressure control, heart failure or other major events.

CARDIOVASCULAR

ASCOT – Anglo-Scandinavian Cardiac Outcomes Trial: Blood Pressure-Lowering Arm (***Lancet***, 2005; **366**: 895–906)

Preliminary results from the large ASCOT open label trial were presented in 2005. Some 19 000 higher risk patients with hypertension were randomised either to atenolol 50–100 mg, with bendroflumethazide 1.25–2.5 mg if needed, or to amlodipine 5–10 mg, with perindopril 4–8 mg per day if needed. The groups did not differ for the primary outcome which was non-fatal MI and fatal coronary heart disease. But ASCOT was still stopped early because the amlodipine-based arm had significantly lower rates of all cause mortality and all coronary events. Amlodipine plus perindopril also seemed to prevent onset of diabetes and may be a promising combination.

It was better than atenolol plus bendroflumethiazide for reducing strokes, cardiovascular mortality and all cause mortality (*Lancet*, 2005; **366**: 895–906).

Thiazides are still well-supported as first line therapy but this research supports existing data that beta blockers should not be used first line for hypertension without other compelling indications (*Evidence-Based Medicine*, 2006; **11**: 42).

Further analysis discovered that addition of atorvastatin to amlodipine can reduce fatal and non-fatal cardiac events by more than 50% and stroke by over 25%. The effect is potent, appears within only 3 months and does not appear when atorvastatin is added to atenolol. A theory is that these two drugs work synergistically to help stabilise atherosclerotic plaques (*Eur Heart J*, 2006; **27**: 2982–2988).

Guidelines

In 2006 the guidelines from the British Hypertension Society and NICE were updated with regards to advice on medications.

British Hypertension Society guidelines for hypertension management 2004 (BHS-IV): summary (***BMJ***, 2004; **328:** 634–640)

These guidelines from the British Hypertension Society (www.bhsoc.org):
- recommend routine screening at least every 5 years for all adults and annually if high–normal blood pressure
- emphasise formal assessment of total risk of cardiovascular disease
- advise use of multifactorial interventions, including statins and aspirin, to reduce risk
- recommend a treatment algorithm based on the AB/CD rule

Risk assessment

A new chart has been produced to calculate risk of cardiovascular disease. The aim is now to assess 10 year risk of all cardiovascular disease events rather than risk of CHD alone.

It has been simplified since 1999 by including only three age strata and now there is no separate chart for type-2 diabetics because their risk of cardiovascular disease is taken to be equivalent to people who have had an MI. Therefore they follow the secondary prevention approach.

Drug treatment

Targets are 140/85 mmHg for most patients but for diabetics and those with established cardiovascular disease a lower target of 130/80 mmHg is recommended.

Medication is recommended in patients with:
- sustained grade 2 hypertension (>160/100 mmHg)
- grade I hypertension (systolic blood pressure 140–159 or diastolic blood pressure 90–99 mmHg, or both), if there is any complication of hypertension, target organ damage or diabetes, or if there is an estimated 10 year risk of cardiovascular disease of 20%

The AB/CD algorithm

Clinical trials have shown that treatment algorithms deliver better blood pressure control than current clinical practice. We also know most people need more than one drug for blood pressure control. This algorithm classifies hypertensives into 'high renin' or 'low renin'.

A – ACE inhibitors or ARBs

B – beta blockers

C – calcium channel blockers

D – diuretics

A and B inhibit the renin–angiotensin system whereas C and D do not affect that system making them more effective first line agents for older white people or black people. New guidance downgrading beta blockers came in during 2006 in agreement with NICE (*see below*).

Particular caution is advised when using beta blockers and diuretics in patients at especially high risk of developing diabetes, e.g. strong family history of diabetes, obesity, impaired glucose tolerance, features of the metabolic syndrome, or of South Asian and African–Caribbean descent.

A paper by the BHS President in the *BMJ* (2006; **332**: 833–836) discusses ethnic variations and tells how hypertension could be usefully divided, like diabetes, into Type 1 and Type 2. Hypertension in black people is more prevalent than in whites and the different pathogenesis denotes the need for different approaches.

Hypertension: management in hypertension in adults in primary care

NICE – Updated June 2006 (www.nice.org.uk)

This set of guidelines from NICE also emphasises the need for formal risk assessment to include all cardiovascular treatments. They recommend monitoring of blood pressure over 140/90 mmHg, formal assessment of risk to identify those with a 10 year cardiovascular risk of >20%, and lifestyle advice. However, they follow the ALLHAT trial in that drug therapy can often begin with a low-dose thiazide.

In response to current research, NICE has removed beta blockers from their birthright of first line treatment for hypertension. Good evidence has indicated they are less effective than alternatives in the elderly at preventing stroke and in reducing the risk of diabetes (especially if also taking a thiazide).

For those aged 55 or for black patients a calcium channel blocker or thiazide should be used. For those under 55, ACE inhibitors are first line.

CARDIOVASCULAR

Recent Papers

USE OF GUIDELINES

Treating hypertension with guidelines in general practice
Campbell NC, Murchie P
BMJ, 2004; **329**: 523–524

This editorial examines the reception given to the guidelines in primary care. Increasingly stringent targets make our control of blood pressure statistically poor. The lower the targets the worse we are! It is controlled in only one-third of patients who are on medication.

Although there is much evidence regarding types of medication, targets are less evidence-based and are felt to be somewhat arbitrary. The lower the blood pressure the better, but additional drugs have diminishing returns with fifth and sixth drugs offering little improvement.

Current targets are felt to be unachievable in most patients. The authors recommend an informed dialogue with patients who have differing opinions in what they will accept in terms of adverse effects and risk. The patient's opinions and role in taking medication must be considered as they are the final arbiters of our success. Effective communication is essential.

Applicability to primary care of national clinical guidelines on blood pressure lowering for people with stroke: cross sectional study
Mant J, McManus RJ, Hare R
BMJ, 2006; **332**: 635–637

British Hypertension Society guidelines for lowering BP after stroke or TIA to 140/85 are based on the PROGRESS trial. But the research was on hospital patients.

This Birmingham study found the following in a primary care population with confirmed stroke and TIA:

- they averaged 12 years older than those in the trials – important because over the age of 80, reduction in risk of stroke through lowering BP may be offset by an increase in mortality
- they were twice as likely to be women
- the median time elapsed since stoke was 2.5 years rather than 8 months – important as risk of further cerebrovascular event declines with time

These factors undermine the applicability of the research to primary care in a very important area.

CARDIOVASCULAR

LIFESTYLE MODIFICATION

Randomised controlled factorial trial of dietary advice for patients with a single high blood pressure reading in primary care
Little P, Kelly J, Barnett J *et al.*
BMJ, 2004; **328**: 1054

The authors looked at the watchful waiting period of hypertension before definitive diagnosis in nearly 300 people following a high reading of blood pressure over 160/90 mmHg. Usual advice was given to all but some were randomised in a 2×2×2 factorial design to additional brief interventions: an information booklet, diet prompt sheets, and advice to use a low sodium–high potassium salt.

These strategies have worked in tightly controlled secondary care settings but have had less exposure to assessment in general practice.

The interventions had no effect on blood pressure but they did prompt patients to change their diet, which is likely to be important in the overall management of blood pressure.

There was even a suggestion that the advice to use a low sodium–high potassium diet had an adverse effect on anxiety levels at one month.

MEDICATION

Should beta blockers remain first choice in the treatment of primary hypertension? A meta-analysis
Lindholm LH, Carlberg B, Samuelsson O
Lancet, 2005; **366**: 1545–1553

Beta blockers are not as effective as other antihypertensive drugs in the absence of overt heart disease, according to this Swedish meta-analysis (also reviewed in *Evidence-Based Medicine*, 2006; **11**: 85).

They have been a popular first choice for treating hypertension over the years but this has recently come under renewed scrutiny and they may not have the same excellent benefits that they have in secondary prevention.

They identified seven RCTs involving 27000 subjects with primary hypertension that compared beta blockers with placebo or no treatment, and 13 trials with 106000 participants that compared beta blockers with other antihypertensives.

The risk of stroke was reduced by 19% when compared with placebo, less than half that previously assumed. When compared with other antihypertensive medications, beta blockers were associated with a 16% higher risk of stroke. It is suggested that reduction in brachial BP may not reflect reductions in central systolic BP as well as other antihypertensives.

The authors conclude that beta blockers should not be used as first line drugs when there are thiazides, calcium channel blockers, and ACE inhibitors, which seem to have advantages. Nor should they be used as a reference in trials. Beta blockers should be reserved for where there are comorbidites such as post-MI, heart failure, arrhythmia, and stress. Sudden discontinuation should be avoided – reduce the dose while substituting the alternative.

CARDIOVASCULAR

Low dose diuretics are the best first line antihypertensive treatment. *Evidence-Based Medicine,* 2004; **9**: 12

The following article is presented

Health outcomes associated with various antihypertensive therapies used as first-line agents: a network meta-analysis
Psaty BM, Lumley T, Furberg CD *et al.*
JAMA, 2003; **289**: 2534–2544

This review supported the use of low-dose diuretics as first-line treatment in hypertension. A review of 42 randomised controlled trials over a mean of 3–4 years showed thiazides to be as effective or more effective than all other antihypertensive agents in preventing major cardiovascular disease endpoints. Diuretics were shown to be unsurpassed in decreasing cardiovascular outcomes. But as most hypertensives require more than one drug for control there is still a question over the best combinations.

Thiazide diuretic prescription and electrolyte abnormalities in primary care
Clayton JA, Rodgers S, Blakey J *et al.*
Br J Clin Pharmacol, 2006; **61**: 87–95

In this large study in UK general practice, only one-third of those on thiazides had a record of their electrolytes being tested and 20% of those tested were hypokalaemic and/or hyponatraemic.

The incidence of morbidity from hyponatraemia relates to the absolute level and speed of change. Thiazide-induced hyponatraemia typically occurs within 2–12 days of drug initiation. Chronic hyponatraemia is generally asymptomatic until the sodium concentration falls below 125 mmol/l. Approximately 1% of the patients in this study dropped their sodium concentration below that level and it is likely that they will have been symptomatic and perhaps required hospitalisation.

Just over 1% of the patients tested had severe hypokalaemia (potassium <3.0 mmol/l). In the majority the thiazide was discontinued and in those who continued the thiazide, the potassium concentration was normal when repeated. The evidence linking thiazide-induced hypokalaemia and cardiac complications is conflicting.

Still, this is reminder to increase testing and monitoring and use low doses wherever possible.

Gout, not induced by diuretics? A case-control study from primary care
Janssens HJEM, van de Lisdonk EH, Janssen M *et al.*
Ann Rheum Dis, 2006; **65**: 1080–1083

Fear of provoking gout have led some to be shy of using diuretics but this case-control study reassures us. Patients with their first case of gout were matched by age and gender with controls. The relative risk of gout in those who had ever had a diuretic was 1.56 but this was accounted for by higher associations of gout with those suffering from hypertension and heart failure. (There was no association with MI.)

The authors tell us there is no need to avoid diuretics or substitute them in those with or at risk of gout. We should be focussing on hypertension and cardiovascular morbidity when we see a patient with gout.

CARDIOVASCULAR

ACE inhibitors reduced cardiovascular events and all cause mortality in elderly people with hypertension. *Evidence-Based Medicine,* 2003; **8**: 144
The following article is presented
A comparison of outcomes with angiotensin-converting-enzyme inhibitors and diuretics for hypertension in the elderly
Wing LM, Reid CM, Ryan P *et al.*
N Engl J Med, 2003; **348**: 583–592

This Second Australian National Blood Pressure Study [ANBP2] looked at over 6000 elderly Australians between 65 and 84 years of age. It was a high quality study which came out shortly after ALLHAT, with an apparently contradictory conclusion.

They found in this group that ACE inhibitors were more effective than diuretics for reducing a composite outcome of all cardiovascular events and all-cause mortality.

The choice of drugs was left to the general practitioners in this study. Certainly there were differences between the studies. ALLHAT included patients as young as 55 and fewer than 50% were white compared with 95% of ANBP2. We know that ACE inhibitors are less effective in the black population.

The commentator points out that large studies such as these tend to find statistically significant differences between treatments that actually have very little clinical difference between them. He refers to the 'tedious arguments about the superiority of one drug over another' in reference to our generally lousy performance in controlling hypertension, and he sees no reason why the superiority of diuretics should not stand as a first-line approach. Perhaps it is time to return to a rational approach based on history and a patient's response to treatment.

Systematic review: antihypertensive drug therapy in black patients
Brewster LM, van Montfrans GA, Kleijnen J
Ann Intern Med, 2004; **141**: 614–627

This systematic review looked at the use of various antihypertensives in the black population. It took in 30 trials and around 20000 black patients.

Interestingly beta-blockers and ACE inhibitors were no more effective than placebo in reducing blood pressure. Calcium-channel blockers came out with consistently improved antihypertensive efficacy. The analysis suggests that these might therefore be the best first-line agent for black hypertensives followed by diuretics.

Cardiovascular outcomes showed the usual improvements as long as the target blood pressure was achieved. However, there was some evidence in the black population that the risk of diabetes may have increased with thiazides and some evidence of an increase in cardiovascular events with ACE inhibitors.

CARDIOVASCULAR

COMBINATION THERAPY

Value of low dose combination treatment with blood pressure lowering drugs: analysis of 354 randomised trials
Law MR, Wald NJ, Morris JK *et al.*
BMJ, 2003; **326**: 1427

This fascinating meta-analysis takes the argument in an entirely new direction. The authors examined 354 randomised trials in 40 000 treated patients on thiazides, beta blockers, ACE inhibitors, ARBs, and calcium channel blockers. They found:
- all five categories of drug produced similar reductions in blood pressure and the effects were additive
- the average reduction was 9.1 mmHg systolic and 5.5 mmHg diastolic at standard dose and only 20% lower at half standard dose
- the drugs reduced blood pressure more so from higher levels

Regarding side-effects:
- symptoms attributable to thiazides, beta blockers, and calcium channel blockers were strongly dose related, but were not dose-related for ACE inhibitors (mainly cough)
- angiotensin II receptor antagonists caused no apparent side-effects
- using two drugs in combination, side-effects were less than additive
- adverse metabolic effects (such as changes in cholesterol or potassium) were negligible at half standard dose

The authors conclude that combination low-dose drug treatment increases efficacy and reduces adverse effects. Three drugs at half standard dose are estimated to lower blood pressure by 20/11 mmHg on average and thereby reduce the risk of stroke by 63% and IHD events by 46% at age 60–69. Low-dose combination therapy should be considered first line. Three such drugs are preferable to one or two drugs at standard dose. Drug selections should still be tailored for the patient.

Angiotensin-converting enzyme inhibitors and calcium channel blockers for coronary heart disease and stroke prevention
Verdecchia P, Reboldi G, Angeli F, *et al.*
Hypertension, 2005; **46**: 386–392

This review of 28 trials compared ACE inhibitors and calcium channel blockers (CCBs) in terms of serious cardiovascular end-points and stroke. This included a total of 179 000 patients suffering 9500 cardiac cases and 6000 cases of stroke.

Protective effects are mainly due to effects on BP where any of the four classes of drug perform well. However, two classes appear to have additional benefits beyond these effects:
- ACE inhibitors appeared superior to CCBs for prevention of MI and cardiac death
- CCBs appeared superior to ACE inhibitors for prevention of stroke

The authors propose the combination of ACE inhibitor and calcium blocker as a promising rationale for a broad spectrum of cardiovascular prevention.

Blood pressure control by home monitoring: meta-analysis of randomised trials
Cappuccio FP, Kerry SM, Forbes L et al.
BMJ, 2004; **329**: 145

> Home blood pressure monitoring is feasible and acceptable. We know that the white coat effect is important in the diagnosis and treatment of hypertension and is not a research artefact. This meta-analysis of 1359 hypertensives in 18 randomised controlled trials showed that systolic blood pressure was lower in hypertensives who used home blood pressure monitoring. The proportion achieving targets increased over that of clinic monitoring. Differences are small but we know small blood pressure differences matter. The authors conclude that home blood pressure monitoring improves hypertensive control and could be considered as a useful adjunct in practice to involve patients more closely in the management of their blood pressure.

Self monitoring of blood pressure at home
Stergiou G, Mengden T, Padfield PL et al.
BMJ, 2004; **329**: 870–871

> This editorial reminds us that the 2004 British Hypertension Society guidelines provide a threshold level for diagnosis when self-monitoring hypertension at 135/85 mmHg.
>
> Self-monitoring allows multiple readings over time devoid of the white coat effect and possibly better cardiovascular outcomes. It may improve control by increasing compliance and could reduce health costs by reducing visits.
>
> However, inaccuracy of electronic devices is a problem and self-monitoring may increase anxiety or lead to patients adjusting their own doses. It requires training with information and advice on interpretation.
>
> The first direct comparison of 24-hour ambulatory BP measurement against home measurement found that home BP measurement is just as effective at guiding treatment. They remind us it is more convenient and better accepted by patients but training is required and validated devices must be used (*Am J Hypertens*, 2006; **19**: 468–476).

Prediction of stroke by self-measurement of blood pressure at home versus casual screening blood pressure measurement in relation to the Joint National Committee 7 classification: the Ohasama study
Asayama K, Ohkubo T, Kikuya M et al.
Stroke, 2004; **35**: 2356–2361

> This large study of 1702 patients for 11 years showed an additional value for home blood pressure monitoring in predicting stroke. Interestingly the home-based approach showed a smoother stepwise correlation between blood pressure and cardiovascular risk, whereas readings in the clinic could not differentiate such risk unless they were at the extremes of high or low readings. The review in *Evidence-Based Medicine* (2005; **10**: 92) concludes that this indicates home BP readings are another dataset to help to predict target organ damage.

CARDIOVASCULAR

The same group have also found that conventional BP measurement fails to identify some individuals at high or low risk, but these cases may be 'unmasked' by the use of ambulatory BP (*J Am Coll Cardiol*, 2005; **46**: 516–517).

Targets and self monitoring in hypertension: randomised controlled trial and cost effectiveness analysis
McManus RJ, Mant J, Roalfe A, *et al.*
BMJ, 2005; **331**: 493

A Birmingham study compared usual care to visits by patients to the practice to use the facilities to monitor their own BP, the location of the measurements providing a nice safety net in case of persistently high readings. They showed that self-monitoring is feasible in a community setting, is popular with patients and has negligible costs. It can bring the benefits of home monitoring to individuals without the means to purchase their own equipment. After a year there were no differences between the groups except that patients who self monitored lost more weight. The authors recommend GPs should offer this option to their hypertensive patients.

An accompanying editorial agrees that the professional measurement data we use can be applied to self monitoring. This study showed cost-effectiveness while reaching targets more effectively than usual care through absence of the white coat effect and possibly better adherence. Whether it can be sustained over time is yet to be shown. Self selection by enthusiastic participants may mean it is not suitable for all (*BMJ*, 2005; **331**: 466–467).

Further Research

- Debate continues on whether hypertension causes headache. A meta-analysis of 94 randomized placebo-controlled trials. All the different antihypertensives got in on the act. Headaches were prevented in 1 in 30 of those treated. As the only thing they have in common is lowering BP, this implies that high BP causes headaches. This conflicts with some observational evidence but whether it is true or not, this should not detract from the practical benefits of lowering blood pressure to prevent headaches the authors argue (*Circulation*, 2005; **112**: 2301–2306).

LIPIDS

What we know already:

- Statins reduce further coronary events and improve survival in patients with coronary heart disease
- Absolute reductions in cholesterol are greatest where pretreatment levels are higher and this group receives most benefit
- Meta-analysis makes it clear that lowering LDL cholesterol is predicted to decrease all stroke in the general population by 10% for a 1 mmol/l reduction due to benefits in thromboembolic rather than haemorrhagic stroke
- Safety profile is very good – on meta-analysis 1% fewer treated patients than placebo patients reported problems. The only serious effects are rare – rhabdomyolysis and liver failure from hepatitis
- Less than half of those taking statins achieve target levels of cholesterol
- About half the patients that might benefit receive statins and a one-third are on suboptimal doses. There is significant underprescribing in the elderly
- The main barriers to prescribing within general practice are organisational: confusing guidelines, errors and omissions by GPs, problems communicating with secondary care and reluctance by patients to take medication
- Uncertainty regarding choice and dose of statin remains
- Impact on other conditions such as dementia and osteoporosis has been uncertain
- Statins represent the largest drug cost to the NHS – £738 million in 2004

Key trials

There are some classic trials regarding lipids that it is important you should know.

Primary prevention

WOSCOPS – The West of Scotland Coronary Prevention Study (1995)
WOSCOPS was a randomised controlled trial involving 6595 men aged 45–64 years with high total cholesterol levels (above 6.5 mmol/l) and no previous history of MI or CHD. They received either pravastatin or placebo and were followed up for 5 years.

Treating 1000 patients for 5 years would prevent 7 deaths from CHD and 20 non-fatal MIs.

Pravastatin was shown to reduce:
- total cholesterol by 20%
- death from CHD by 31%
- death from any cause by 22%
- revascularisation procedures by 37%

The Air Force/Texas Coronary Atherosclerosis Prevention Study (1998)
This trial involved men and women without a history of cardiovascular disease. It ran-

CARDIOVASCULAR

domised 5608 men and 997 women, with average cholesterol levels of 5.7 mmol/l, to either placebo or lovastatin, and followed up for over 5 years.

Lovastatin reduced the risk of:
- New cardiovascular disease by 54% in women and 34% in men
- Revascularisation procedures by 33%

The group treated with a statin benefited most when individual cardiovascular risk was higher but cholesterol level alone was found to be a poor indicator of that risk.

Secondary Prevention

The 4S Trial – The Scandinavian Simvastatin Survival Study (1994)

This large randomised double-blinded trial of 4444 men (81%) and women (19%) was a milestone in the secondary prevention of cardiovascular disease. Patients between 35 and 70 years who already had angina or a previous MI and had a cholesterol between 5.5 and 8.0 mmol/l were given either simvastatin or a placebo. Doses were adjusted over a median of 5.4 years follow up.

There were no significant differences in non-cardiovascular death, including death from cancer, trauma or suicide, and the drug was well tolerated.

In the simvastatin group, total cholesterol, LDL cholesterol, and triglycerides reduced by 25%, 35% and 10%, respectively; HDL cholesterol increased by 8%.

Simvastatin was shown to reduce the risk of:
- total mortality by 30%
- coronary death by 42%
- major coronary events by 34%
- revascularisation procedures by 37%

Ten-year follow up confirmed that the survival advantage persists. Importantly there was no validation of concerns regarding cancer. No difference was noted in its incidence or mortality between the simvastatin group and the placebo group (*Lancet*, 2004; **364**: 771–777).

CARE – Cholesterol and Recurrent Events (1996)

This was a 5-year mission to explore the effect of pravastatin (or placebo) on over 4000 men and women under 75 years. They were all post-MI patients who had a total cholesterol under 6.2 mmol/l (average 5.4 mmol/l).

Pravastatin was found to reduce the risk of:
- Cardiac event (both fatal and non-fatal) by 24%
- Stroke by 28%
- Revascularisation procedures by 26%

LIPID – The Long-term Intervention with Pravastatin in Ischaemic Disease (1998)

This was similar to CARE but with over 9000 subjects. They were under 75 years with cholesterol under 7 mmol/l. The trial was a double-blinded, randomised controlled trial and compared the effects of 40 mg of pravastatin with those of placebo with a mean follow-up period of 6.1 years.

Pravastatin was found to reduce the risk of:
- cardiac events (both fatal and non-fatal) by 24%
- MI by 29%

- overall mortality by 22%
- stroke by 19%
- revascularisation procedures by 20%

For every 1000 patients assigned to pravastatin, death from any cause would be avoided in 30 patients, death due to coronary disease avoided in 19, and death due to stroke avoided in 8.

The Heart Protection Study (*Lancet*, 2002)

This was an important trial (also mentioned in the diabetes chapter) that looked at over 20 000 patients aged 40–80 years. Men accounted for 75% and subjects either had vascular disease (whether coronary, cerebral or peripheral) or a risk factor such as diabetes. All were therefore at high risk and had a broad range of baseline total cholesterols averaging 5.9 mmol/l. The benefits of simvastatin in this group were conclusive on all counts. In addition, there was no difference in nonvascular mortality or cancer incidence.

Doubt has even been cast on the need to test lipids before starting statins in these groups as 40 mg of simvastatin has been shown to be so beneficial and targets so questionable. However, testing could increase concordance with therapy as well as identify particularly high triglycerides or low HDLs for special attention.

Recent papers

GENERAL USE OF STATINS

Switching statins
Moon JC
BMJ, 2006; **332**: 1344–1345

Around 85% of all statins prescribed are simvastatin or atorvastatin. In May 2003 simvastatin's patent expired and the cost reduced eightfold for the 40 mg dose and 20-fold for the 20 mg dose. Simvastatin 40 mg can cost less than £1 per month per patient when purchased in bulk.

Simvastatin 40 mg and atorvastatin 10 mg and 20 mg have been shown to be equally effective. Meta-analysis using simvastatin 40 mg and atorvastatin 10 mg showed no significant differences in mortality, death from coronary heart disease, or stroke.

The only important difference is cost.

The first line statin is simvastatin 40 mg, which is substituted when a newly admitted patient has been taking atorvastatin 10 mg or 20 mg

It is time, the authors argue, for the UK to implement therapeutic substitution of simvastatin 40 mg nationally by switching patients currently taking atorvastatin 10 mg and 20 mg, and prescribing generic simvastatin. If simvastatin is not tolerated or considered inappropriate, the alternative is pravastatin 40 mg, another cheap generic statin. This could save the NHS £1 billion over the next 5 years. Atorvastatin remains on patent until 2011.

CARDIOVASCULAR

Lifetime cost effectiveness of simvastatin in a range of risk groups and age groups derived from a randomised trial of 20 536 people
Heart Protection Study Collaborative
BMJ, 2006; **333**: 1145

Analysis of the Heart Protection Study data showed that 40 mg of simvastatin is cost-saving in most age groups and vascular risk groups studied.

Extrapolating the data beyond the 5 year period of study and also estimating lifetime cost per life year gained and per QALY gained, found that this same 40 mg could be cost-effective for people 5 years either side of the 40–80 years age range of the study.

Costs per life year gained ranged from £450 to £2500 for people with a 5% five year risk of a major vascular event. That is about half the risk proposed by NICE but well within the costs they usually allow.

PREVENTING STROKE

Cholesterol lowering with simvastatin reduced stroke in patients with, or at risk of, vascular disease. *Evidence-Based Medicine,* 2004; 9: 143
The following article is presented
Effects of cholesterol-lowering with simvastatin on stroke and other major vascular events in 20 536 people with cerebrovascular disease or other high-risk conditions
Collins R, Armitage J, Parish S *et al.*
Lancet, 2004; **363**: 757–767

This further analysis of the landmark Heart Protection Study adds more complete data to the question of the effect of statins on the risk of stroke. Remember, subjects had a medical history of vascular disease or diabetes and were given simvastatin or placebo. Benefits in stroke reduction were significant by the second year and an overall 30% reduction in ischaemic stroke was measured in these high-risk individuals. The groups did not differ for haemorrhagic stroke.

This subgroup analysis confirms the finding of the overall study and also of other studies that have shown similar benefits independent of baseline cholesterol or type of statin. The study further supports the expansion in use of these drugs and the commentator recommends starting them in all patients who can tolerate them after non-haemorrhagic stroke or TIA, regardless of age, gender, blood pressure or anything else.

Statins reduce stroke but not stroke mortality. *Evidence-Based Medicine,* 2005; 10: 73
The following paper is reviewed
Statins in stroke prevention and carotid atherosclerosis: systematic review and up-to-date meta-analysis
Amarenco P, Labreuche J, Lavallee P, *et al.*
Stroke, 2004; **35**: 2902–2909

Meta-analysis of 26 RCTs showed that statins reduce stroke but may not reduce fatal stroke. The effect depends on the degree of LDL cholesterol lowering – each 10% reduction corresponded to a risk reduction of all stroke of 16%. There was

CARDIOVASCULAR

no effect on haemorrhagic stroke. Entry criteria were diverse but most patients had coronary artery disease or dyslipidaemia. In these patients, the fact that statins reduce risk of stroke (as well as cardiovascular problems) provides additional motivation for using them.

Sharing a common pathology with coronary artery disease, statin use after ischaemic stroke is almost certainly cost effective for most patients and is becoming more widespread even if it is just to prevent MI.

High-dose atorvastatin after stroke or transient ischemic attack
SPARCL Investigators – Stroke Prevention by Aggressive Reduction in Cholesterol Levels
N Engl J Med, 2006; **355**: 549–559

We know statins reduce the number of strokes in those at increased risk for cardiovascular disease. But are they as effective after a recent stroke or TIA where heart disease is absent?

SPARCL randomly assigned 4731 patients with LDL cholesterol under 5 mmol/l and no known heart disease, but who had had a recent stroke or TIA, to high dose (80 mg) atorvastatin per day or placebo.

Follow up at 5 years showed modest but clear benefit. High doses of the statin:
- reduced the chances of another stroke over 5 years
- slightly increased haemorrhagic stroke
- reduced the risk of major cardiovascular events
- had a similar mortality in the two groups

MANAGEMENT STRATEGY

Intensive versus moderate lipid lowering with statins after acute coronary syndromes
Cannon CP, Braunwald E, McCabe CH *et al.*
N Engl J Med, 2004; **350**: 1495–1504

Aggressive lowering of lipids improves outcomes after hospitalisation for acute coronary syndrome. This paper from the PROVE IT-TIMI trial (Pravastatin or Atorvastatin Evaluation and Infection Therapy – Thrombolysis in Myocardial Infarction) looked at cardiovascular end-points for over 4000 recent admissions. It found that aggressive treatment with atorvastatin 80 mg, lowered the LDL cholesterol to 1.6 mmol/l compared to 2.6 mmol/l with the standard dose treatment, albeit with a different drug – pravastatin 40 mg.

The PROVE IT and the Myocardial Ischaemia Reduction with Aggressive Cholesterol Lowering (MIRACL) C-reactive protein sub-study also showed that high-dose atorvastatin (80 mg) led to significantly lower markers of inflammation. It is proposed that this mechanism accounts for the very early benefits, within 30 days, of aggressive statin therapy. The improvements in LDL cholesterol probably take the credit for the reduction in longer-term events.

CARDIOVASCULAR

Association between different lipid-lowering treatment strategies and blood pressure control in the Brisighella Heart Study
Borghi C, Dormi A, Veronesi M *et al.*
Am Heart J, 2004; **148**: 285–292

This Italian study randomised 1356 subjects to four different lipid-lowering strategies: low-fat diet, cholestyramine, gemfibrozil, or simvastatin. They were observing effects on blood pressure to investigate whether previous studies suggesting that statins lower blood pressure were valid. A significant decrease in blood pressure was observed particularly in those with higher blood pressure. Statins were more effective than non-statins. As a result of this 'therapeutic crossover' of effects, the authors promote the use of statins to assist hypertensive control in hypercholesterolaemic patients.

Further Research

- A recent landmark study of 167 US patients to assess the addition of Niaspan (nicotinic acid) to a statin showed that the combination reduced atherosclerosis by 68%. The ARBITER 2 group measured carotid intima medial thickness and although not powered to show cardiovascular end-points indicated a strong trend towards reduction in cardiovascular events, which will doubtless attract further study. Most people suffered the common side-effect of flushing but could cope with it and compliance did not suffer. *Circulation*, 2004; **110**: 3512–3517.

- A search of over 1000 patients showed no cases of abnormal transaminase values that were attributable to statins. Only two moderately abnormal CK values were potentially attributable to statin use. There were no documented adverse sequelae associated with these results. This study therefore questions the usefulness of routine measurement of transaminase and CK levels in all patients taking statins. *Arch Intern Med*, 2003; **163**: 688–692. However, the 80 mg dose of simvastatin carries a risk of myopathy of approximately 1 in 250. *Am J Cardiol*, 2005; **96**: 69–75.

- Suggestions that statins promote bone formation and increase bone strength persist. In a meta-analysis of the available evidence, observational studies suggest that the risk for hip and non-spine fractures is lower among older women taking statins, but analyses of cardiovascular trials fail to support this. The authors call for controlled trials of the effect. *Arch Intern Med*, 2004; **164**: 146–152. A large study with 91 000 subjects, 95% male veterans, has shown that statin use was associated with a reduction in fracture risk of 36%. *Arch Intern Med*, 2005; **165**: 2007–2012.

- In elderly people, low levels of total cholesterol and LDL cholesterol levels are significantly associated with higher mortality. This could reflect frailty, malnutrition, or subclinical disease. *J Am Geriatr Soc*, 2005; **53**: 219–226.

- They are also associated with poorer performance on a variety of cognitive measures. Cholesterol is important in brain function. *Psychosom Med*, 2005; **67**: 24–30.

CARDIOVASCULAR

- Analysis of the long-running. high quality Women's Health Initiative does not support fears that women taking statins are at a higher risk of breast cancer. Contrary to earlier studies, there may even be a protective effect. *J Natl Cancer Inst*, 2006; **98**: 700–707.

CARDIOVASCULAR

CORONARY HEART DISEASE

What we know already:

- Coronary heart disease is already the major cause of illness and death in Western countries
- Some 80–85% of men and women with CHD have at least one of the big four conventional risk factors – smoking, diabetes, hyperlipidaemia, and hypertension
- Lifestyle measures that reduce risk of cardiovascular disease include smoking cessation, regular exercise and maintenance of normal weight
- Good evidence supports an association between coronary heart disease and depression, social isolation or lack of social support, as well as catastrophic life events
- Dietary measures include reducing intake of total and saturated fats, increasing consumption of fish, reducing salt, limiting alcohol consumption, and eating at least five portions per day of fresh fruit and vegetables
- Meta-analysis shows that exercise-based cardiac rehabilitation reduces all cause and cardiac mortality
- Multidisciplinary disease management programmes for patients with coronary heart disease improve processes of care, reduce admissions to hospital, and enhance quality of life or functional status
- Cardiac liaison nurses offering people the choice of home or hospital-based rehabilitation and nurse-led clinics bridge the gap between primary and secondary care. They help optimise secondary prevention to reach long-term government targets
- National guidelines for prevention of CHD recommend the use of absolute risk profiles to guide treatment. They set explicit standards for secondary prevention and cardiac rehabilitation
- Coronary heart disease mortality has halved since 1981 in the UK, resulting in 68 000 fewer deaths in 2000

Guidelines

The British Hypertension Society has published guidelines on use of aspirin and statins in patients at risk of cardiovascular complications.
- Aspirin: use 75 mg daily if patient is aged 50 years with blood pressure controlled to <150/90 mmHg and target organ damage, diabetes mellitus, or 10 year risk of cardiovascular disease of 20% (measured by using the new Joint British Societies' cardiovascular disease risk chart)
- Statin: use sufficient doses to reach targets if patient is aged up to at least 80 years, with a 10 year risk of cardiovascular disease of 20% (measured by using the new Joint British Societies' cardiovascular disease risk chart) and with total cholesterol concentration 3.5 mmol/l

Recent Papers

INCIDENCE

Explaining the decline in coronary heart disease mortality in England and Wales between 1981 and 2000
Unal B, Critchley JA, Capewell S
Circulation, 2004; **109**: 1101–1107

This study from Liverpool looked at the reasons for the decline in coronary mortality that has benefited England and Wales since the 1970s. It used a model to assess the uptake and effectiveness of cardiological treatments and the effect of trends in risk factors. Coronary heart disease mortality rates decreased between 1981 and 2000 by 62% in men and 45% in women in the 25 to 84 years age group. This resulted in 68 230 fewer deaths in 2000. Some 42% of this reduction was attributed to improved treatments in individuals (such as thrombolysis, improved treatments in heart failure and in secondary prevention measures) and 58% to population risk factor reductions (smoking, blood pressure and cholesterol).

The authors summarised that more than half the reduction in coronary heart disease mortality was attributable to reductions in major risk factors, principally smoking. This was despite negative trends in levels of obesity, physical activity and diabetes.

They emphasised the importance of a comprehensive strategy that promotes primary prevention, particularly for smoking and dietary change, and that maximises population coverage of effective treatments, especially for secondary prevention and heart failure.

Modelling the decline in coronary heart disease deaths in England and Wales, 1981–2000: comparing contributions from primary and secondary prevention
Unal B, Critchley JA, Capewell S
BMJ, 2005; **331**: 614

The same authors used a validated model to estimate how much of the recent cardiovascular improvements were attributable to control of risk factors in apparently healthy people (primary prevention) and in patients with CHD (secondary prevention).

Changing the risk factors of the healthy was responsible for four times the mortality benefit than these changes in those with established CHD, that is 81% versus 19% of lives saved.

The risk factors they were referring to were smoking, cholesterol, and blood pressure.

Comprehensive population-wide strategies for tobacco control and healthier diets are what really matters.

A remarkably similar picture is reported from Ireland between 1985 and 2000, with coronary artery disease falling by 47% and with half attributable to specific treatments for the disease and its risk factors, and half attributable to lifestyle changes especially smoking. However, with rises in obesity, diabetes and sedentary lifestyles, these trends are offset by around 13% or 500 deaths. And things may well get worse. *J Epidemiol Comm Health*, 2006; **60**: 322–323.

CLINICAL ISSUES

CARDIOVASCULAR

Trends in rates of different forms of diagnosed coronary heart disease, 1978–2000: prospective, population based study of British men
Lampe FC, Morris RW, Walker M, *et al.*
BMJ, 2005; **330**: 1046

A big drop in the rate of major coronary events in the last two decades has been largely offset by the increase in diagnosing angina according to a study of nearly 8000 middle-aged men.

The rate of major coronary events fell by an average of 3.6% a year, whereas the rate of first diagnosed angina increased by an average of 2.6% a year. These effects almost balance each other out when looking for an impact on the overall incidence of CHD. But the apparent increase in angina may well may be due to increased diagnosis of previously hidden disease and more aggressive management. The figure may settle in the future so we can see that tackling risk factors prevents angina as well. Until then, this study confirms prevention of more serious events such as MI.

It also highlights the need for continued emphasis on the primary prevention of coronary heart disease and a good angina service.

DETECTION

Comparison of methods to identify individuals at increased risk of coronary disease from the general population
Wilson S, Johnston A, Robson J *et al.*
BMJ, 2003; **326**: 1436–1438

It is impossible to accurately assess coronary risk without measuring lipids. As screening the entire population is not considered cost-effective, this study set out to evaluate the guidelines on measurement of cholesterol according to the National Service Framework (NSF) for coronary heart disease and to compare alternative strategies for identifying people at high risk of coronary disease.

The NSF criteria, Sheffield tables, an age threshold of 50 years, and fixed cholesterol values, were compared to a 'gold standard' prediction from the Framingham equation which identified 1053 individuals (with no previous vascular history) with a ten year coronary event risk in excess of 15%.

The NSF guidelines selected 43% of the study population for cholesterol measurement and identified 81% of those at 15% or greater risk. Improved screening is therefore indicated.

The Sheffield tables selected 73% and identified 99.9% of those at high risk. The cost of this high sensitivity was a false positive rate of 68%.

Estimated risk assessments using fixed cholesterol values selected just 18% and identified 76% of those at 15% or greater risk.

An age threshold of 50 years selected 46% identified 93% of the high-risk group.

The authors conclude that measuring the cholesterol concentration of everyone aged 50 years and over is a simple and efficient population screening tool. Its simplicity and transparency should increase uptake to screening and outweigh the costs of extra cholesterol testing.

CARDIOVASCULAR

Haemostatic/inflammatory markers predict 10-year risk of IHD at least as well as lipids: the Caerphilly collaborative studies

Yarnell JW, Patterson CC, Sweetnam PM et al.
Eur Heart J, 2004; **25**: 1049–1056

This Belfast study looked at predictive values of three haemostatic/inflammatory risk markers – fibrinogen, plasma viscosity and white cell count – for subsequent ischaemic heart disease.

Two UK populations totalling 4860 men were followed up at 10 years. Haemostatic/inflammatory risk factors showed an independent, graded relationship to coronary events that was at least as strong as that given by plasma lipids. They could help risk stratification in the future as well as provide new targets for intervention.

High attributable risk of elevated C-reactive protein level to conventional coronary heart disease risk factors: the Third National Health and Nutrition Examination Survey

Miller M, Zhan M, Havas S
Arch Intern Med, 2005; **165**: 2063–2068

C-reactive protein (CRP) is a marker of systemic inflammation that is predictive of CHD events reflecting a hostile internal environment built on cigarettes and TV dinners. However, elevated CRP is rare in the absence of other abnormal risk factors so it may have limited clinical utility as an additional screening tool.

C-reactive protein in the prediction of cardiovascular and overall mortality in middle-aged men: a population-based cohort study

Laaksonen DE, Niskanen L, Nyyssonen K
Eur Heart J, 2005; **26**: 1783–1789

Or you could believe these researchers instead who feel that CRP has an independent role.

CRP levels in this study predicted both cardiovascular and overall mortality in middle-aged men, independent of other risk factors. They also proposed new cut-off points (in tertiles) which were better at predicting mortality among men without CVD at baseline.

MEDICATION

Effect of combinations of drugs on all cause mortality in patients with ischaemic heart disease: nested case-control analysis

Hippisley-Cox J, Coupland C
BMJ, 2005; **330**: 1059–1063

Combinations of statins, aspirins, and beta blockers are associated with the greatest reduction in all cause mortality – about 83% – in patients with a first diagnosis

CARDIOVASCULAR

of ischaemic heart disease. The was the first large study to assess the effects of drugs combined in this way and identified 13 000 cases of ischaemic heart disease in a new UK database, QRESEARCH. Controls were matched for ischaemic heart disease, age, sex, and year of diagnosis and were alive at the time their matched case died.

The addition of an ACE inhibitor provided no additional benefit.

A strategy to reduce cardiovascular disease by more than 80%
Wald NJ, Law MR
BMJ, 2003; **326**: 1419–1423

Papers from this important issue of the *BMJ* bang the drum for the Polypill. Wald and Law propose this neologism as a panacea for heart disease.

They have synthesised over 750 trials with 400 000 participants and the argument goes like this.
- The strategy was to reduce simultaneously the four cardiovascular risk factors (low density lipoprotein cholesterol, blood pressure, serum homocysteine, and platelet function) regardless of pretreatment levels.
- Develop a single daily pill combining effective drugs to achieve a large effect in preventing cardiovascular disease with minimal adverse effects.
- Changing all four risk factors together reduces IHD events by 88% and stroke by 80%.
- The recommended combination is a statin (e.g. atorvastatin 10 mg or simvastatin 40 mg), three blood pressure lowering drugs (e.g. a thiazide, a beta-blocker, and an ACE inhibitor) each at half standard dose, folic acid (0.8 mg), and aspirin (75 mg).
- The components of the Polypill would cause adverse symptoms in 8–15% of people (depending on the precise formulation). Aspirin has the most side-effects but the advantages for thrombotic stroke outweigh those of increased haemorrhagic stroke.
- Withdrawal due to side-effects would occur in 1–2 per 100 and fatal side-effects in less than 1 in 10 000 users.
- There may be some contraindications to the Polypill, e.g. beta-blockers in asthma, aspirin if not tolerated.

With these caveats, they propose giving this combination pill to anyone at high risk but also to **all** over 55s. One-third of people taking this pill from age 55 would benefit, gaining on average about 11 years of life free from an IHD event or stroke.

They propose that this would have a greater impact on the prevention of disease in the Western world than any other single intervention.
- Cost would be low with generic ingredients that are all off-patent.
- There is no need to measure risk.
- There is no need for investigations.
- They propose a new model where we recognise that in Western society risk is high in all of us.
- Targeting single risk factors has so far produced only modest reductions in disease so there is much to gain and little to lose.

All the ingredients are proven effective in randomised controlled trials except folic acid whose evidence is observational but still compelling. The maximum observed effect of folic acid lowers serum homocysteine by about 25% and reduces IHD events by about 16% and stroke by 24%.

A combination of three low-dose drugs from different groups has greater efficacy and fewer adverse effects than using one or two drugs in standard dose.

The blood pressure reduction with three drugs in combination at half standard dose is about 11 mmHg diastolic, reducing coronary events by 46% and stroke by 63%.

Other than the statin, omitting a single component has a relatively minor effect. Aspirin prevents 32% of IHD events when used alone but only prevents an additional 5% when added to other ingredients of the Polypill.

The most important BMJ for 50 years?
Smith R
BMJ, 2003; **326**

Richard Smith's playful editorial piece describes the Polypill as 'genius'.

The use of multiple low-dose antihypertensives to lessen side-effects and maximise benefit is praised.

The inexpensive ingredients make it good news for the developing world but not for pharmaceutical companies. Perhaps a large generic company in India could supply us? (It has been claimed that manufacturers in India plan to forge ahead without further study in order to bring a Polypill to market quickly.)

Yes, there are issues of medicalisation but then the plan does circumvent the need for screening so nicely. And then of course what are we going to do with all the cardiologists and cardiac surgeons?

A cure for cardiovascular disease?
Rodgers A
BMJ, 2003; **326**: 1407–1408

This editorial agrees that large reductions in risk are likely with the Polypill.

The argument that three blood pressure lowering agents at half the standard dose are the best way to achieve large reductions in blood pressure is found convincing.

The author agrees that the drugs involved, contrary to modern perceptions, have remarkably few side-effects and pharmacological reasons for stopping treatment are rare. He calls for more information on the adverse effects of the combination but recognises that all the drugs involved have been extensively studied.

A wide debate on the new paradigm is called for. Treating risk rather than risk factor threshold is the new concept here and treating vast asymptomatic populations using age alone as a variable is controversial to say the least. It will involve a challenge to cardiovascular disease being a 'natural' cause of death.

Further trials will also be needed to look at issues such as tolerability and adherence as well as technical issues of production.

CARDIOVASCULAR

SECONDARY PREVENTION

Secondary prevention of coronary heart disease in older patients after the national service framework: population based study
Ramsay SE, Whincup PH, Lawlor DA *et al.*
BMJ, 2006; **332**: 144–145

Since the implementation of the NSF for prevention of coronary heart disease in 2000, prescription of drugs to men and women with established heart disease has improved markedly according to this review in 24 general practices. We know these drugs can produce relative reductions in the risk of CHD by 75% or more, so improvements were a priority for the framework.

Statins improved most and doubled in usage but, even by 2003, only about 80% of men and women with a history of MI were talking antiplatelets, two-thirds were receiving statins, and less than half were taking beta blockers and ACE inhibitors.

So, considerable opportunities for improvement remain especially for those with angina.

Secondary prevention clinics for coronary heart disease: four year follow up of a randomised controlled trial in primary care
Murchie P, Campbell NC, Ritchie LD *et al.*
BMJ, 2003; **326**: 84–86

This evaluation of nurse-led secondary prevention clinics in primary care looked at 19 Scottish practices and 1343 patients with coronary heart disease. Although the study (also reviewed in *Evidence-Based Medicine*, 2003; **8**: 158) was limited in power, it showed that attention to medical and lifestyle issues in this intervention seemed to lead to significantly fewer total deaths and probably fewer coronary deaths. These advantages persisted in the medium term, as follow up was over an average of nearly 5 years, and have added to the knowledge base by showing survival advantages. Patients should attend clinics sooner rather than later.

A cost analysis of this study appeared in *BMJ*, 2005; **330**: 707:
- the intervention cost £136 per patient
- during the four year follow-up, 28 fewer patients died in the intervention group
- there was a gain of 0.11 mean life years per patient
- cost was just over £1000 per QALY

Nurse-led clinics for the secondary prevention of CHD seem to be cost effective in primary care.

Recent developments in secondary prevention and cardiac rehabilitation after acute myocardial infarction
Dalal H, Evans PH, Campbell JL
BMJ, 2004; **328**: 693–697

This review focuses on the importance and failure so far to make secondary prevention happen. Overlap exists between secondary prevention work and

CARDIOVASCULAR

comprehensive cardiac rehabilitation which offers post-MI patients behavioural / psychological support and education in addition to an exercise plan.

More work is needed to improve:

- Exercise-based rehabilitation after MI
- Uptake of antiplatelets, statins, ACE inhibitors and beta-blockers
- Monitoring of risk factors
- Structured long-term care assisted by validated registers of high-risk patients
- Nurse-led secondary prevention clinics and home-based plans
- The 'implementation gap' requiring enhanced communication and coordination between primary and secondary care
- Monitoring for psychological complications such as depression

Factors involved in deciding to start preventive treatment: qualitative study of clinicians' and lay people's attitudes

Lewis DK, Robinson J, Wilkinson E
BMJ, 2003; **327**: 841–845

This Liverpool study interviewed four general practitioners, four practice nurses, and 18 lay people on their views about benefits of preventative drug treatment for coronary heart disease.

- Both clinicians and lay people in this study found it difficult to make logical decisions about preventive treatment.
- There was a general acceptance that resources are finite and should be targeted where they are most effective.
- Most lay people wanted to be involved in determining their own treatment.
- Many preferred lifestyle change to medication.
- There is a danger that increased pressure on GPs may marginalise patients' preferences denying the true dialogue between clinicians and patients that is necessary before starting lifelong preventive treatment.

PREHOSPITAL THROMBOLYSIS

Prospective observational cohort study of time saved by prehospital thrombolysis for ST elevation myocardial infarction delivered by paramedics

Pedley DK, Bissett K, Connolly EM *et al.*
BMJ, 2003; **327**: 22–26

Prehospital thrombolysis has been shown in the landmark GREAT study – the Grampian Region Early Anistreplase Trial – to have a long-lasting benefit on morbidity and mortality in rural areas. This study used a model where paramedics assessing chest pain liaised with hospital doctors by telemetry in an area that was about to lose its coronary care unit. Median call to needle time was 52 minutes compared to 125 minutes for hospital thrombolysis. Infarction was later confirmed in 89% of the paramedic group and 92% of the hospital-assessed group. The results showed the method to be safe and necessary for rural areas to meet the targets of the NSF for early thrombolysis (less than 60 minutes). Some 64% receiving prehospital thrombolysis achieved this compared to 4% treated in hospital.

CARDIOVASCULAR

Further Research

- Data from the British Women's Heart and Health Study indicate that heart disease is more common in British women over 60 than previously thought and is being underdiagnosed and undertreated. One in five had some sort of vascular disease. One in two was hypertensive. One in four was obese. One in two had a cholesterol over 6.5 mmol/l, and 12% smoked. Only 40% were taking aspirin and only around 20% were on a statin.

- Despite improvements following the implementation of NSF for CHD, a study in 17 GP practices in the UK showed there was still room for improvement in older patients over seventy years who were less likely to be taking a statin, beta blockers post MI or have well controlled BP. *Br J Gen Pract,* 2005; **55**: 369–375.

- In a US study, discontinuation of therapy at 6-months occurred in 8% of those taking aspirin, 12% of those taking beta blockers, 13% of those taking statins, and 20% of those taking ACE inhibitors. Male sex and prior heart failure were associated with improved compliance with ACE inhibitors. *Am J Med,* 2004; **117**: 73–81.

- Patients with stable coronary artery disease who are already on intensive standard therapy (antiplatelets, statins, beta blockers and others) show no clinical benefit from additional treatment with an ACE inhibitor (trandolapril), when left ventricular function was preserved, according to the PEACE Trial – Prevention of Events with ACE Inhibition. *New Engl J Med,* 2004; **351**: 2058–2068. This might be surprising but *Evidence-Based Medicine* (2005; **10**: 78) comments that the subjects of PEACE were a lower risk group than those in the HOPE trial. At the moment though, there is no need for ACE inhibitor in uncomplicated CHD.

- Another meta-analysis of six trials showed ACE inhibitors not to be clearly better than any other antihypertensive at preventing heart failure in hypertensive patients. *Am J Cardiol,* 2004; **93**: 240–243.

- *Chlamydia pneumoniae* has been found in atherosclerotic plaques and infection may play a role in CHD. A trial looking at suggestions that a 14 day course of azithromycin might benefit cardiac morbidity found the reverse. CLARICOR was randomised and placebo-controlled and with a longer follow up than other equivocal analyses, and found an increased mortality with this approach, and definitely no suggestion of any protective effect. *BMJ,* 2006; **332**: 22–27.

HEART FAILURE

What we know already:

- Heart failure accounts for 5% of admissions to medical wards, with enormous healthcare costs from high re-admission rates
- Hypertension precedes heart failure in over 90% of cases and the treatment of hypertension can prevent more than 40% of heart failure events
- Diagnosis by clinical assessment of symptoms and signs is difficult and is incorrect in more than half of cases. Unrecognised hypervolaemia is common as blood volume does not correlate well with physical signs and JVP may be the most useful
- It is largely poorly managed in general practice and the National Service Framework (NSF) for CHD stresses that the substandard care of patients with heart failure is unacceptable
- Even in hospital, there are major deficiencies of prescription of ACE inhibitors and beta blockers and even recording of an ECG
- Some suggest that a NSF for chronic heart failure is urgently needed as only a systematic overhaul and a multidisciplinary approach can stop heart failure being the 'Cinderella of cardiology'
- B-type natriuretic peptide is a red flag in heart failure indicating volume overload and a stretched ventricle. Levels above 500 pg/ml are accepted as diagnostic but it is a strong prognostic indicator regardless of the stage of heart failure. Each 100 pg/ml increase in BNP was associated with a 35% increase in the relative risk of death. Even in asymptomatic patients, BNP > 20 pg/ml was associated with twice the risk of death
- Evaluation of BNP in the emergency department leads to quicker treatment, fewer hospitalisations, a shorter length of stay and lower costs, actually improving outcomes
- Even when ejection fraction is preserved, in so-called diastolic heart failure, there is also substantial mortality

Key trials

MERIT-HF: Effect of metoprolol in chronic heart failure: Metoprolol Randomised Intervention Trial in Congestive Heart Failure (MERIT-HF). Lancet, 1999; 353: 2001–2007

Nearly 4000 patients with class II–IV heart failure, stable on optimum standard therapy (any combination of diuretics and ACE inhibitor) were assigned increasing doses of slow release metoprolol. The study was halted at mean follow up of 1 year as all-cause mortality was significantly lower in metoprolol group (34% risk reduction). There were significantly fewer cardiovascular deaths and the drug was well tolerated.

It improved survival in stable patients, preventing 1 death per 27 patients treated per year.

CHARM: Effects of candesartan on mortality and morbidity in patients with chronic heart failure: the CHARM-Overall programme. Lancet, 2003; 362: 759–771

This was a prospective study of 7599 patients with chronic heart failure (NYHA class II–IV) given placebo or candesartan – an angiotensin II receptor blocker (ARB).

- Cardiovascular death significantly reduced in the candesartan group (18% vs. 20%).
- Hospital admission due to heart failure was significantly reduced (20% vs. 24%).
- Non-cardiovascular death was not significantly different but overall mortality was reduced.
- Benefit was greatest where there was reduced left ventricular ejection fraction and occurred even if the patients were already on an ACE inhibitor.

ValHEFT (The Valsartan Heart Failure Trial) has shown similar benefits for losartan but a retrospective analysis implied that adding an ARB on to an ACE inhibitor and a beta blocker was associated with an increased mortality. CHARM is a prospective study and contradicts this saying it is safe in mild to moderate left ventricular failure.

***RALES: The effect of spironolactone on morbidity and mortality in patients with severe heart failure. N Engl J Med**, 1999; **341**: 709–717.*

In patients with severe heart failure, an aldosterone blocker might be the preferred agent to add to an ACE inhibitor and a beta blocker rather than an ARB based on the results of the Randomized Aldactone Evaluation Study (RALES). However, only a relatively small proportion of patients were receiving both an ACE inhibitor and a beta blocker. Direct comparative studies of an ARB and an aldosterone blocker in patients with left ventricular failure on this regime are needed.

Guidelines

NICE – *Management of Chronic Heart Failure in Adults in Primary and Secondary Care* (http://www.nice.org.uk)

NICE guidance now recommends:
- Full evaluation of all patients suspected of having heart failure using 12-lead ECG or testing B-type natriuretic peptide (BNP), to exclude a diagnosis of heart failure
- ACE inhibitors should be given in the presence of left ventricular dysfunction
- Diuretics are used for symptoms
- Beta blockers licensed for use in cases of heart failure are used in a carefully monitored 'start low, go slow' manner after treatment with diuretics and ACE inhibitors, regardless of whether or not symptoms persist
- All patients with chronic heart failure should be monitored at least every six months with clinical assessment of function, fluid status, cardiac rhythm, medication review, and measurement of urea, electrolytes, and creatinine

Recent Papers

DETECTION

Barriers to accurate diagnosis and effective management of heart failure in primary care: qualitative study
Fuat A, Hungin APS, Murphy JJ
BMJ, 2003; **326**: 196–200

A focus group of 30 UK GPs was interviewed to assess their beliefs and practices relating to managing heart failure in primary care.
- Uncertainty in making a diagnosis led to poor uptake of evidence-based strategies.
- Doctors are still struggling to make a symptomatic rather than pathophysiological diagnosis.
- Lack of confidence in therapeutic approaches led to reluctance to initiate treatment. They were concerned about using ACE inhibitors in the elderly and confused about the resurgence of beta blockers and spironolactone. They found the research rapidly changing and had doubts about the applicability to primary care.
- Lack of time and availability of diagnostic tests and fear of overloading secondary care were noted.
- Local organisational factors such as access to echocardiography and, most importantly, interpretation of its results as well as interaction with cardiologists were a significant barrier.
- Individual negative experiences and personal preferences could at times adversely affect judgement.

The authors point out that science has outstripped the ability and capacity of NHS delivery systems. Rapidly changing treatment options have confused doctors and drugs previously regarded as dangerous, such as beta blockers, are back in vogue. They call for new, conjoint models of care to straddle primary and secondary care. The study strengthens the case for multidisciplinary heart failure clinics as outlined in the NSF for coronary heart disease.

Public awareness of heart failure in Europe: first results from SHAPE
Remme WJ, McMurray JJ, Rauch B, et al.
Eur Heart J, 2005; **26**: 2413–2421

The Study of Heart failure Awareness and Perception in Europe (SHAPE), found poor community awareness of what heart failure actually is.
- Only 3% could correctly identify heart failure from a description of typical symptoms and signs.
- Most thought that these patients should reduce all physical activity.
- Most thought it was less serious than it is.
- One-third also wrongly thought heart failure was a normal consequence of getting older.
- Nearly one-third thought modern drugs could not prevent the condition.

It could be time to rebrand heart failure and sell it to the public.

CARDIOVASCULAR

Medical history, physical examination, and routine tests are useful for diagnosing heart failure in dyspnoea. *Evidence-Based Medicine,* 2006; **11**: 58
The following paper is reviewed
Does this dyspnoeic patient in the emergency department have congestive heart failure?
Wang CS, FitzGerald JM, Schulzer M et al.
JAMA, 2005; **294**: 1944–1956

A review of 18 high quality studies on patients with acute dyspnoea showed that the findings useful for ruling in heart failure were (in decreasing order) pulmonary venous congestion and interstitial oedema on CXR, a third heart sound, a history of heart failure, and jugular venous distension.

For ruling out heart failure the best findings were a serum BNP <100 pg/ml, absence of cardiomegaly and pulmonary venous congestion on CXR, crepitations, exertional dyspnoea, and a negative history of heart failure.

Prevalence and prognostic implications of electrocardiographic left ventricular hypertrophy in heart failure: evidence from the CHARM programme
Hawkins NM, Wang D, McMurray JJ et al.
Heart, 2007; **93**: 59–64

ECG is a simple, cheap tool which has been shown to be a significant independent predictor of worsening clinical outcome in heart failure even when systolic function is preserved.

Further analysis of the CHARM study showed that LVH was present on ECG in 15% of those patients with heart failure, with and without reduced left ventricular fraction. It proved to be associated with a 78% increase in cardiovascular death and major cardiovascular events overall.

A relationship with hypertension had previously been recognised but was inconclusive in heart failure.

Portable echocardiography
Ashrafian H, Bogle RG, Rosen SD et al.
BMJ, 2004; **328**: 300–301

This editorial looks at the role of a new tool – portable echocardiography. This may have a role in our reorganisation as traditional models are failing heart failure patients. In trained hands, and this training may only take a few hours, it can provide basic assessment of ventricular function, measurement of the ventricular chambers, and identification of structural lesions. This could allow us to initiate changes in treatment. Sensitivity for detection of cardiac abnormalities is higher than that of clinical examination and reaches 70–90% compared with conventional echocardiography.

It is a relatively reliable technique but some studies have shown that important findings do get missed. It is recognised that if used, records should be stored in anticipation of a second opinion. Perhaps portable echocardiography is best restricted to fewer more specialist technicians with ongoing feedback from specialists as part of a team which recognises its limitations.

CARDIOVASCULAR

Management of chronic heart failure in the community: role of a hospital based open access heart failure service

Shah S, Davies MK, Cartwright D et al.
Heart, 2004; **90**: 755–759

This Birmingham study evaluated an open access heart failure service based at a teaching hospital. They assessed nearly 1000 GP referrals of patients with suspected heart failure.

- Only 31% were found to have left ventricular systolic dysfunction (LVSD denotes an ejection fraction < 50% on echocardiography).
- Risk factors for this were male sex, age over 60 years, diabetes, ischaemic heart disease or atrial fibrillation.
- Abnormal ECG and cardiothoracic ratio > 0.5 were good predictors of LVSD.
- A normal ECG had a negative predictive value of 80%
- A cardiothoracic ratio of < 0.5 on CXR had a negative predictive value of 82%.
- A combined negative predictive value of 88% make ECG and CXR good predictors with which to identify lower risk patients.
- The authors suggest that this type of model is a cost-effective service to community referrals.

MEDICATION

Adverse effects of beta-blocker therapy for patients with heart failure: a quantitative overview of randomised trials

Ko DT, Hebert PR, Coffey CS et al.
Arch Intern Med, 2004; **164**: 1389–1394

Beta blockers have become popular for heart failure, substantially improving survival in patients with LVSD and reducing heart failure and hospitalisation. But concerns about side-effects linger. This overview of randomised trials showed beta blocker therapy was associated with small but significant absolute risks of hypotension (11 per 1000), dizziness (57 per 1000), and bradycardia (38 per 1000). There was no significant fatigue associated with therapy and fewer patients were withdrawn from beta blocker therapy than from placebo.

This information should alleviate concerns about prescribing this life-saving therapy to patients with heart failure.

A similar Medline search and analysis (reviewed in *Evidence-Based Medicine,* 2003; **8**: 15) looked at patients on beta blockers for reasons of MI, hypertension, or heart failure. They noted an increase in withdrawals because of fatigue or sexual dysfunction. Beta blockers did not increase depressive symptoms.

Reviewers of the Ko study in *Evidence-Based Medicine* (2005; **10**: 42) ask that because the upper age limit was 67 years, how generalisable are these results to older patients who have so much to gain and are already on many other drugs? And which beta blocker should we choose?

A meta-analysis with 12 000 subjects looking at all-cause mortality data from

CLINICAL ISSUES

CARDIOVASCULAR

five completed trials revealed that elderly and non-elderly heart failure patients both derive considerable and similar mortality reduction from the use of beta-blockers (*Am J Cardiol,* 2005; **95**: 896-898).

Detrimental effects of beta-blockers in COPD: a concern for nonselective beta-blockers
van der Woude HJ, Zaagsma J, Postma DS, *et al.*
Chest, 2005; **127**: 818–824

This study may look as though it is in the wrong chapter but unless we think of our heart failure patients who also suffer with COPD, we may offer them a treatment that does them a great disservice. The authors compared different beta blockers – propranolol, metoprolol and celiprolol and showed different types of beta blockers have different pulmonary effects:
- propranolol reduced FEV_1, increased airway hyperresponsiveness, and reduced the effect of formoterol
- metoprolol increased airway hyperresponsiveness but did not affect FEV_1
- celiprolol seemed safe at the doses used with no pulmonary effects

Angiotensin receptor blockers and myocardial infarction
Verma S, Strauss M
BMJ, 2004; **329**: 1248–1249

This is a useful editorial summarising the current controversy over the role of angiotensin receptor blockers looking at their effects in the following trials.
- VALUE – this trial showed a 19% increase in fatal and non-fatal MI compared to amlodipine in high-risk hypertensives.
- CHARM-Alternative – showed a 36% increase in MI with candesartan despite lowering blood pressure.
- CHARM-Preserved – reduced admissions for chronic heart failure but did not prevent death.
- SCOPE – candesartan showed a non-significant increase in fatal and non-fatal MI in the elderly despite lowering blood pressure.
- LIFE – showed no reduction in MI.
- RENAAL – in diabetics with nephropathy, losartan offer renal protection but no reduction in cardiovascular mortality.

So ARBs reduce blood pressure but may increase MI. ACE inhibitors on the other hand have consistently produced at least a 20% reduction in MI in high risk patients. Large trials are awaited (ONTARGET/TRANSCEND) but in the meantime the authors warn, should we get fully informed consent before using these drugs and forget about thinking of them as ACE inhibitors without the cough?

However, a systematic review in 2005 of all available data on ARBs shows a neutral impact on MI. While more data are awaited, we need not worry about the risk of MI if we think our patients need an ARB in preference to an ACE inhibitor. *BMJ,* 2005; **331**: 873.

Angiotension receptor blockers do not differ from ACE inhibitors in chronic heart failure or acute MI. *Evidence-Based Medicine,* 2005; **10**: 76.
The following paper is reviewed
Meta-analysis: angiotensin-receptor blockers in chronic heart failure and high-risk acute myocardial infarction
Lee VC, Rhew DC, Dylan M, *et al.*
Ann Intern Med, 2004; **141**: 693–704

A review of 24 RCTs found that in patients with chronic heart failure, ARBs do not differ from ACE inhibitors for all cause mortality or hospital admission.

The commentary reminds us that there is no evidence that ARBs are any better, and ARBs cost much more than generic ACE inhibitors. They tell us 'ARBs *are* great drugs; their misfortune is that ACE inhibitors are too' and suggest that the pharmaceutical industry so keen to show superiority for their latest offerings are 'probably close to giving up'.

Association between performance measures and clinical outcomes for patients hospitalized with heart failure
Fonarow GC, Abraham WT, Albert N *et al.* for the OPTIMIZE-HF Investigators
JAMA, 2007; **297**: 61–70

Performance indicators used to assess quality of care on discharge from hospitals for heart failure may need updating.

Patients with left ventricular dysfunction who were discharged on an ACE inhibitor or ARB were significantly less likely to die or be admitted within 60–90 days in this US study. However, there were no such associations for four other indicators routinely used – a measure of left ventricular dysfunction, smoking cessation interventions, treating atrial fibrillation with warfarin, and providing written advice on heart failure.

Beta blockers, despite clearly being associated with a reduction in mortality when prescribed on discharge, were not used as a quality measure in this US study.

Better indicators of more clinical relevance could improve outcomes.

Further Research

- Digoxin is useful in heart failure but the level should be kept low. Previously the DIG (Digitalis Investigation Group) trial seemed to show that digoxin did not increase survival but did help to keep patients out of hospital. A new analysis shows the optimal range in men to be 0.5–0.8 ng/ml. Mortality is lower in this group. Mortality was higher than placebo with higher levels of digoxin. *JAMA*, 2003; **289**: 871–878.

- Early combined statin and beta blocker therapy reduces mortality after MI complicated by some degree of heart failure. Benefits of these drugs are additive, according to the Optimal Trial in Myocardial Infarction with the Angiotensin II Antagonist Losartan (OPTIMAAL). Risk reduction was about 25% for statin treatment alone, 30% for beta blockers alone, and close to 50% for the combination of statins and beta blockers compared with no treatment. Still only around half were given these drugs on discharge from hospital. *Am J Cardiol*, 2004; **93**: 603–606.

- A US study showed almost one-third of patients with LVSD were not prescribed an ACE inhibitor upon discharge from hospital, sacrificing a 14% relative reduction in mortality in the first year alone. Overhesitation in prescribing to the elderly (who have most to gain) may be to blame. *Circulation*, 2004; **110**: 724–731.

- Assays of BNP and N-terminal pro-BNP variant in primary care reduced referrals to a cardiology clinic by 25% in nearly 300 patients in South Durham who had symptoms and signs suggestive of heart failure. *Br J Gen Pract*, 2006; **56**: 327–333.

STROKE

What we know already:

- Stroke is the second leading cause of death in the world and the largest single cause of major disability in the UK
- Each year 100 000 people in England and Wales have a stroke. Thirty per cent die in the first month and a third are still significantly disabled at one year. Five per cent require long-term residential care
- The cost to the NHS is around £2.3 billion per year
- Haemorrhagic strokes account for 20% but are more likely to be fatal
- The UK has poor survival rates for stroke and low research funding
- Stroke units are the gold standard of care, improving mortality and recovery from stroke, but are under-resourced
- Survival rates 10 years following a stroke are higher for those who went to a stroke unit rather than general ward – possibly due to early reduction in disability
- Therapeutic benefits have been shown for aspirin, antihypertensives, statins and treatment for atrial fibrillation
- The National Service Framework for Older People Standard 5 outlines the recommended approach to stroke
- The Face Arm Speech Test which assesses facial droop, arm strength, and normal conversation, can accurately diagnose stroke with good agreement between paramedics and physicians. FAST may facilitate rapid triage of stroke to urgent specialist care

Key trials

The Heart Protection Study and other major trials have confirmed that stroke risk halves for every 10 mmHg fall in diastolic pressure even at conventional normotensive values. The effect is regardless of baseline BP and there seems to be no demonstrable floor to this benefit.

The HOPE study (2000)
This involved 9297 subjects from 19 countries. They were all high-risk but had controlled BP.
- Ramipril reduced fatal stroke by 61% and non-fatal stroke by 24%, independent of BP. The reduction in BP was quite small (3.8 / 2.8 mmHg) but the reduction in stroke risk was greater than expected at 32%
- The effect of 10 mg ramipril is stronger than 2.5 mg, so titrating the dose upwards will be important to realise maximum benefit
- It is unknown how much of this benefit will translate to other ACE inhibitors
- Patients already taking aspirin have less benefit and this interaction needs further study
The authors of HOPE recommend that patients at high risk of stroke should be treated with ramipril for primary and secondary prevention irrespective of their initial BP levels.

PROGRESS (2001)
In the perindopril protection against recurrent stroke study, a combination of perindopril and the diuretic indapamide reduced the risk of stroke over 4 years by 28%, with BP reduction of 9/4 mmHg. This benefited intracerebral haemorrhage perhaps more than ischaemic events.

Recent Papers

INCIDENCE

Change in stroke incidence, mortality, case-fatality, severity, and risk factors in Oxfordshire, UK from 1981 to 2004 (Oxford Vascular Study)
Rothwell PM, Coull AJ, Giles MF et al.
Lancet, 2004; **363**: 1925–1933

A UK study showed that incidence of stroke in Oxfordshire fell by 40% over the past 20 years. This is likely to be due to the increased use of preventive treatments and reduction in risk factors.

The authors looked at changes in incidences of stroke and TIA rates between two previous local studies, the Oxford Community Stroke Project which ran between 1981 and 1984, and the Oxford Vascular Study (OXVASC) which ran from 2002 to 2004.

Although 28% more strokes were expected in OXVASC due to an increase in the elderly population (33% increase in those aged 75 or older), the observed number actually fell.

Incidence declined by more than 50% for primary intracerebral haemorrhage but was unchanged for subarachnoid haemorrhage.

Major increases in treatment with antiplatelets, lipid-lowerers, and antihypertensives were noted. So were substantial reductions in smoking, total cholesterol, and mean systolic and diastolic blood pressures.

There is still significant undertreatment allowing for improvements in the future but it is nice to see we are doing something right.

Population based study of early risk of stroke after transient ischaemic attack or minor stroke: implications for public education and organisation of services
Coull AJ, Lovett JK, Rothwell PM
BMJ, 2004; **328**: 326

This prospective cohort study showed that the risk of stroke after TIA or minor stroke is much higher than commonly quoted. Nine Oxfordshire practices identified 87 patients with a new TIA or minor stroke. The estimated risk of stroke in these patients was 8–12% at seven days, 11–15% at one month, and 17–18.5% at three months. We know that 15% of ischaemic strokes are preceded by a TIA and with British guidelines recommending assessment of TIA within 2 weeks, a significant number will have had a stroke by the time they are seen. This means urgent preventative treatment is needed and a structure put in place that allows patients to be seen in a matter of hours or days rather than weeks. Public education is needed so patients present early.

CARDIOVASCULAR

A simple score (ABCD) to identify individuals at high early risk of stroke after transient ischaemic attack
Rothwell PM, Giles MF, Flossmann E *et al.*
Lancet, 2005; **366**: 29–36

This team from Oxford have validated a simple scoring system to predict the risk of stroke in the 7 days following a TIA. The system is called ABCD and has a maximum of 6 points according to:

- Age (≥60 years = 1),
- Blood pressure (systolic > 140 mmHg or diastolic ≥90, or both = 1),
- Clinical signs (unilateral weakness = 2, speech disturbance but no weakness = 1, other = 0)
- Duration of symptoms (≥60 minutes = 2, 10–59 = 1, < 10 = 0).

The seven day risk of stroke was 0.4% for those who scored less than 5, 12% for patients who scored 5, and 31% for patients who scored 6. A score of 6 should be treated as a medical emergency, they suggest.

Commentary in *Evidence-Based Medicine* (2006; **11**: 27) reminds us that other factors sometimes considered predictive of risk, such as crescendo pattern, carotid stenosis and multiplicity, were not considered, and without further validation the score is not quite ready for clinical use. And whom should we admit? There is no intervention proven to decrease stroke risk in the short term, so perhaps only those who are being considered for thrombolysis. How often is that happening in your local hospital? That aside, once the cause is established, early initiation of secondary prevention should logically decrease ongoing risk.

Underinvestigation and undertreatment of carotid disease in elderly patients with transient ischaemic attack and stroke: comparative population based study
Fairhead JF, Rothwell PM
BMJ, 2006; **333**: 525–527

An expansion of the OXVASC population looked at secondary care services in Oxfordshire.

They found that patients over 80 years who suffer a TIA or minor ischaemic stroke have a steep increase in incidence of symptomatic carotid stenosis (> 50% stenosed). However, that age group is substantially underinvestigated with carotid imaging and undertreated with carotid endarterectomy.

Accusations of ageism have appeared and in investigating whether or not this is ageism, the authors found there is good evidence of benefit for endarterectomy in the elderly and they have little increased risk from the surgery. The decision not to refer or go through with imaging the carotids could be made in primary or secondary care. The study could not tell us. But it could say this was not likely to be due to contraindication or the patient's own choice.

CARDIOVASCULAR

Ageism in services for transient ischaemic attack and stroke
Young J
BMJ, 2006; **333**: 508–509

This author tells us about the overt and covert rationing inherent in a system such as the health service where underfunding has allowed ageism to flourish, he argues. Evidence of the intervention conferring greater benefit in the elderly because of their higher absolute risk for stroke makes this unethical and unsustainable.

Avoiding disabling stroke at any age is a priority. We can use educational measures to tell doctors the best practice, streamline local services, and redesign stroke services in a similar way to CHD programmes to reduce such ageism.

MEDICATION

Secondary prevention for stroke and transient ischaemic attacks
Muir KW
BMJ, 2004; **328**: 297–298

This editorial discusses the current state of play with secondary prevention for stroke and TIA arguing that concepts of hypertension and hypercholesterolaemia may have become irrelevant or even harmful in this group.

Almost all stroke / TIA patients, it is stated, will benefit from treatment for cholesterol and blood pressure regardless of actual levels.

Given the benefits of these medications, clinicians must improve diagnostic accuracy as only half of those referred as TIAs have actually had one. Other neurological diagnoses are made in 30%.

Concerns over polypharmacy, drug interactions and co-morbidities could mean that these opportunities are lost and patients are sentenced to disabling or fatal strokes.

The data in the previous synopsis has shown the higher than commonly quoted rate of stroke after TIA. Whether secondary preventative medication such as antiplatelets, antihypertensives and statins can work in this very early period will be assessed in new trials – FASTER (Fast Assessment of Stroke and Transient ischaemic attack to prevent Early Recurrence) and PRoFESS (Prevention Regimen for efFEctively avoiding Second Strokes). The phrase 'just a TIA' may become a casualty to a new era of aggressive treatment. A TIA should be taken seriously for the warning that it is.

LONG-TERM CARE

Training care givers of stroke patients: randomised controlled trial
Kalra L, Evans A, Perez I et al.
BMJ, 2004; **328**: 1099

This randomised controlled trial looked at the benefit of providing training to informal caregivers of 300 stroke patients.

Training was given in basic nursing and facilitation of personal care. The intervention was successful in lowering the burden for the caregiver. The training group and, interestingly, their stroke patients both had reductions in anxiety and depression and improvements in quality of life. The mortality, institutionalisation and disability of the patients were unaffected.

Caregivers can be a somewhat neglected group. This straightforward training in stroke-related problems and lifting and handling, in just a handful of sessions, was successful in improving psychosocial outcomes in both carers and patients at three months and after one year.

There was also significant reduction of costs of health and social care during the year. This was mainly due to lower hospital costs as well as a trend to use less respite care.

Alternative strategies for stroke care: cost-effectiveness and cost-utility analyses from a prospective randomized controlled trial
Patel A, Knapp M, Perez I *et al.*
Stroke, 2004; **35**: 196–203

We know that stroke units improve outcomes in mortality and institutionalisation but this study looked at cost-effectiveness and included all healthcare and informal care costs.

It assigned 447 victims of stroke to three methods of care; stroke unit, stroke team, or domiciliary care. Follow up was over a year and average healthcare and social care costs for the year were £11 450 for stroke unit, £9527 for stroke team, and £6840 for domiciliary care.

Most of the costs were related to the initial period of care following the stroke. The authors conclude that the benefits of more intensive interventions come at a significantly higher cost.

Further Research

- An American study had paramedics give neuroprotective magnesium sulphate to focal strokes before arrival in hospital. The results of the Field Administration of Stroke Therapy-Magnesium (FAST-MAG) pilot trial showed this is a viable proposition and a further placebo-controlled study will now assess the value of this intervention in the first hour or two after stroke. *Stroke*, 2004; **35**: 106–108.

CARDIOVASCULAR

DIABETES

What we know already:

- Diabetes is a chronic progressive disease that affects 1.3 million people in England with perhaps another million cases undetected
- It is responsible for 5% of all NHS expenditure
- By 2025, it has been estimated that 300 million people will be diabetic – a global pandemic
- Even if obesity levels remain constant which seems unlikely, the most important factor is the increasingly elderly demographic
- A population strategy for screening for type 2 diabetes does not appear to fulfil WHO criteria – universal screening is impractical and too expensive. High-risk groups should be sought more intensively and screened opportunistically
- Various diabetic risk scores looking at combinations of risk factors in specific populations have been developed. A US study found a cost-effective strategy for diabetes screening was to target hypertensives over the age of 55
- Poor control of risk factors is widespread particularly in the young. One US study found that only 7% of the participants were within recommended targets for HbA1c, cholesterol and blood pressure
- Patients with type 2 diabetes do not view their condition as seriously as the healthcare professionals who are trying to help them manage it
- Many health workers feel as though diabetes is difficult to treat and requires more time and resources than they have available
- Beta blockers can be used for diabetics in cardiac failure without worrying about worsening glycaemic control. Outcomes in mortality were not as great as in non-diabetics but were still a healthy 16%. Use unless absolutely contraindicated or not tolerated
- Routine prescription of statins in type 2 diabetes particularly in older patients should now be considered
- Supplementation of a sulfonylurea with a glitazone or metformin yields similar benefits on HbA1c (around 1%) and on fasting glucose, but may have benefits for lipid profiles and urinary albumin-to-creatinine ratio (a marker of microalbuminuria)
- Nephropathy has been shown to be an independent risk factor for early cardiovascular death in diabetic patients
- Microalbuminuria is associated with a twofold to fourfold increase in the risk of deaths; overt proteinuria and hypertension compound the risk
- Those who have a coffee intake of seven cups per day have been found to be at least 50% less likely to develop diabetes than those drinking one or two cups per day. The mechanism is unknown

Key trials

The United Kingdom Prospective Diabetes Study (UKPDS)

This was a landmark study of over 5000 diabetics. It was published in 1998 and showed the value of tight blood pressure control in type 2 diabetics. Heart failure was reduced by 56% and strokes by 44%. Although reduction in myocardial infarction alone was not significant, when combined with other vascular end points (i.e. sudden death, stroke, and peripheral vascular disease) reduction was 34%.

Tight control also had considerable benefits on the development of retinopathy and proteinuria.

Other lessons were that:

- Drug treatment is markedly better than diet in terms of any diabetic related end-point
- Metformin should be the drug of choice especially in the obese as it is the only oral hypoglycaemic agent proved to reduce cardiovascular risk in this group
- The group treated with metformin had no hypoglycaemia and less weight gain
- Intensive glycaemic control resulted in reduced microvascular complications and fewer diabetic end-points than less intense control but no difference in mortality
- Further analysis showed that the level of glycaemic control is more important than the nature of the therapy and that even small reductions in HbA1c will prevent diabetic deaths

DCCT (Diabetes Control and Complications Trial)
Another landmark study showed that intensive efforts in glycaemic control benefited type 1 diabetics by reducing microvascular complications. But it also increased the number of hypoglycaemic episodes and the need for monitoring.

HOPE (Heart Outcomes Prevention Evaluation) and microHOPE study
This 5 year study included 9297 patients who were aged 55 years or older with a history of vascular disease or diabetes, plus one other cardiovascular risk factor. It included 3577 mainly type 2 diabetics and participants were given the ACE inhibitor ramipril or placebo.

Systolic blood pressure decreased by 2–3 mmHg in the ramipril group and reduced combined myocardial infarction, strokes, and deaths from cardiovascular diseases by 25%. The relative risk reduction for myocardial infarction was 22%, stroke 33%, and cardiovascular death 37%. It was reported in 2005 that the benefits observed in HOPE were maintained during 2.6 years of post-trial follow-up for cardiovascular death, stroke, and hospitalisation for heart failure.

The Microalbuminuria, Cardiovascular, and Renal Outcomes in HOPE (MICRO-HOPE) substudy showed that ramipril treatment was also associated with a reduced risk of developing nephropathy. It was concluded that ACE inhibitors should be first-line treatment for blood pressure control in diabetics and may have a role in normotensive patients.

As well as protecting against complications of diabetes, ramipril also significantly lowered the number with a new diagnosis of diabetes by 34%.

Two meta-analyses (*Diabetes Care*, 2005; **28**: 2261–2266 and *J Am Coll Cardiol*, 2005; **46**: 821–826) confirmed that either ACE inhibitors or ARBs at a pre-diabetic stage reduce the incidence of type 2 diabetes by approximately 25%. These medications may find an increasing role in areas such as metabolic syndrome, impaired fasting glucose and those with a family history of diabetes.

DREAM (the Diabetes REduction Assessment with ramipril and rosiglitazone Medication)
Looking prospectively into the possibility that ACE inhibitor treatment with ramipril may prevent new diabetes, DREAM has so far failed to confirm that it reduced the risk of diabetes in non-diabetic patients at high risk of the disease.

CARDIOVASCULAR

However, rosiglitazone at 8 mg per day substantially reduced the incidence of type 2 diabetes and increased the likelihood of regression to normoglycaemia (*Lancet*, 2006; **368**: 1096–1105).

Heart Protection Study
This was a randomised placebo-controlled trial designed to determine whether the lipid-lowering agent simvastatin reduced mortality and vascular events in 20 536 high risk patients aged 40–80 years with and without coronary disease. Patients had a broad range of baseline cholesterol levels. It showed that in high-risk patients including diabetics without previous coronary heart disease, simvastatin reduced all-cause mortality, coronary deaths, strokes and major vascular events. The authors suggest a role for routine use of statins in high-risk diabetics regardless of cholesterol level.

Guidelines

The National Service Framework (NSF) on Diabetes laid out 12 standards of care for all aspects of the management of diabetes in December 2001 and produced a delivery strategy in January 2003. These are available on the Department of Health's website.

NICE has a series of guidelines for type 1 and type 2 diabetes. It recommended in August 2003 that treatment with thiazolidinediones (glitazones) for type 2 diabetes should be reserved for those who cannot tolerate the combination of metformin and a sulphonylurea. They should replace the less well tolerated drug. Insulin treatment should not be delayed when treatment with metformin and a sulphonylurea has failed.

Recent Papers

Excess risk of fatal coronary heart disease associated with diabetes in men and women: meta-analysis of 37 prospective cohort studies
Huxley R, Barzi F, Woodward M
BMJ, 2006; **332**: 73–78

Meta-analysis of 37 studies has shown that the relative risk for CHD associated with diabetes is 50% higher in women than it is in men. This may be due to a more adverse risk profile in women who do tend to have higher BP and worse lipids, particularly if diabetic. There could also be a treatment bias at play that favours men.

Combining fasting plasma glucose and glycosylated haemoglobin improved the accuracy for detecting patients with diabetes. *Evidence-Based Medicine,* 2003; **8**: 186
The following article is presented
Diagnostic strategies to detect glucose intolerance in a multiethnic population
Anand SS, Razak F, Vuksan V *et al.*
Diabetes Care, 2003; **26**: 290–296

Measuring a combination of FPG and HbA1c was better than FPG alone in detecting diabetes but still lacks satisfactory diagnostic properties for impaired glucose tolerance according to this study.

The gold standard investigation is still the oral glucose tolerance test (OGTT) which may offer better sensitivity and specificity for development of the macrovascular and microvascular complications of diabetes. The burden of screening is, however, enormous so do we use FPG levels, an OGTT, determination of HbA1c, or close follow up with repeated determinations of FPG?

There may currently be no clear cut answers but some conclusions may be made.

- Persons should be targeted according to their risk of diabetes taking into consideration ethnic origin, obesity, and family history.
- A formal index should be developed and validated for that purpose.
- People at high risk of diabetes and cardiovascular complications should be closely followed even if fasting glucose is normal.
- Whether to use a screening tool which combines FPG values and HbA1c or something else may depend on the local population, as well as cost.
- Serious ongoing effort should be made in these patients to target lifestyle changes and identify risk factors.

PREVENTION

Prevention of diabetes
Heneghan C, Thompson M, Perera R
BMJ, 2006; **333**: 764–765

There are two strategies for preventing diabetes – lifestyle interventions and drugs.

Intensive support and ongoing training can prevent diabetes in those with impaired glucose tolerance as well as improve control of those already diagnosed. But less than intensive support begins to fail and effects are difficult to replicate in the real world.

Which brings us on to drugs.

Metformin and orlistat have all been shown to reduce the incidence of diabetes. Rosiglitazone and ramipril have also been investigated.

The authors advise caution regarding the DREAM research (*see above*) in that their study population was composed of people with impaired glucose tolerance rather than abnormal fasting glucose. A subtle point, but it is fasting glucose that we usually end up using in real life to screen for diabetes in the UK. There was also a query over the wisdom of using a combined end point of dia-

Clinical Issues

CARDIOVASCULAR

betes and death. Combining end points is done when risk reductions are likely to be similar, but this is not the case here and analysis should be performed separately.

It will not be clear whether rosiglitazone prevents diabetes until further analysis after a washout period.

The prevention of type 2 diabetes: general practitioner and practice nurse opinions
Williams R, Rapport F, Elwyn G et al.
Br J Gen Pract, 2004; **26**: 531–535

This was a qualitative study based on 21 practices in Wales. Opinions from focus groups of general practitioners and practice nurses were sought with regard to the role of primary care in the detection and management of people at risk of developing type 2 diabetes.

Primary care is likely to have a role in this large task. Indeed some were actively engaged in detection, management and follow-up of these individuals whereas others felt this was more the remit of other agencies in the area of health promotion and education.

The questionable validity of 'screening' was a factor and even those who had started case-finding had reservations about their resources to do the job well. Factors such as low motivation of patients to change their lifestyle were mentioned, as was perceived overmedicalisation of precursor conditions of impaired glucose tolerance and impaired fasting glycaemia.

Opinions were strongly held and suggest that if general practice is to absorb this role, given the current pressures on primary care, healthcare practitioners will need to be motivated and sufficiently well resourced.

MEDICATION

Efficacy of lipid lowering drug treatment for diabetic and non-diabetic patients: meta-analysis of randomised controlled trials
Costa J, Borges M, David C et al.
BMJ, 2006; **332**: 1115–1124

The risk of MI in patients with diabetes is as high whether nor not they have had an MI in the past and dyslipidaemia is a consistent finding in those with type 2 diabetes.

This meta-analysis of 12 studies found that lipid-lowering drugs are even more effective in preventing major coronary events in diabetics than in non-diabetics when the baseline risk of diabetes is factored in.

The paper supports the use of statins in secondary prevention but also for primary prevention of cardiovascular disease in diabetics. Target cholesterol thresholds remain to be clarified – particularly for primary prevention.

CARDIOVASCULAR

Diabetes and lipid lowering: where are we?
Reckless JPD
BMJ, 2006; **332**: 1103–1104

> NICE endorses use of statins in people with an absolute risk of 20% over 10 years as effective and cost-effective, particularly when using generics. This editorial clarifies the situation now that we are sure that statins cut cardiovascular risk in type 2 diabetes.
> - All patients with diabetes should be considered for, and most likely receive, a statin if their LDL cholesterol is ≥ 2 mmol/l
> - Less research is available about type 1 diabetes, but statins are indicated for those aged 40 years or over
> - The role of fibrates is not as clear. They will remain second line agents and fenofibrate beats gemfibrozil as the agent of choice

---

Metformin does not increase risk of lactic acidosis or increase lactate levels in type 2 diabetes. *Evidence-Based Medicine,* 2004; **9**: 111
The following article is presented
Risk of fatal and nonfatal lactic acidosis with metformin use in type 2 diabetes mellitus: systematic review and meta-analysis
Salpeter SR, Greyber E, Pasternak GA *et al.*
Arch Intern Med, 2003; **163**: 2594–2602

> This meta-analysis of 194 studies (126 RCTs and 68 cohort studies, $n = 56\,692$, mean age 57 years, 61% men) found that metformin is not associated with an increased risk of lactic acidosis or with an increase in lactate levels. Although its predecessor phenformin was removed from the market because of this side effect, this analysis did not find a single case associated with metformin directly. The original study suggests that this may be due to a different chemical structure to the original drug which inhibits hepatic gluconeogenesis without altering turnover of lactate or lactate oxidation.
>
> One point in the study is that although patients with absolute contraindications might have been excluded from the trials, we do know that metformin is still commonly prescribed to such apparently contraindicated patients.

Contraindications to the use of metformin
Jones GC, Macklin JP, Alexander WD
BMJ, 2003; **326**: 4–5

> This editorial confirms that no mortality has been accredited to metformin alone. As it has a short half-life and is excreted solely through the kidney, accumulation rarely occurs except in advanced renal failure. A trigger such as tissue hypoxia is usually required. This article proposes revised guidelines for its use including:
> - Stop if serum concentration of creatinine is higher than 150 μmol/l
> - Withdraw during periods of suspected tissue hypoxia (e.g. due to myocardial infarction, sepsis)
> - Withdraw two days before general anaesthesia and reinstate when renal function is stable
> - Withdraw after contrast medium containing iodine

CARDIOVASCULAR

With these provisos the authors promote the use of metformin to be as widespread as possible in type 2 diabetes.

Glycemic control continues to deteriorate after sulfonylureas are added to metformin among patients with type 2 diabetes

Cook MN, Girman CJ, Stein PP *et al.*
Diabetes Care, 2005; **28**: 995–1000

Adding sulfonylureas to metformin improves glycaemic control but it does nothing for the ongoing trend of glycaemic deterioraton. This can begin as early as 6 months after the end of monotherapy, and is probably due to a declining capacity to secrete insulin. This adds to support for earlier use of glitazones.

In another study, a direct comparison of monotherapy found pioglitazone to be superior to gliclazide in sustaining glycaemic control in type 2 diabetics over a 2nd year period (*Diabetes Care*, 2005; **28**: 544–550).

Effects of angiotensin converting enzyme inhibitors and angiotensin II receptor antagonists on mortality and renal outcomes in diabetic nephropathy: systematic review

Strippoli G, Craig M, Deeks J *et al.*
BMJ, 2004; **329**: 828

Many papers extol the virtues of early treatment with angiotensin converting enzyme (ACE) inhibitors or angiotensin II receptor blockers (ARBs). They find fewer cardiovascular deaths and less nephropathy and recommend early treatment. This systematic review of 43 trials looked at the effects of ACE inhibitors and ARBs on renal outcomes and all cause mortality in patients with diabetic nephropathy.

This article found the evidence for interchangeability between these drugs to be inconclusive and that ACE inhibitors should be used in preference. Although we know the two classes of drugs have equivalent effects on renal outcomes, the prevention of early death is only clear for ACE inhibitors as there has been a lack of adequate head to head trials.

Given the limits of the original data, commentary for this paper in *Evidence-Based Medicine* (2005; **10**: 77) concluded that the evidence only supports the use of ACE inhibitors in type 1 diabetes with nephropathy and the use of ACE inhibitors or ARBs in type 2 diabetes with nephropathy.

A *Drug and Therapeutics* review agreed that use of one of these medications is a quality target in microalbuminuria and while evidence is limited where there is no nephropathy, ACEs and ARBs are still a reasonable choice for hypertensive control in diabetics (*Drug Ther Bull*, 2005; **43**: 41–45).

A small Japanese study suggests that using both these medications in half doses may exploit different mechanisms to increase the renoprotective effect (*Am J Hypertens*, 2005; **18**: 13–17).

An intensive intervention reduced cardiovascular and microvascular events in type 2 diabetes and microalbuminuria. *Evidence-Based Medicine,* 2003; **8**: 142
The following article is presented
Multifactorial intervention and cardiovascular disease in patients with type 2 diabetes
Gaede P, Vedel P, Larsen N *et al.*
N Engl J Med, 2003; **348**: 383–393

> **Question: In patients with type 2 diabetes and microalbuminuria, is a targeted intensive multifactorial intervention more effective than conventional treatment?**
>
> This Danish study looked at 160 patients for nearly 8 years. They were equally divided into intensive or conventional treatment groups. Half received strict treatment goals with a stepwise implementation of behaviour modification (low fat diet, exercising three to five times a week, and smoking cessation) and medication that targeted hyperglycaemia, hypertension, dyslipidaemia, microalbuminuria, and secondary prevention of cardiovascular disease. All received an ACE inhibitor or angiotensin II-receptor antagonist as well as aspirin and vitamins. The other half received conventional treatment of risk factors from their GP according to national guidelines. Improvement in the intensive group for cardiovascular events and microvascular events was shown to reach 50%, illustrating the massive potential of multifactorial intensive interventions. The commentator draws attention to the need for three things:
> * systems that allow primary prevention
> * earlier detection
> * aggressive intervention
> The need for community specialists as well as good electronic management systems should be part of these new models of care.

Self monitoring

Blood glucose self-monitoring in non-insulin-treated type 2 diabetes: a qualitative study of patients' perspectives
Peel E, Parry O, Douglas M *et al.*
Br J Gen Pract, 2004; **54**: 183–188
and
Home blood glucose monitoring in type 2 diabetes
Reynolds RM, Strachan MWJ
BMJ, 2004; **329**: 754–755

> These articles highlight the controversy of home blood glucose monitoring in type 2 diabetics. Proponents argue that it empowers the patient to recognise their own patterns but there is evidence of an adverse effect on quality of life with more worry and distress the more the patients test. Glycaemic control has not been shown to be better than in those who monitor urine glucose. NICE only recommends the measure as part of integrated self-care and does not advocate routine

CARDIOVASCULAR

testing. Monitoring in special circumstances such as pregnancy, steroid treatment or intercurrent illness does seem useful however.

Patients feel that it heightens their awareness of the necessary lifestyle changes but it also amplifies a sense of failure and self-blame when control is not so good.

The role of home testing needs to be assessed further. More education and discussion with patients may help home blood glucose monitoring find its place in type 2 diabetes.

A Cochrane review in April 2005 failed to find enough studies of a sufficiently rigorous standard to allow a conclusion on the validity of self-monitoring of blood or urine glucose in non-insulin controlled diabetics.

Additional research from the Fremantle Diabetes Study found no significant differences in HbA1c in those who performed self-monitoring of blood glucose and those who did not. Although it may be useful if they eventually need insulin, it seems that home testing is not something we should be routinely encouraging (*Diabetes Care*, 2006; **29**: 1764–1770).

Further Research

- The DIAD Study – Detection of Ischaemia in Asymptomatic Diabetics – investigated type 2 diabetics who were asymptomatic for cardiovascular disease looking for signs such as diagnostic ECG changes or perfusion abnormalities. Their tests detected signs of coronary disease in 22% perhaps supporting a role for more intensive medication. *Diabetes Care*, 2004; **27**: 1954–1961.

- Inhaled insulin is faster acting than injectable insulins and has been shown to improve overall glycaemic control and HbA1c levels in type 2 diabetics during a 12 week trial in over 300 patients who were poorly controlled on tablets. In common with other insulin therapies, hypoglycemia and mild weight gain occurred. *Ann Intern Med,* 2005; **143**: 549–558.

- An 11-year prospective study of 28812 postmenopausal women has confirmed a link between coffee consumption and a reduced risk of diabetes. Women with the highest intake were 22% less likely to develop diabetes than those with the lowest. This was largely regardless of weight or age and was accounted for largely by intake of decaffeinated rather than regular coffee. We still don't know what the magic ingredient might be but it ain't caffeine. *Arch Intern Med,* 2006; **166**: 1311–1316.

CARDIOVASCULAR

ASTHMA

What we know already:

- About 300 million people worldwide have asthma and with increasing urbanisation and western lifestyles, a further 100 million cases are expected by 2025
- Asthma accounts for one in every 250 deaths worldwide. It accounts for 8% of self-reported poor health in 18–64 year olds and 18 million working days are lost annually to asthma
- Nearly half of all asthmatics feel limited in their daily life as a result of their condition, putting asthma above diabetes but below arthritis as a chronic health problem
- Up to 1.4 million asthmatics in the UK are thought to have suboptimal control
- Emerging evidence indicates that after years of increasing prevalence, the healthcare burden of asthma seems to be levelling off in the UK and falling in some countries
- Reasons are unclear and probably multifactorial, perhaps relating to improved use of inhaled corticosteroids and changes in the incidence of atopy
- Only about one-third of people attend asthma clinics for their annual review
- The START trial – Inhaled Steroid as Regular Therapy in Early Asthma – has demonstrated that early budesonide is effective and cost-effective in early asthma for all ages
- Leukotriene receptor antagonists have been found in systematic review to be less effective as a single agent than low doses of inhaled steroid
- Self-management plans are becoming the cornerstone of high quality care
- Specialist interventions such as nurse-led clinics targeted at schools and deprived areas can moderately improve uptake of review and symptom control but are expensive
- A greater focus on psychological aspects of illness should be a central part of any long-term therapeutic strategy

Guidelines

British guideline on the management of asthma. British Thoracic Society/Scottish Intercollegiate Guidelines Network. *Thorax*, 2003; **58**: 1–94. Online 2005 update at www.sign.ac.uk.

Recent Papers

Systematic review of prevalence of aspirin induced asthma and its implications for clinical practice
Jenkins C, Costello J, Hodge L
BMJ, 2004; **328**: 434–437

This review states that aspirin aggravates asthma in adults much more commonly than the 10% previously thought. Aspirin-induced asthma is a distinct syndrome characterised by the onset of asthma 30 minutes to 3 hours after the ingestion of aspirin in sensitive people.

The prevalence of aspirin-induced asthma was as high as 21% in adults and 5% in children when determined by oral provocation testing. When assessed by verbal history, it was much lower – adults 3%, children 2%.

Sensitive patients usually suffer cross-reactivity with other NSAIDs: ibuprofen, 98%, naproxen, 100%, and diclofenac, 93%. The incidence of cross-sensitivity to paracetamol among such patients was only 7%.

The authors recommend:
- packs of aspirin and NSAIDs should carry standardised warnings to asthmatics
- avoidance of aspirin and NSAIDs indefinitely in anyone who has had a reaction or has high risk features, i.e. severe asthma symptoms, nasal polyps, urticaria, or chronic rhinitis
- in those under 40 years, or those who have not used aspirin and NSAIDs recently without incident, only use if necessary and ensure the first dose is under medical supervision
- when there is uncertainty and clinical necessity, oral provocation testing should be performed

LONG-TERM MANAGEMENT

The addition of peak expiratory flow monitoring to symptom-based self management did not enhance outcome in children with asthma. *Evidence-Based Medicine,* 2005; **10**: 87
The following paper is reviewed
Peak flow monitoring for guided self-management in childhood asthma: a randomized controlled trial
Wensley D, Silverman M
Am J Respir Crit Care Med, 2004; **170**: 606–612

The addition of routine peak expiratory flow monitoring to symptom-based self management does not improve outcome over symptom-based self-management alone, according to this study in 90 children aged 7–14 years whose asthma was stable. (It is too tricky a process in the under sevens.)

Patient education must be developmentally appropriate. As children grow, their care changes from parent-centred to patient-centred. There may still be a role for peak flow in some children to help them perceive early exacerbations.

Targeted routine asthma care in general practice using telephone triage
Gruffydd-Jones K, Hollinghurst S, Ward S *et al.*
Br J Gen Pract, 2005; **56**: 918–923

This study looked at nearly 200 patients in South-East England over 12 months and found that a trained asthma nurse could successfully use telephone interviews to routinely follow up cases. The vast majority liked the system and costs were reduced by over one-third compared to usual face-to-face care, adding to previous studies which find a role for this type of intervention.

MEDICATION

Steroids

Doubling the dose of inhaled corticosteroid to prevent asthma exacerbations: randomised controlled trial
Harrison TW, Oborne J, Newton S
Lancet, 2004; **363**: 271–275

> This paper is one of several high quality trials that show that doubling the dose of inhaled corticosteroids fails to prevent asthma attacks. They gave asthmatics a steroid or placebo inhaler to use in a flare-up. Over 12 months, half reached for it. No difference in symptoms scores or the need for oral steroids was detected. Recommendations to double up on inhaled steroids are absent from the latest guidelines. Doses that are more than double are as yet uninvestigated.

Use of inhaled corticosteroids during pregnancy and risk of pregnancy induced hypertension: nested case-control study
Martel MJ, Rey E, Beauchesne MF, et al.
BMJ, 2005; **330**: 230

> Around 5% of women take drugs for asthma in pregnancy. This 10-year study of over 4500 pregnancies in asthmatics reassures us that there is no association between the use of inhaled steroids and pregnancy-induced hypertension or pre-eclampsia.
>
> Markers of poor asthma control and use of oral steroids were each associated with increased risks of these two conditions.

Combination therapy

Combined budesonide and formoterol for maintenance and relief provided better asthma control than budesonide for maintenance and terbutaline for relief.
Evidence-Based Medicine, 2006; **11**: 138
The following paper is reviewed
Budesonide/formoterol in a single inhaler for maintenance and relief in mild-to-moderate asthma: a randomized, double-blind trial
Rabe KF, Pizzichini E, Ställberg B et al.
Chest, 2006; **129**: 246–256

> Budesonide/formoterol in a single inhaler simplifies and improves asthma therapy for both maintenance and symptom relief beyond that of budesonide at a higher dose with terbutaline for relief. This forces patients to take extra doses of steroid when they need their reliever – something that often goes by the wayside in favour of extra rescue medication when symptoms worsen.
>
> The combination more than halved the risk of severe exacerbations, led to 90% fewer asthma-related hospitalisations and 77% fewer treatment days with oral steroids.
>
> It is not clear however which ingredient should receive the credit.

RESPIRATORY

The correlation between asthma control and health status: the GOAL study

Bateman ED, Bousquet J, Keech ML and the GOAL Investigators
Eur Respir J, 2007; **29**: 56–62

The GOAL Investigators Group – Gaining Optimal Asthma ControL – looked at patients with uncontrolled asthma. It previously showed that step-wise increase of a salmeterol/fluticasone inhaler achieved 'Total Control' of symptoms (defined as being symptom-free for at least 7 out of 8 weeks) in a greater proportion and at lower steroid doses than fluticasone alone. They conclude that the noble aim of 'Total Control' is achievable and was achieved here in 41% compared to 28% with fluticasone alone.

A further study made an assessment using the Asthma Quality of Life Questionnaire and demonstrated improved quality of life with the GOAL method to levels approaching normality. This improvement was even distinguishable between those with Total Control and those with otherwise high levels of control.

Addition of salmeterol to usual asthma pharmacotherapy may increase respiratory related deaths or life threatening experiences. *Evidence-Based Medicine,* 2006; **11**: 139

The following paper is reviewed

The Salmeterol Multicenter Asthma Research Trial: a comparison of usual pharmacotherapy for asthma or usual pharmacotherapy plus salmeterol

Nelson HS, Weiss ST, Bleecker ER *et al.*
Chest, 2006; **129**: 15–26

The SMART study used more than 26 000 asthma patients in over 6000 sites in the US and sent a few alarm bells ringing when it had to be stopped early. The addition of salmeterol to usual asthma therapy (including steroids) was associated with an increase in asthma-related and respiratory death – an effect which may be more pronounced in African–Americans. Caution is advised when using long acting beta-2 agonists while research continues.

Effect of long-acting β-agonists on severe asthma exacerbations and asthma-related deaths

Salpeter SR, Buckley NS, Ormiston TM *et al.*
Ann Intern Med, 2006; **144**: 904–912

Results from a meta-analysis involving nearly 20 000 people from 19 trials have shown that long-acting beta-2 agonists may be responsible for up to 80% of the 5000 asthma-related deaths in the US annually.

Compared to placebo, both salmeterol and formoterol increased risk of asthma hospitalisations to similar degrees, alongside their well-documented ability to relieve asthma symptoms. Effects were similar for children and adults alike.

Regular use may increase bronchial hyperactivity. Symptoms may worsen without warning and impaired response to the usual beta agonist's use may cause the trouble.

Although death from asthma is rare, users of long-acting beta agonists were 3.5 times more likely to die from asthma and 2.5 times more likely to be hospitalised.

Further Research

Children

- Stressful life events in children aged 6–13 years with chronic asthma lead to both acute and delayed exacerbations. Symptoms increased nearly five-fold within 2 days of a severely negative life event such as illness, death, separation and divorce. There was also almost twice the rate of expected exacerbations around 6 weeks later. Heightened sensitivity to this is needed by health professionals. *Thorax*, 2004; **59**: 1046–1051.

- A cohort of 199 children followed until age 32–42, showed that half do not outgrow asthma. Complete remission was defined as no symptoms, no medication, normal lung function and no bronchial hyperresponsiveness. Only 22% achieved this. A further 30% reached clinical remission (no symptoms). *Thorax*, 2004; **59**: 925–929.

- Early steroid treatment helps asthma. This study also quantified that in children under 11 years, 3-year growth was reduced in the budesonide group by an average of 1.34 cm. *Lancet*, 2003; **361**: 1071–1076.

- Although inhaled steroids reduce the burden of asthma symptoms they do not have a disease-modifying effect that persists after discontinuation. Those at high risk of persistent asthma were randomised to fluticasone or placebo in this study and growth was slowed only during use of the steroid. *N Engl J Med,* 2006; **354**: 1985–1997

Other

- Smokers display steroid insensitivity. Prednisolone improves asthma control in never-smokers, but not in smokers (*Am J Respir Crit Care Med,* 2003; **168**: 1308–1311). Smokers have six times as many exacerbations and barely respond to our most proven weapon. *Thorax,* 2005; **60**: 282–287.

- A 20-year longitudinal study of over 3000 patients with active asthma found they were about 12 times more likely to develop COPD than nonasthmatics, even after controlling for smoking. The authors suggest these previously distinct entities may share common pathology. *Chest*, 2004; **126**: 59–65.

CHRONIC OBSTRUCTIVE PULMONARY DISEASE

What we know already:

- COPD is our fourth most common cause of death and is largely a disease of vulnerable smokers
- COPD is diagnosed if the patient has an FEV_1 of less than 70% of predicted normal and an FEV_1/FVC ratio of less than 70% with less than 15% reversibility
- Annual NHS costs of COPD in the UK have been estimated at around one billion pounds
- Admission for acute exacerbations have increased by 50% in the last decade and sit at around 90 000 admissions per year
- An average stay of 11 days means one million bed days a year in the UK
- Spirometry improves detection rates of COPD and its use is promoted in the new contract
- Only smoking cessation and oxygen alter the natural history of the disease
- Pulmonary rehabilitation is effective in the short to medium term in improving exercise tolerance, smoking cessation, symptoms and quality of life
- Suitable rehabilitation programmes are by no means universally available so physicians continue to prescribe expensive pharmacotherapy that is considerably less effective for a disease that by definition is resistant to drug treatment
- Beta agonist inhalers – both short and long acting and particularly in combination with a steroid – modestly improve lung function and symptoms
- Salmeterol can give symptomatic and physiological improvements in severe COPD despite 'non-reversibility' on spirometry
- There are no high quality data to support the use of theophylline or aminophylline to treat exacerbations of COPD for either symptoms or lung function

Guidelines

National clinical guideline on management of chronic obstructive pulmonary disease in adults in primary and secondary care. National Collaborating Centre for Chronic Conditions for NICE. *Thorax*, 2004; **59**(suppl 1): 1–232.

Global strategy for the diagnosis, management, and prevention of chronic obstructive pulmonary disease. GOLD – Global Initiative for Chronic Obstructive Lung Disease. World Health Organization, November 2006. These guidelines now refer to COPD as 'preventable and treatable' in order to present a positive outlook and stimulate effective programmes.

Recent Papers

Guidelines for chronic obstructive pulmonary disease
MacNee W
BMJ, 2004; **329:** 361–363

This article examines the 2004 NICE guidelines as an update to the 1997 British Thoracic Society guidelines.

Diagnosis of COPD is to be based on a good history with confirmation of airflow limitation by spirometry. Controversially and unlike other guidelines, no recommendation is made to measure the post-bronchodilator change in spirometry to assist in identifying reversibility and it uses symptoms to guide treatment rather than a percentage drop in FEV_1. Evidence-based use of medication is extensively reviewed and a role given to mucolytics. The role of pulmonary rehabilitation is firmly established and advocated, as are recommendations for the availability of ambulatory oxygen.

Developing COPD: a 25 year follow up study of the general population
Løkke A, Lange P, Scharling H *et al.*
Thorax, 2006; **61**: 935–939

This extensive study analysed information and lung function tests from over 8000 men and women aged over 30 years to determine the 25-year absolute risk of developing COPD in the general population.

- The percentage of men with normal lung function ranged from 96% of never smokers to 59% of continuous smokers.
- They estimate that COPD goes undiagnosed in 80% of those with the condition. More than one-third of those with COPD were still smoking.
- Sufferers were more likely to be older, manual workers, male and more socio-economically deprived.
- The 25-year incidence of moderate and severe COPD was 20.7% and 3.6%, respectively.
- Deaths from COPD constituted 3.7% of all deaths and, as expected, there were almost no COPD deaths during the first 10 years of follow up.
- COPD is becoming as common in women as in men. Although women may be slightly more susceptible to tobacco, men smoke more to make up for this difference.
- Absolute risk is an easier concept to convey to patients and at around 25% the absolute risk of developing COPD among continuous smokers is larger than previously estimated.

RESPIRATORY

DETECTION

A randomized controlled trial on office spirometry in asthma and COPD in standard general practice
Lusuardi M, De Benedetto F, Paggiaro P et al.
Chest, 2006; **129**: 844–852

The charmingly named SPACE program – Spirometry in Asthma and COPD: a Comparative Evaluation – was a 9 month prospective Italian study that failed to demonstrate that spirometry can help GPs identify asthma and COPD earlier.

Evaluation of possible cases was made with and without spirometry by 570 trained GPs. Specialists were blinded while checking the diagnoses but found no improvement in accuracy where spirometry had been used.

High initial ratings by the GPs in terms of feasibility and usefulness tailed off dramatically and one-quarter failed to respond to the study by the end.

An accompanying editorial suggests the method is best offered only to smokers with dyspnoea on exertion. Clearly, work is needed on the model of clinical back-up that best supports the role of spirometry in primary care.

Effect of primary care spirometry on the diagnosis and management of COPD
Walker PP, Mitchell P, Diamantea F et al.
Eur Respir J, 2006; **28**: 945–952

This study offered an open access service to a primary care area in the UK between 1999 and 2003 in which over 1500 patients were referred for spirometry and reversibility testing.
- 53% had pre-bronchodilator airflow obstruction.
- 19% of subjects responded fully to reversibility testing.
- Half of those in whom obstruction persisted received a diagnosis of COPD.
- COPD was significantly undertreated prior to spirometry.
- Testing led to considerable increases in prescribing of anti-cholinergics, beta agonists and inhaled steroids.

This well-organised service is a good model of how spirometry can be useful in uncovering COPD, improving treatment and avoiding misdiagnosis by using reversibility testing.

Unrecognised heart failure in elderly patients with stable chronic obstructive pulmonary disease
Rutten FH, Cramer MJ, Grobbee DE et al.
Eur Heart J, 2005; **26**: 1887–1894

A Dutch study of over 400 patients with a diagnosis of COPD but without a diagnosis of heart failure underwent an extensive diagnostic work-up. They found that 20% had previously unrecognised heart failure. Of these half had systolic failure, half had 'isolated' diastolic failure and none had right-sided heart failure.

They conclude that unrecognised heart failure is common in elderly patients with stable COPD. Detection must be improved to allow access to proven therapies.

MANAGEMENT

Evaluating the effectiveness of combination therapy to prevent COPD exacerbations: the value of NNT analysis
Halpin DM
Int J Clin Pract, 2005; **59**: 1187–1194

> Prevention of exacerbations of COPD has the potential to prevent hospital admissions and deaths while improving quality of life and reducing fear over these dreaded episodes. This analysis indicates that use of a budesonide/formoterol combination inhaler (instead of a formoterol-only inhaler) means that the NNT needed to prevent one such exacerbation is only 2. Given the enormous healthcare costs of COPD admissions, this is an appealing finding.

Inhaled corticosteroids slow the progression of airflow limitation in COPD.
Evidence-Based Medicine, 2004; **9**: 75
The following paper is reviewed
Inhaled corticosteroids reduce the progression of airflow limitation in chronic obstructive pulmonary disease: a meta-analysis
Sutherland ER, Allmers H, Ayas NT *et al.*
Thorax, 2003; **58**: 937–941

> Inhaled corticosteroid therapy is a controversial area. This is not much helped by the fact that two meta-analyses attempting to clarify things reviewed almost the same data and turned out differently. They came to almost the same conclusion but this is the one that reached statistical significance. This meta-analysis did find that giving inhaled corticosteroids for more than 2 years reduces the progression of airflow limitation. The results were small at a benefit of only 7.7 ml/year of FEV_1 gained. More severe patients benefited more. The commentator argues that this benefit may be as close to irreversibility as we get and that we should focus our efforts on something that really does work like smoking cessation as well as making sure we do not mistake asthma for COPD.

LONG-TERM CARE

Hospital at home for patients with acute exacerbations of chronic obstructive pulmonary disease: systematic review of evidence
Ram FSF, Wedzicha JA, Wright J *et al.*
BMJ, 2004; **329**: 315

> This was a systematic review of seven trials looking at the recent innovation of hospital at home. In terms of end-points of re-admission and death, it was found to be as safe as hospital care. Cost analysis suggests savings can be made particularly as many patients have extended hospital stays due to social circumstances rather than just severity of symptoms.
>
> The review does not claim that it is suitable for all – only one in four of the COPD patients presenting to hospital could be managed at home with the support of a respiratory nurse. Some were anxious and refused to take part. There were difficulties in analysing the value of different interventions as they were not

RESPIRATORY

uniform between the trials but as the popularity of the initiative grows and finds its place, the optimal level of support should be identifiable.

Oxygen treatment at home
Gibson GJ
BMJ, 2006; **332**: 191–192

Long-term oxygen for hypoxaemic COPD improves survival. This paper refers to the February 2006 changes in the supplying of oxygen to patients in England and Wales.

Although GPs can still prescribe oxygen, this is likely to be more for emergency and palliative care purposes.

More detailed assessment of new candidates for oxygen at home and ambulatory oxygen will be coordinated by hospital respiratory and paediatric services, in liaison with companies that service regional NHS contracts.

Those suitable for ambulatory oxygen are usually those well-motivated patients who desaturate on exertion and demonstrate improvement when breathing oxygen during exercise – estimated as half of those currently receiving long-term oxygen therapy on the NHS.

The intention is for the changes to be cost-neutral, with the costs of the increased staffing required for these more detailed evaluations hopefully offset by savings in inappropriate prescribing. It will be tricky, however, to get those who have had oxygen inappropriately prescribed to understand that shortage of breath does not necessarily mean shortage of oxygen, but this rationalisation should provide an improved service. Children, for example, need frequent reassessments as they grow and many will probably benefit from ambulatory oxygen.

GP discussion of prognosis with patients with severe chronic obstructive pulmonary disease: a qualitative study
Halliwell J, Mulcahy P, Buetow S *et al.*
Br J Gen Pract, 2004; **54**: 904–908

Health professionals do not discuss prognosis with COPD patients as openly as with cancer patients. This New Zealand study interviewed 15 GPs and five respiratory consultants and identified seven areas to focus on in order to overcome this.

The areas were: identifying and using opportunities presented to discuss prognosis, discussing prognosis early, being respectful and caring, awareness of the implications of diagnosis, use of uncertainty to facilitate discussion, building of the doctor–patient relationship, and working as a team.

RESPIRATORY INFECTION AND ANTIBIOTICS

What we know already:

- Sore throat and otitis media are two of the commonest reasons for children to visit doctors
- Clinical examination is unreliable for differentiating between viral and bacterial infection
- Antibiotics have not been shown to be useful routinely in infections such as pharyngitis, otitis media, rhinitis and sinusitis.
- Marginal benefits on long-term complications may not be translated into cost-effectiveness
- Simple prediction tools using clinical measures such as temperature, presence of exudates, enlarged cervical lymph nodes and absence of cough are imperfect but can help predict beta haemolytic streptococcal pharyngitis in combination with knowledge of local prevalence
- Expected recovery from cough is consistently overestimated by clinicians. At 2 weeks, one in four is not recovered and one in eight may have a complication – such as rash or painful ears. Informing parents will align expectations
- GPs may perceive more pressure to prescribe than actually exists and reducing prescribing prevents future requests for consultation
- Antibiotic prescribing has been reducing for the last 10 years due to considerable reductions in the burden of disease rather than more targeted prescribing
- A fall of 50% in the prescribing of antibiotics to children by GPs has not led to an increase in hospital admissions for peritonsillar abscess or rheumatic fever
- The pace and development of new antibiotics has not kept up with growth in antibiotic resistance and we may be approaching the end of the antibiotic era

Guidance

UK Antimicrobial resistance strategy and action plan. *Dept of Health, 2000.*
This report describes how surveillance, prudent use of antimicrobials and infection control are the key elements to controlling resistance and maintaining the effectiveness of antibiotics.

Recent Papers

SYMPTOMATIC TREATMENT

Effect of dextromethorphan, diphenhydramine, and placebo on nocturnal cough and sleep quality for coughing children and their parents
Paul IM, Yoder KE, Crowell KR *et al.*
Pediatrics, 2004; **114**: e85–e90

Cough syrup medicated with dextromorphan or diphenhydramine is no better than sugar water in suppressing night-time cough in children. They are very commonly used but this small study in 100 children compared both these cough medicines with sugar syrup alone. The sleep of both parents and children improved equally on all three approaches, showing the natural self-limiting course of the illness and/or the power of placebo.

The authors advise clinicians to consider the potential for adverse effects (dextromorphan is a drug of abuse) and the costs of the drugs before recommending them to families.

Mechanisms of the placebo effect of sweet cough syrups
Eccles R
Respir Physiol Neurobiol, 2006; **152**: 340–348

Misunderstandings that cough linctuses can shorten or 'cure' a respiratory illness persist. This research on over-the-counter cough medicines proposes that their main mode of action is through their pleasing sweet taste and the placebo effect. All but two of 60 medicines examined were sweetened and ingredients such as lemon and citric acid may promote reflex salivation as well as secretion of airway mucus.

ANTIBIOTIC RESISTANCE

Old drugs for new bugs
Pitlik S
BMJ, 2003; **326**: 235–236

A re-emergence of susceptibility to older semi-retired antibiotics may give us another weapon in our antibacterial strategy.

Examples are use of co-trimoxazole for MRSA and chloramphenicol to treat typhoid fever that has become increasingly resistant to quinolones.

Whether these 'forgotten' drugs will be effective on a large enough scale remains to be seen. It is possible that sensitivity of the bacteria to these antibiotics may 'recover' rapidly by reactivation of resistance-encoding genes. *In vitro* surveillance will inform us whether cycling of antibiotics could be an effective policy.

Antibiotics, resistance, and clinical outcomes
Woodhead M, Fleming D, Wise R
BMJ, 2004; **328**: 1270–1271

Some research shows that even when evidence of resistance to an antibiotic in the general population seems to be weak, exposure to antibiotics can be strongly related to resistance within the same individual. For example, resistance of gram-negative bacilli to trimethoprim occurs more in those who have been prescribed it.

Group level data may therefore be seriously misleading and these new analyses of individual data appear to be essential.

Delayed prescriptions
Arroll B, Kenealy T, Goodyear-Smith F *et al.*
BMJ, 2003; **327**: 1361–1362

This editorial provides a nice summary of its subject matter. Prescriptions written with the proviso that they are not used immediately have been shown to be very useful in curbing our overprescriptive tendencies. Early studies showed that only around 30% of delayed prescriptions were cashed in after 3 days with no adverse effects. When not given prescriptions for antibiotics, 13% returned for them and got them in the end.

A summary of the few controlled trials that have been done draws these conclusions:

- patients seem willing to tolerate a fair level of symptoms in order to avoid antibiotics
- it seems they are even keener to avoid their children having antibiotics for otitis media where symptoms levels were higher
- reductions in prescribing are greater when the patient is made to return to the surgery to collect the prescription
- more use of delayed prescriptions may reduce repeat visits
- some GPs worry it makes them look incompetent
- doctors like the ability to include the patient in the decision, as well as reductions in costs and side effects
- patients are not concerned about antibiotic resistance
- systems for collecting the prescriptions may need to be well-organised within practices
- qualitative research suggests that once their patients were weaned off the expectation of antibiotics, the need for delayed prescriptions became redundant. This may be a useful intermediate step rather than going 'cold turkey'

Do delayed prescriptions reduce antibiotic use in respiratory tract infections? A systematic review
Arroll B, Kenealy T, Kerse N
Br J Gen Pract, 2003; **53**: 871–877

This systematic review found five controlled trials on the subject. Antibiotic usage was lowered by 44% when a delayed prescription was given for the common cold and by 75% for otitis media.

Duration of the delay for prescriptions ranged widely up to 1 week, but the consistency of the studies show it is an effective means of reducing antibiotic usage for acute respiratory infections.

This paper is also reviewed in *Evidence-Based Medicine* (2004; **9**: 108). The review praises the fact that respiratory diagnoses have been looked at separately from conditions such as UTI where there may be higher expectations of treatment. Delayed prescribing is described as a useful additional tool in the consultation which may help bridge the expectation gap. It may help to avoid 'uncomfortable resolu-

RESPIRATORY

tions' to the consultation although the barrier to receiving the drugs could come over as 'untrusting and paternalistic'.

Delayed prescribing of antibiotics for upper respiratory tract infection
Little P
BMJ, 2005; **331**: 301–302

Widespread adoption of delayed prescribing since 1997 may explain the reduction in the proportion of prescriptions delivered to the pharmacist in recent years.

Asking the patient to return for the prescription means few ending up taking antibiotics but given the higher reconsultation rates, this is not clearly preferable. This editorial explains that we cannot turn our back on antibiotics for uncomplicated respiratory infections. After all, there are expectations and occasionally complications. Delayed prescriptions are a compromise that seem to re-educate patients gently. Don't leave it any longer than 72 hours to recheck an otitis media for the need for antibiotics and you should be fine.

SORE THROAT

Why do general practitioners prescribe antibiotics for sore throat? Grounded theory interview study
Kumar S, Little P, Britten N
BMJ, 2003; **326**: 138–141

This rather 'touchy-feely' interview analysis of 40 GPs comes in at a different angle. Here the general practitioners seem to take the credit for reductions in prescribing patterns.

All the doctors agreed that antibiotics are mostly unnecessary. They identified external pressures, such as research, local advice and published reports, that had influenced them to reduce antibiotic prescribing.

They were more likely to prescribe for sicker and more deprived patients and justified this because of concerns about complications. They all felt their decision-making was 'rational and systematic, informed by personal clinical experience and research evidence and influenced by advice from policy makers and local microbiologists'. The doctors were mostly comfortable with their decisions and happy they were not prescribing just to maintain the doctor–patient relationship.

The paper describes at length anecdotes which illustrate the processes underlying prescribing practices, behaviours, beliefs and decision-making in sore throat. It reads as an interesting diary of feelings about sore throat, although the highly conversational style makes some of it a bit hard to swallow.

The conclusion that we as 'general practitioners have reduced prescribing for sore throat in response to research and policy initiatives' could be true but given the content of the paper it is at the very least a leap of faith.

Penicillin for acute sore throat in children: randomised, double blind trial
Zwart S, Rovers MM, de Melker RA et al.
BMJ, 2003; **327**: 1324

The authors have previously reported superiority of penicillin for 7 days over 3 days or placebo in adults with sore throat and group A streptococcus. Turning to children, this important paper assessed effectiveness of penicillin for 3 or 7 days compared with placebo. Some 156 children, mean age 10 years, with sore throat and at least two of the four Centor criteria (history of fever, absence of cough, swollen cervical lymph nodes, and tonsillar exudate) were recruited. Seriously ill children were excluded.

Penicillin treatment for 3 or 7 days did not abbreviate symptoms of sore throat more than placebo. This was true in the total group and the 96 with group A streptococci. The authors point to the likelihood of a higher carrier rate of streptococcus which could limit the value of throat swabs in this group.

Treatment did not affect school attendance or recurrences of sore throat.

Where group A streptococcus was identified, 3 days of penicillin actually lengthened the symptoms by about a day. The authors blame a reduction in natural immune response without a successful eradication.

Seven days' treatment was twice as effective as 3 days or placebo at eradicating streptococci, however.

Complications were principally 'imminent quinsy' (rather than the true major complication of quinsy) and there were no other major complications.

They conclude that nearly all Western children with sore throat can be treated safely without penicillin and the few sequelae that do arise can be treated successfully when they occur.

A commentary on the paper by Little in the same issue of the *BMJ* concludes that these more unwell children (two Centor criteria) do not benefit from antibiotics. It questions the validity of the Centor criteria, which are developed to predict streptococcal infection when asymptomatic carriage rates are high. There is uncertainty over how many of the criteria to use and whether they actually predict potential benefit from treatment in some subgroups. This study showed that seven children with two Centor criteria need to be treated to prevent one worsening illness. It could be a good case for delayed prescriptions, which have been shown not to result in complications in streptococcal pharyngitis.

COUGH

Information leaflet and antibiotic prescribing strategies for acute lower respiratory tract infection. A randomized controlled trial
Little P, Rumsby K, Kelly J et al.
JAMA, 2005; **293**: 3029–3035

This UK study included over 800 adults and children with cough and at least one other symptom referable to the lower respiratory tract (coloured sputum, chest pain, dyspnoea, or wheezing). Asthma and COPD were excluded. The authors found:

RESPIRATORY

- antibiotics provided little or no benefit for patients with cough and lower respiratory tract symptoms, including fever and green sputum
- cough lasted about 3 weeks in most patients regardless of treatment method, and for at least a month in 25%
- providing a verbal explanation about the expected course is required for patient satisfaction
- the duration of 'moderately bad' symptoms was shorter in the immediate antibiotic group, but only by one day
- elderly patients were less likely to benefit from antibiotics
- results for vulnerable subgroups and those with green sputum were no more convincing

Three day versus five day treatment with amoxicillin for non-severe pneumonia in young children: a multicentre randomised controlled trial
ISCAP Study Group
BMJ, 2004; **328**: 791

This trial from India recruited over 2000 children under 5 years. Participants had cough, rapid respiration or difficulty in breathing. Asthmatics were excluded. It found the two approaches in the title equally effective with cure rates at 90%. Adherence to the treatment was 94% for the 3 day course and 85% for the 5 day course. Rates of relapse were similar in both groups. Respiratory syncitial virus was isolated in 23% and associated with failure of antibiotics. For non-severe community-acquired pneumonia in the community, 3 days of antibiotics were as effective as 5 days but cheaper and with greater adherence to treatment.

Effectiveness of discontinuing antibiotic treatment after three days versus eight days in mild to moderate–severe community acquired pneumonia: randomised, double blind study
el Moussaoui R, de Borgie CA, van den Broek P et al.
BMJ, 2006; **332**: 1355

This study looked at patients with mild to moderate cases of community-acquired pneumonia who were admitted to hospital for intravenous amoxicillin. It found that stopping antibiotics after 3 days was no worse than switching to orals to complete a traditional course of treatment lasting 7–10 days.

Reducing lengths of prescriptions are likely to benefit antibiotic resistance as total consumption corresponds well to resistance rates of pathogens.

Patients needed to show substantial improvement after 3 days to be considered for the trial.

Community acquired pneumonia in primary care
Goossens H, Little P
BMJ, 2006; **332**: 1045–1046

This editorial highlights the lack of evidence which could help us target antibiotics towards high risk patients.

There is a lack of adequately powered studies giving us good prediction rules for adverse outcomes in community-acquired pneumonia. Doctors still use their own arbitrary criteria and seldom have the advantage of a chest X-ray or microbiology. Times may change. Rapid nucleic acid detection assays and amplification techniques are showing promise as diagnostic tools in LRTI and molecular diagnostics is expected to boom in the next decade. When we get rapid answers at an affordable price we will no longer have to rely on nineteenth century methods and can hope to be able to combat resistance and preserve our remaining antibiotics.

Whooping cough in school age children with persistent cough: prospective cohort study in primary care
Harnden APR, Bruggemann AB, Mayon-White R et al.
BMJ, 2006; **333**: 174–177
and
Whooping cough in general practice
Butler C, Francis N, Dinant G
BMJ, 2006; **333**: 159–160

This article and accompanying editorial describes the underdiagnosis of *Bordetella* infection in school-age children of 5–16 years.

Precisely diagnosing the cause of persistent cough is difficult for GPs. Children often end up with empirical prescriptions for asthma inhalers or getting an unneeded chest X-ray.

GPs rarely diagnose or consider pertussis in these children, but in this cohort of 172 children in the UK who had a persistent cough lasting more than 2 weeks (and who consented to a blood test for serology and kept a cough diary), 37% had evidence of a recent *Bordetella* pertussis infection even though 85% of these had been fully immunised as children. Cough persisted for a median of 16 weeks.

Doctors do now recognise that acute cough persists longer than previously thought, irrespective of treatment, and ideally would be able to provide a confident diagnosis.

Unfortunately, laboratory testing is currently not considered very practical nor clinically important as there is little evidence that prescribing erythromycin reduces symptoms or prevents transmission.

GPs will need to think about this diagnosis even in immunised children and stop thinking of it just as a condition of very young children who whoop. New non-invasive salivary tests may help.

Now that we have a pre-school booster for pertussis, the reservoir of infection may reduce but perhaps we also need a booster in adolescents, as they have in the US.

Prednisolone versus dexamethasone in croup: a randomised equivalence trial
Sparrow A, Geelhoed G
Arch Dis Childhood, 2006; **91**: 580–583

Oral dexamethasone is used to treat croup but sometimes doctors substitute prednisolone. This Australian study of 133 children with an average age of 37 months compared single doses of equivalent potency in children with mild to moderate croup and suggests that this is not a legitimate thing to do.

Some 29% of the prednisolone group needed further medical care compared to

RESPIRATORY

just 7% of the dexamethasone group, probably due to its longer half-life. More doses of prednisolone may be needed if using this drug.

RELATED INFECTIONS

Sinusitis

POEM: Antibiotics are no better than placebo for symptoms of sinusitis. *BMJ,* 2003; **327**: 8 Nov
This is based on the following article
Effect of amoxicillin-clavulanate in clinically diagnosed acute rhinosinusitis. A placebo-controlled, double-blind, randomized trial in general practice
Bucher HC, Tshudi P, Young J *et al.*
Arch Intern Med, 2003; **163**: 1793–1798

This was a randomised, placebo-controlled, double-blind trial with 252 adults from 24 general practices. Recruits had a history of purulent nasal discharge and maxillary or frontal pain for at least 2 days. All had pus documented on rhinoscopy. Symptomatic treatments were used alongside co-amoxiclav or placebo. Cure rates at 1 week (30%) and 2 weeks (75%) were similar in both groups.

The antibiotics failed to quicken relief of symptoms of rhinosinusitis but did increase adverse effects.

Rhinitis

Are antibiotics effective for acute purulent rhinitis? Systematic review and meta-analysis of placebo controlled randomised trials
Arroll B, Kenealy T
BMJ, 2006; **333**: 279

Some GPs prescribe for a purulent nasal discharge – a familiar feature of a common cold. This review showed that although a small benefit is possible, the number needed to treat overlapped the number needed to harm – usually in terms of gastrointestinal effects. As most patients get better anyway antibiotics should not be first line treatment.

Conjunctivitis

Antibiotics for upper respiratory tract infections and conjunctivitis in primary care
Rietveld RP, Bindels PJE, ter Riet G
BMJ, 2006; **333**: 311–312

In Western countries, withholding antibiotics for minor complaints such as otitis media, rhinitis, conjunctivitis and sore throat can be considered harmless, because complications such as rheumatic fever, mastoiditis and quinsy have become rare and are not associated with the placebo groups in clinical trials.

RESPIRATORY

The downside of side-effects, antibiotic resistance and a loyal following of future consultations for trivia make the benefits small and often absent. Delayed prescriptions are a good way of reducing the number of prescriptions in those who cannot contain themselves when asked to go away empty handed.

Topical chloramphenicol was not effective in children with acute infective conjunctivitis. *Evidence-Based Medicine,* 2006; **11**: 18
The following paper is reviewed
Chloramphenicol treatment for acute infective conjunctivitis in children in primary care: a randomised double-blind placebo-controlled trial
Rose PW, Harnden A, Brueggemann AB *et al.*
Lancet, 2005; **366**: 37–43

This study of 326 children in 12 primary care practices in Oxfordshire found that whether or not chloramphenicol drops or placebo drops were used, there was no difference in cure rates at 7 days for conjunctivitis. This is especially important as the study was done in primary care, unlike the specialist clinics that produced studies that did show benefit. Perhaps disease in this group was milder but more relevant to the sort of patients seen by GPs. Although a self-limiting disease, pressure often comes from nurseries that prevent children with red eyes from attending.

A randomised controlled trial of management strategies for acute infective conjunctivitis in general practice
Everitt HA, Little PS, Smith PWF
BMJ, 2006; **333**: 321

A study of over 300 adults and children with infective conjunctivitis were treated with immediate chloramphenicol, no antibiotics or delayed treatment. They found delayed prescribing to be a cost-effective strategy as it reduced antibiotic use (by around half compared to immediate antibiotics) and reduces medicalisation (as fewer intended to consult for the same thing in the future). Duration and severity of symptoms were reduced to a similar degree as in the immediate group and 30% of those who were allotted to the 'no antibiotics' group came back later and got them anyway.

It might be right to prescribe when early symptoms are severe and when social issues such as day care for children are highlighted, but chloramphenicol is now available over the counter in the UK so primary care strategies may be sidelined.

Otitis

Wait-and-see prescription for the treatment of acute otitis media: a randomized controlled trial
Spiro DM, Tay K, Arnold DH *et al.*
JAMA, 2006; **296**: 1235–1241

Delayed prescriptions may also take off in the US. Children with otitis media had similar short and medium term outcomes whether or not they were given antibiotics immediately or with a delayed prescription. Use of antibiotics reduced from

RESPIRATORY

87% to 37% with no differences in ear pain, fever or use of analgesics. More parents said they would do without next time.

Nonsevere acute otitis media: a clinical trial comparing outcomes of watchful waiting versus immediate antibiotic treatment
McCormick DP, Chonmaitree T, Pittman C
Pediatrics, 2005; **115**: 1455–1465

This article tries to interest US community physicians in some watchful waiting for otitis media. Some 223 children were randomised to antibiotics or watchful waiting for non-severe otitis media. The groups were similar in terms of satisfaction, physician contacts and days off school, but antibiotics came out three times more expensive.

For a successful watchful waiting strategy, a measure of severity is needed (a scoring system in this case), parent education, management of symptoms and good access to follow up. The antibiotic group did have fewer treatment failures and improved symptomatic relief but also had more adverse events and resistant bacteria in the nasopharynx at day 12.

THE WHEEZY CHILD

Commonly used pharmacological treatments for bronchiolitis in children do not seem to be effective. *Evidence-Based Medicine,* 2004; **9**: 141
The following paper is reviewed
Pharmacologic treatment of bronchiolitis in infants and children: a systematic review
King VJ, Viswanathan M, Bordley WC *et al.*
Arch Pediatr Adolesc Med, 2004; **158**: 127–137

In children with bronchiolitis, little consensus exists about optimal management strategies although medicines such as bronchodilators and corticosteroids are commonly used. This systematic review set out to look at the effectiveness of commonly used treatments for bronchiolitis in infants and children and reviewed 44 studies of the most common interventions – epinephrine, β-2-agonist bronchodilators, corticosteroids and ribavirin.

The only positive effects that seemed to be shown were possibly a temporary relief of symptoms immediately after a bronchodilator nebuliser. It is postulated that these short-term benefits might improve feeding and reduce restlessness and therefore be appealing but results are inconsistent at best. Inhaled budesonide even seemed to prolong symptoms. There was generally an impressive absence of good quality evidence to support a routine role for any of these drugs in bronchiolitis. No convincing effects on hospital admissions or length of stay were illustrated.

A sufficiently large, well-designed pragmatic trial of the commonly used interventions for bronchiolitis is called for.

Corticosteroids do not reduce hospital length of stay or respiratory distress in infantile acute viral bronchiolitis. *Evidence-Based Medicine,* 2005; **10**: 20
The following review is presented
Glucocorticoids for acute viral bronchiolitis in infants and young children
Patel H, Platt R, Lozano JM *et al.*
***Cochrane Database Syst Rev,* 2004**

A Cochrane review of 13 RCTs in infants and young children with acute viral bronchiolitis proclaimed that systemic corticosteroids are no better than placebo for respiratory distress or shortening hospital stays. Neither is any drug, according to Cochrane reviews. Most infants are only admitted to hospital due to inability to predict which children will have apnoea or respiratory failure.

Further Research

- Meta-analysis suggests that exposure to at least one course of antibiotics in the first year of life may predispose to asthma later in childhood with more courses possibly increasing the risk. More work is needed to verify this. *Chest*, 2006; **129**: 610–618.

- Human metapneumovirus (hMPV) first isolated in 2001 is an important new virus particularly in young children. Over a 25 year period, 20% of children, mean age 12 months, with a lower respiratory infection tested positive for metapneumovirus. It usually presented as bronchiolitis, but also as croup and exacerbations of asthma. *N Engl J Med*, 2004; **350**: 431–433.

- A placebo-controlled trial in 720 children with mild croup showed that a single dose of dexamethasone (0.6 mg per kg) resulted in small but real benefits, shortening symptoms and improving sleep while reducing parental stress. As oral dexamethasone is already established in moderate to severe croup, the authors state it should be given to all children with croup of any severity. *N Engl J Med*, 2004; **351**: 1306–1313.

RESPIRATORY

INFLUENZA

What we know already:

- Over 3000 deaths occur each year from influenza related causes
- Two interventions can lessen the impact of flu: immunisation with inactivated vaccines and treatment and prophylaxis with antivirals
- Vaccination reduces admissions, mortality and morbidity in high-risk groups. Health policies target high-risk individuals
- Fears over immunising COPD patients are unfounded. Although an increase in prescriptions for oral steroids given on the day of influenza vaccination has been observed, there is no increased risk of adverse outcomes
- Older antivirals, such as amantadine and rimantadine, are limited by rapid emergence of resistance, lack of effectiveness against influenza B, and central nervous system side-effects
- Neuraminidase inhibitors are recommended in identified outbreaks of influenza in the community and are effective prophylaxis, resulting in a relative reduction of 70–90% in the odds of developing flu
- For treatment of flu, systematic review shows that zanamivir or oseltamivir reduce duration of symptoms by between 0.4 and 1.0 days. Given within 48 hours, they provide around 30–40% relative reduction in the odds of complications requiring antibiotics
- Most of the elderly have difficulty using inhalers of zanamivir, particularly loading and priming Diskhalers. This limits their use of this delivery system
- Influenza is an important cause of acute respiratory illness in young children. Attack rates among preschool children often exceed 40% in epidemic years
- Common childhood complications include febrile convulsions, otitis media, bronchiolitis, and croup, and lead to heavy prescribing of antibiotics
- Near patient testing has shown a sensitivity of 44% and a specificity of 97% in children. Being good at ruling in influenza might assist optimal management, improve surveillance of flu, and satisfy parents denied antibiotics. However, the test cannot rule out influenza

Recent Papers

IN THE ELDERLY

Effect of influenza vaccination on excess deaths occurring during periods of high circulation of influenza: cohort study in elderly people
Armstrong BG, Mangtani P, Fletcher A *et al.*
BMJ, 2004; **329**: 660–663

Mortality being a rare end-point, it has been difficult to prove the effectiveness of influenza vaccine on mortality directly. This meta-analysis therefore looked at observational studies and found the effectiveness of influenza vaccine regarding all cause mortality to be 68%.

The study took a novel approach by measuring effectiveness as the degree to which less circulating influenza was related to fewer deaths in vaccinated people (rather than directly comparing mortality in vaccinated and unvaccinated people). Some 24 535 people aged over 75 were followed up for more than 4 years with reference to levels of circulating influenza. During a flu outbreak, all cause mortality, predominantly respiratory, was lower in those who had received the vaccine than in those who had not. In fact, in vaccinated people, mortality was low enough to escape an association with the higher levels of circulating influenza completely.

Detection and control of influenza outbreaks in well-vaccinated nursing home populations
Monto AS, Rotthoff J, Teich E *et al.*
Clin Infect Dis, 2004; **39**: 459–464

The other very important part of influenza research is outbreak control. In the first place, this requires early detection of a definite rise in incidence of influenza-positive cases.

Over two seasons in nursing homes in Michigan, close influenza surveillance was performed and oseltamivir was used in all homes with influenza transmission. They found that control of the outbreak depended on how quickly it was recognised and the extent of antiviral use. This was done well in five out of eight homes showing that oseltamivir prophylaxis was a useful part of initial outbreak strategies.

Rapid antigen detection tests for outbreak recognition had a specificity of 92% but a sensitivity of only 77%. In addition, it is worth noting staff levels of vaccination averaged around only 50%.

Annual revaccination against influenza and mortality risk in community-dwelling elderly persons
Voordouw AC, Sturkenboom MC, Dieleman JP *et al.*
JAMA, 2004; **292**: 2089–2095

This is the first study to look at the benefits of annual influenza revaccination in elderly persons.

Overall, a first vaccination was associated with a non-significant annual reduction in the risk of death by 10% but revaccination in subsequent years was associated with a further reduced annual mortality risk of 15%. This improved to 28% in epidemic periods.

Overall, at a vaccination coverage around 70%, influenza vaccination is estimated to prevent 1 death for every 302 vaccinees or 1 for every 195 revaccinations.

Vaccinating year on year increases reductions in the risk of death in this older population.

RESPIRATORY

IN CHILDREN

The underrecognized burden of influenza in young children
Poehling KA, Edwards KM, Weinberg GA *et al.*
N Engl J Med, 2006; **355**: 31–40

US authorities recommend a yearly influenza vaccination for toddlers between the age of 6 months and 2 years based on high levels of hospitalisation for influenza. This study demonstrates that the burden of influenza is actually very much higher in the community – by a factor between 10 and 250 times.

The commonest symptoms were fever (95%), cough (96%) and runny nose (96%). Doctors recognised the illness in only 28% of inpatients and 17% of outpatients. This may be a missed opportunity if we want to prevent complications and outbreaks.

Influenza vaccination in asthmatic children: effects on quality of life and symptoms
Bueving HJ, van der Wouden JC, Raat H *et al.*
Eur Respir J, 2004; **24**: 925–931

This Dutch study looked at whether influenza vaccination affects quality of life, symptomatology and spirometry in nearly 700 asthmatic children. If they reached a pre-defined level of respiratory symptoms a nurse turned up and performed a pharyngeal swab and spirometry and reassessed 1 week later.

Compared with a placebo vaccination:
- influenza vaccination improved health-related quality of life in the weeks of illness related to influenza-positive swabs
- there was no effect on symptoms during those weeks
- no differences were found for quality of life/symptoms throughout the year

They conclude the influenza vaccination had a moderately beneficial effect on quality of life in influenza-positive weeks of illness in children with asthma.

ARTHRITIS and NSAIDs

What we know already:

- Musculoskeletal conditions accounted for up to 20% of all general practitioner consultations. Around 5% require referral for a specialist opinion
- Rheumatoid arthritis is a persistent chronic disease affecting 0.5% of people worldwide
- Standard symptomatic treatment has done little to alter disease progression
- DMARDs – disease-modifying antirheumatic drugs – inhibit cytokine production and newer drugs are revolutionising therapeutic approaches by showing ever earlier benefits
- Evidence of minor levels of inflammation for up to 10 years prior to presentation make it possible to screen for a disease that is becoming virtually preventable
- Earlier imaging with MRI and high resolution ultrasonography can facilitate definitive diagnosis of characteristic features much earlier
- Primary carers needs to consider early referral in all new cases to minimise lifelong incapacity
- Osteoarthritis is the most common form of arthritis and accounts for 11% of all sick days and £1.2 billion of annual expenditure
- Osteoarthritis is the major cause of disability in the elderly, most commonly affecting the knee and prevalence is rising with the changing demographic
- Although NSAIDs are slightly better than paracetamol for reducing osteoarthritis-related pain, or pain at rest, the downside is not outweighed when symptoms are mild
- Treatment guidelines for knee osteoarthritis recommend starting pain relief with paracetamol and later substituting with NSAIDs, but in the UK 15% of patients use paracetamol, while 50% use NSAIDs regularly
- NSAIDs have a 2–4% annual incidence of serious gastrointestinal ulcer and complications – four times higher than in non-users. They also cause fluid retention and worsen renal insufficiency
- Adverse cardiovascular safety profiles have limited use of COX-2 inhibitors (Rofecoxib was withdrawn from the market in 2004 due to concerns regarding increased mortality from heart failure)
- Taking some NSAIDs for more then 2 years appears to reduces the risk of Alzheimer's disease but may be ineffective in established disease and is not a recommended indication

Recent Papers

RHEUMATOID ARTHRITIS

Medication

Retardation of joint damage in patients with early rheumatoid arthritis by initial aggressive treatment with disease-modifying antirheumatic drugs: five-year experience from the FIN-RACo study
Korpela M, Laasonen L, Hannonen P et al.
Arthritis Rheum, 2004; **50**: 2072–2081

Aggressive initial treatment of early RA with the combination of three DMARDs (methotrexate, sulfasalazine, hydroxychloroquine) for the first 2 years is better than just using one DMARD on its own. Triple therapy with combinations of DMARDs improved long-term radiology (over at least 5 years) in peripheral joints in patients with early and clinically active RA. Adding other DMARDs in after 2 years does not make up the difference when the window of opportunity has been lost and does not increase remission rates. Predictors of worse joint damage were disease duration before diagnosis, ESR, and the presence of serum rheumatoid factor at baseline.

Etanercept (Enbrel) in patients with rheumatoid arthritis with recent onset versus established disease: improvement in disability
Baumgartner SW, Fleischmann RM, Moreland LW et al.
J Rheumatol, 2004; **31**: 1532–1537

Another study confirmed the importance of an early start to DMARD therapy. Of the two groups used, one had not received methotrexate and one had failed treatment with one or more DMARDs. Both groups improved on treatment with etanercept. The effect occurred as early as week two and persisted for the 3 years of the study. Those with recent onset of RA showed greater benefit than those with established disease. Prompt early treatment of RA minimises longer-term disability.

Combination of infliximab and methotrexate therapy for early rheumatoid arthritis: a randomized, controlled trial
St Clair EW, van der Heijde DM, Smolen JS et al.
Arthritis Rheum, 2004; **50**: 3432–3443

In early active RA, combining methotrexate with infliximab – anti-TNF (tumour necrosis factor) alpha monoclonal antibody – provides greater clinical, radiographic, and functional benefits than methotrexate alone. However, a significant proportion of patients can achieve remission using methotrexate alone so the balance of side effects (mainly a higher incidence of serious infections such as pneumonia) should be considered.

MUSCULOSKELETAL

Prednisolone plus a disease modifying antirheumatic drug improved outcomes in early rheumatoid arthritis. *Evidence-Based Medicine,* 2006; **11**: 79
The following paper is reviewed
Low-dose prednisolone in addition to the initial disease-modifying antirheumatic drug in patients with early active rheumatoid arthritis reduces joint destruction and increases the remission rate: a two-year randomized trial
Svensson B, Boonen A, Albertsson K *et al.*
Arthritis Rheum, 2005; **52**: 3360–3370

This Swedish study of 259 patients who were starting treatment with a DMARD (usually methotrexate or sulphasalazine) for the first time were also given either 7.5 mg of prednisolone or placebo. Radiographic joint damage and functional disability decreased more with prednisolone with no increase in adverse events.

The study was not blinded and only had 2 years follow up but was well executed. The 5% of patients with highly active disease and 115 with osteoporosis were excluded – a reminder that steroids are not ideal for all.

Concerns remain over the aggravation of cardiovascular risk factors by prednisolone and intensive anti-osteoporotic treatment is warranted. Although in this study most patients were treated with a single DMARD, this is increasingly unlikely to be the case in real life with more intensive drug combinations yielding positive results.

Mortality in patients with rheumatoid arthritis treated with low-dose oral glucocorticoids. A population-based cohort study
Sihvonen S, Korpela M, Mustonen J *et al.*
J Rheumatol, 2006; **33**: 1740–1746

Mortality increases where low-dose oral glucocorticoids are used for more than 10 years in rheumatoid arthritis patients. The risk of mortality increased by 14% for each year and by 69% over 10 years compared to those not on steroids. The main reason was cardiovascular death but there were also more deaths due to infections and intestinal perforations due to amyloidosis.

Long-term management

Effect of a treatment strategy of tight control for rheumatoid arthritis (the TICORA study): a single-blind randomised controlled trial
Grigor C, Capell H, Stirling A *et al.*
Lancet, 2004; **364**: 263–269

This Glasgow study showed the superiority of intensive outpatient management of rheumatoid arthritis using antirheumatic drugs and intra-articular steroid injections over routine care. Monthly assessments were used to step up drug therapy and identify joints for injecting. Anti-TNF therapy was not used in this study. There were very substantial improvements in disease activity, radiographic change, physical function, and quality of life. And at no additional cost.

MUSCULOSKELETAL

Patient initiated outpatient follow up in rheumatoid arthritis: six year randomised controlled trial
Hewlett S, Kirwan J, Pollock J et al.
BMJ, 2005; **330**: 171

This study offered over 200 patients with rheumatoid arthritis direct access to hospital rheumatologists on demand to replace the flabby system of regular planned hospital review that accounts for three-quarters of the workload of a rheumatologist. Clinical and psychological outcomes were almost identical compared to those receiving regular planned hospital review. Satisfaction and confidence in the system were significantly higher throughout the 6 years of the study. Direct access patients needed 38% fewer hospital appointments. The number of GP visits for arthritis was unaffected. The authors offer this as a new model of chronic disease management.

OSTEOARTHRITIS

Diagnosis

Several diagnostic aids have moderate to high accuracy for detecting abnormalities in acute knee pain. *Evidence-Based Medicine,* 2004; **9**: 57
The following paper is presented
Evaluation of acute knee pain in primary care
Jackson JL, O'Malley PG, Kroenke K
Ann Intern Med, 2003; **139**: 575–588

This paper looked at the accuracy of clinical decision rules, physical examination, and imaging procedures for finding causes of acute knee pain.

Clinical criteria for osteoarthritis (which were age >50 years, stiffness for < 30 min, crepitus, bony tenderness, bony enlargement, and no palpable warmth) had a sensitivity of 84% and specificity 89%.

X-ray showing presence of osteophytes observed with at least one factor from age >50 years, crepitus, or morning stiffness of <30 min increased sensitivity to 91% with a specificity of 86%. This is pretty good.

The conclusion is that increased use of careful examination with clinical criteria to diagnose osteoarthritis should be able to reduce reliance on imaging.

Treatment

Managing osteoarthritis of the knee
MacAuley D
BMJ, 2004; **329**: 1300–1301

This article also summarises treatment options.
- Physical training can strengthen muscles to relieve symptoms of weakness.
- Endurance exercise benefits mild and moderate osteoarthritis but facilities for exercise training are not commonly available in the UK
- Home-based programmes are also effective.
- Acupuncture may reduce pain and improve both function and quality of life.

MORECAMBE BAY HOSPITALS NHS TRUST

MUSCULOSKELETAL

- Taping, if available, may be useful short term.
- Anti-inflammatory applications are of some help.
- Glucosamine and chondroitin have shown some benefit.
- Intra-articular injections are effective particularly for symptom relief at important times (a meta-analysis showed that steroids injected into the knee are 1.6 times as likely as placebo injections of saline to improve symptoms of osteoarthritis at 2 weeks and may have a longer term effect; *BMJ*, 2004; **328**: 869).
- Ultimately, surgery is effective with total knee replacements a good option.

Glucosamine and chondroitin sulphate did not improve pain in osteoarthritis of the knee. *Evidence-Based Medicine,* 2006; **11**: 115
The following paper is reviewed
Glucosamine, chondroitin sulfate, and the two in combination for painful knee osteoarthritis
Clegg DO, Reda DJ, Harris CL *et al.*
N Engl J Med, 2006; **354**: 795–808

Some analysis has suggested that previous impressions of efficacy of glucosamine and chondroitin were bogus – caused by flaws in study design, small samples and publication bias. But these papers are balanced by papers that support a significant effect. The latest randomised placebo-controlled trial adds to growing opinion that these supplements have little effect on symptoms of osteoarthritis of the knee.

The end point of GAIT (Glucosamine/chondroitin Arthritis Intervention Trial) was a 20% decrease in the WOMAC pain scale in 1583 patients over the age of 40 years. Response to placebo was as high as 60% and the authors conclude that the effects of treatment are unlikely to be clinically important for most patients.

Patients whose pain was moderate or severe may experience some relief but the study was underpowered to verify this.

NSAIDs

Taking stock of coxibs
Drug Ther Bull, 2005; **43**: 1–6

A review of current evidence did not indicate any evidence that coxibs are a 'safer' class of NSAID. They are even different types of drugs. Celecoxib and valdecoxib are sulfonamides. Etoricoxib and the discontinued rofecoxib are methylsulfones and the yet-to-be released lumiracoxib is a phenylacetic acid derivative closer to diclofenac.
- Coxibs may be less likely than conventional NSAIDs to cause dyspepsia, erosion, ulcers and active bleeding.
- Long-term reduction in major GI complications has not yet been demonstrated.
- They see few, if any, situations in which a coxib is unequivocally indicated.
- All NSAIDs, including coxibs, should be avoided, wherever possible, in patients at high risk of gastrointestinal complications.
- Potential hazards limit prescribing a coxib to a patient at cardiovascular risk, especially if taking low-dose aspirin.

MUSCULOSKELETAL

Do coxibs and traditional non-steroidal anti-inflammatory drugs increase the risk of atherothrombosis? Meta-analysis of randomised trials
Kearney PM, Baigent C, Godwin J *et al.*
BMJ, 2006; **332**: 1302–1305

This meta-analysis of 138 published and unpublished trials with 145 000 patients set out to look at three areas: the magnitude of the excess vascular risk associated with COX-2 inhibitors, the risk associated with traditional NSAIDs and the influence of concurrent aspirin.

- Selective COX-2 inhibitors were associated with a highly significant 1.4-fold increase in vascular death largely due to a twofold increase in myocardial infarction.
- This will cause about three extra myocardial infarctions per 1000 patients per year (which could double if everyone who discontinued prescribed COX-2 drugs were fully concordant).
- Determination of whether this was a dose-related effect or indeed differed among users and non-users of aspirin (which chiefly inhibits COX-1 at low doses) was not possible.
- Hazards were not confined to long-term use.
- High doses of traditional NSAIDs (ibuprofen 800 mg t.d.s. and diclofenac 75 mg b.d.) were associated with a similar excess risk of vascular events.
- There was no excess risk associated with high dose naproxen (500 mg b.d.) although there were insufficient data to determine whether it actually protected against cardiovascular effects.

The authors conclude that as numbers of events are relatively small, very large randomised trials will be needed to fill in the gaps.

Life without COX 2 inhibitors
Shaughnessy AF, Gordon AE
BMJ, 2006; **332**: 1287–1288

COX-2 inhibitors were trumpeted as the saviours of safe pain-relief. Now their armour is tarnished and the outpourings of grief continue, how long should we mourn?

As COX-2 inhibitors increase the incidence of myocardial infarction, we should take another look at our alternatives.

Although they rose to prominence on the back of research showing less ulceration, ulceration is neither intrinsically harmful nor a surrogate marker for harm associated with NSAIDs. In addition, gastroscopy findings such as these do not correspond to serious adverse effects and moreover their presence is not related to symptoms of dyspepsia.

Little difference has been shown between COX-2 and the older NSAIDs here. We still have other evidence that provides some insight and options according to this article.

- Misoprostol as co-treatment is effective in older people who need NSAIDs.
- Histamine-2 blockers and proton pump inhibitors are not consistently effective protectors and should not be used routinely except by those who develop a peptic ulcer.
- Topical NSAIDs are safer than oral NSAIDs for osteoarthritis of the knee.

- Paracetamol should be offered first before resorting to other analgesics.
- Opioids can be added later.
- Glucosamine and non-drug options such as therapeutic taping, exercise, and acupuncture are useful in some.

Nonsteroidal anti-inflammatory drugs and risk of first hospital admission for heart failure in the general population

Huerta C, Varas-Lorenzo C, Castellsague J et al.
Heart, 2006; **92**: 1610–1615

This study looked at the association of NSAIDs with nearly 1400 admissions for a first episode of heart failure using the UK General Practice Database.

After controlling for other factors, the risk of a first admission for heart failure following NSAID use was 1.3. The main independent risk factor for admission was a prior clinical diagnosis of heart failure which had a relative risk of 7.3.

The usual aetiological factors such as hypertension, diabetes, renal failure and anaemia as well as obesity, smoking and alcohol use added to the increased risk of hospitalisation. Dose or duration did not appear relevant.

The research supports epidemiological studies that NSAIDs trigger heart failure in susceptible patients even if they have not previously been noted to have heart failure.

TOPICAL NSAIDs

Efficacy of topical non-steroidal anti-inflammatory drugs in the treatment of osteoarthritis: meta-analysis of randomised controlled trials

Lin J, Zhang W, Jones A et al.
BMJ, 2004; **329**: 324

A systematic review in 1998 confirmed that topical NSAIDs were superior to placebo over 2 weeks in the treatment of chronic pain, including pain due to osteoarthritis and tendonitis. This second systematic review in a similar area examined outcomes of stiffness and function (as well as pain) compared to placebo. Superiority was found at 2 weeks but this evaporated by 1 month when use of topical NSAIDs was comparable to placebo.

The authors conclude that there is no evidence to support the long-term use of topical NSAIDs in osteoarthritis.

Longterm efficacy of topical nonsteroidal antiinflammatory drugs in knee osteoarthritis: metaanalysis of randomized placebo controlled clinical trials

Biswal S, Medhi B, Pandhi P
J Rheumatol, 2006; **33**: 1841–1844

This meta-analysis involved 709 patients and looked at the effectiveness of topical NSAIDs. All the studies used showed superiority of the topical agents. The findings show that diclofenac and eltenac gel appear to be effective over the longer-term for pain relief in osteoarthritis of the knee. Other NSAIDs could not be commented upon.

MUSCULOSKELETAL

Pennsaid therapy for osteoarthritis of the knee: a systematic review and metaanalysis of randomized controlled trials
Towheed T
J Rheumatol, 2006; **33**: 567–573

This meta-analysis of trials with Pennsaid – a new topical diclofenac sodium solution containing the absorption enhancer dimethyl sulfoxide – involved 1400 patients in studies up to 12 weeks long. It improved pain, stiffness and physical function better than placebo in osteoarthritis of the knee. One study was a high quality 12 week randomised equivalence trial which showed that topical diclofenac was as effective (with many fewer systemic side effects) as oral diclofenac at 150 mg daily for the same condition.

Systematic review of topical rubefacients containing salicylates for the treatment of acute and chronic pain
Mason L, Moore RA, Edwards JE *et al.*
BMJ, 2004; **328**: 995

This review was not really about NSAIDs but determined the efficacy and safety of topical rubefacients containing salicylates. It excluded the traditional NSAIDs or capsaicin but that still left more than 30 preparations in the UK alone. Rubefacients work by counter irritation. Salicylates have a different mechanism even to other NSAIDs.

There was a dearth of high quality trials and on the whole, proof of good efficacy was in short supply. Topical salicylate may have efficacy in acute pain at 7 days but poor to moderate efficacy in chronic musculoskeletal and arthritic pain at 14 days. The better trials showed little difference from placebo.

Further Research

- Researchers of non-drug treatments for rheumatoid and osteoarthritis fail to report side effects more than half the time. This impedes the ability to judge the benefit–harm balance for options such as surgery, lavage, exercise and psychotherapy as opposed to drug treatments. *Ann Intern Med,* 2005; **143**: 20–25.

- The risk of serious NSAID gastropathy has declined sharply in recent years. In a US report, 24% of this was accredited to lower doses of NSAIDs, 18% was thanks to proton-pump inhibitors and 14% due to the use of less toxic NSAIDs. These improvements are likely to continue with wiser use of safer drugs in minimal effective doses accompanied by appropriate prophylaxis. *Arthritis Rheum,* 2004; **50**: 2433–2440.

BACK PAIN

What we know already:

- Low back pain accounts for 13% of sickness absences in the UK and poses a major socio-economic burden
- It costs the NHS £1billion annually and affects 17 million people in the UK alone
- Those aged 35–55 years are affected most often
- Overall, 1% of people presenting with back pain have a neoplasm, 4% have compression fractures, and 1–3% have a prolapsed disc
- Up to 7% of acute episodes of low back pain develop into chronic pain
- Imaging is not routinely required for back pain of <6 weeks duration without a high suspicion of systemic disease or progressive neurological deficit
- MRI is the most sensitive and specific imaging method for systemic disease. MRI and CT are similarly accurate for degenerative conditions with neurological impairment. Plain X-ray is commonly used but of limited value
- Red flags such as bilateral or alternating leg symptoms, neurological disturbance, sphincter disturbance, and history of malignancy, help to identify those who need investigation
- Pain which was worse in the leg than the back has been shown to have a sensitivity/specificity of 82% / 54% at predicting nerve root compression as confirmed on MRI scan. Pain worse on coughing, sneezing, or straining had figures of 50% / 67%.
- Physiotherapists in the NHS treat 1.3 million people for low back pain annually, but there is only weak evidence for the effectiveness of many of their methods
- Catastrophisation (excessively negative orientation towards pain) and kinesiophobia (fear of movement and injury) predict chronic disability
- Neck pain accounts for 15% of all soft tissue problems in general practice and is a common reason for referral to a physiotherapist
- Little evidence exists for routine use of such interventions and they consume a substantial amount of healthcare resources
- It is becoming clearer that back pain and neck pain share similarities as multifaceted problems requiring multiple approaches

Recent Papers

MUSCULOSKELETAL SERVICES

Improved access and targeting of musculoskeletal services in northwest Wales: targeted early access to musculoskeletal services (TEAMS) programme
Maddison P, Jones J, Breslin A *et al.*
BMJ, 2004; **329**: 1325–1327

The TEAMS experiment took place in an area of Wales with a poorly resourced musculoskeletal service which had long waiting times, many duplicate referrals to other specialities, and GPs who were reluctant to refer due to a perceived lack of service. An improved service was set up establishing clinical triage and a common

MUSCULOSKELETAL

pathway for all musculoskeletal referrals which channelled patients to the appropriate department.

A back pain pathway led by extended role physiotherapists was developed. GPs with special interests (GPwSIs) and physiotherapists were trained to cover uncomplicated musculoskeletal problems in the community.

Over the 18 months of the study:

- the number of referrals more than doubled, revealing the unmet burden of need
- despite this, waiting times for musculoskeletal services fell
- duplicate referrals were abolished
- need for surgery was unchanged
- patients showed a high level of patient satisfaction with the new service

Community-based multidisciplinary clinics run by GPwSIs and specially trained physiotherapists are a popular and effective approach for patients with uncomplicated musculoskeletal problems. Integration of hospital services improves service.

LOW BACK PAIN

Acute low back pain: systematic review of its prognosis
Pengel LM, Herbert RD, Maher C et al.
BMJ, 2003; **327**: 323–325

Evidence has been lacking on how quickly back pain really settles down so this is a useful meta-analysis to assist in counselling patients.

- Pain decreased rapidly in the first month and most patients could return to work.
- Most of the rest will be back at work by 6 months.
- Further improvements occur up to 3 months but little more in the next 9 months.
- Recovery is not as complete as previously advertised. Pain and disability from residual symptoms persist at low levels.
- Most people have a recurrence within 12 months.
- Counselling on prognosis has been shown to reassure and improve functional outcomes.
- Evidence for putative prognostic factors such as distress, and work-related factors such as job satisfaction, comes mainly from weak studies.
- Only one of the included study populations had classic sciatica so there may be further recovery delays in this group.

Clinical course and prognostic factors in acute low back pain: patients consulting primary care for the first time
Grotle M, Brox JI, Veierod MB
Spine, 2005; **30**: 976–982

This study looked in detail at the clinical course of Norwegians presenting with a first episode of acute low back pain of up to 3 weeks duration.

- After 12 weeks, recovery was only 76%.
- Absence from work was 8% at 4 weeks and 6% at three months.

MUSCULOSKELETAL

- Age over 45 years, smoking, more than one neurological sign and high levels of distress were associated with nonrecovery at 3 months.

The authors suggest looking for psychological factors at the initial visit.

In a different Dutch study, GPs took a brief intervention towards actually doing this. They looked at the patients' ideas about the cause of pain, fear-avoidance beliefs and behaviour, catastrophising thoughts, family reactions and occupational factors. They offered information, reassurance and advice in a 20 minute session. Unfortunately no impact on disability, recovery or sick leave was forthcoming (*BMJ*, 2005; **331**: 84).

Predicting persistent disabling low back pain in general practice: a prospective cohort study
Jones GT, Johnson RE, Wiles N *et al.*
Br J Gen Pract, 2006; **56**: 334–341

Good coping strategies such as staying active reduce disabling low back pain. Passive strategies include relying on others for help with the daily tasks and feeling as though they cannot do anything to improve the pain. This study of 922 people with back pain found a threefold increase in persistent disabling pain in those with these high levels of negative coping strategies.

After controlling for severity of symptoms, those who reported a high passive coping score were still at 50% increased risk of a poor outcome.

Implementation of RCGP guidelines for acute low back pain: a cluster randomised controlled trial
Dey P, Simpson CWR, Collins SI *et al.*
Br J Gen Pract, 2004; **54**: 33–37

This cluster randomised trial from North-West England randomised over 2000 patients from 24 health centres to usual GP care or intensive application of the RCGP guidelines. This intervention was supported by educational visits to practices, access to fast-track physiotherapy and a triage service for those with unresolving symptoms.

There was an increased use of the physiotherapy options and back pain units but no change in use of X-rays, sick notes, prescribed drugs or secondary care referrals.

The management of back pain in primary care was largely unchanged by the outreach training strategy attempting to promote greater adherence to the guidelines.

PHYSICAL THERAPIES

Randomised controlled trial of physiotherapy compared with advice for low back pain
Frost H, Lamb SE, Doll HA *et al.*
BMJ, 2004; **329**: 708

Some international guidelines recommend exercise therapy for patients with chronic low back pain (>12 weeks' duration) and some suggest spinal manipulation for acute or subacute low back pain.

MUSCULOSKELETAL

This study measured the effectiveness of routine physiotherapy using methods such as low velocity spinal joint mobilisation techniques, lumbar spine mobility exercises and abdominal strengthening. Patients in the intervention group did feel better in themselves reporting improvements in mental health and physical function. But there was no evidence that it made any actual difference over and above a simple assessment session and advice from a physiotherapist to remain active. Some even received more sessions where the physiotherapist deemed it 'unethical' to withhold further treatment.

Back pain and physiotherapy
MacAuley D
BMJ, 2004; **329**: 694–695

This accompanying editorial asks if we can make referral decisions in the NHS based on these subjective 'benefits'. Also, the treatment was dependent on the physiotherapist using different treatments in no particular pattern.

This is not to say that all physiotherapy is ineffective for back pain. *Ad hoc* treatment in the NHS is ineffective but there may be useful component interventions hidden within. Progressive exercise classes run by a physiotherapist have been shown to be useful, for example. Radiography is not usually necessary. Orthopaedic surgeons are generally uninterested.

NHS physiotherapy is expensive and adds little to an advice sheet. Is it a responsible use of resources? Reinforcing advice to stay active seems to be the best way to go while patients will undoubtedly seek out other treatments when we 'fail' them.

Spinal manipulative therapy is not better than standard treatments for low back pain. *Evidence-Based Medicine,* 2004; **9**: 171
The following article is reviewed
Spinal manipulative therapy for low back pain
Assendelft WJ, Morton SC, Yu EI *et al.*
Cochrane Database Syst Rev, 2004

This Cochrane review quantifies the evidence for spinal manipulative therapy (SMT) in low back pain by comparing different treatment strategies.

They looked at 39 studies with comparisons to sham therapies. The modest short and long-term improvements in low back pain did not differ significantly from three other interventions: GP care/analgesics, physical therapy/exercise, or back school.

The presence of a beneficial effect for SMT is unproven rather than disproven. Small benefits may yet be a cost-effective weapon against the epidemic but at present there is insufficient evidence for routine use.

United Kingdom back pain exercise and manipulation (UK BEAM) randomised trial: effectiveness of physical treatments for back pain in primary care
UK BEAM Trial Team
BMJ, 2004; **329**: 1377

This is a large study of 181 general practices in the Medical Research Council

General Practice Research Framework taken in 63 community settings around 14 centres across the United Kingdom. Some 1334 patients with back pain were randomised to different physical treatments for back pain: a class-based exercise programme ('Back to Fitness'), a package of treatment by a spinal manipulator (chiropractor, osteopath or physiotherapist), or both.

The control group is 'best care' in general practice, placebos being very hard to come by in this area:

- spinal manipulation showed a small to moderate benefit at 3 months and a small benefit at 12 months
- exercise alone improved back function by a small margin at 3 months but not at 12 months
- combined manipulation followed by exercise classes showed a moderate benefit at 3 months and a small benefit at 12 months

An accompanying economic paper showed that manipulation alone is probably the best value for money of these options. The authors argue that the sick leave saved would more than compensate for the chiropractic costs and argue for a major expansion of this role within the NHS. In the meantime they suggest hiring from the private sector.

NECK PAIN

Effectiveness of dynamic muscle training, relaxation training, or ordinary activity for chronic neck pain: randomised controlled trial
Viljanen M, Malmivaara A, Uitti J *et al.*
BMJ, 2003; **327**: 475

Neck pain affects two-thirds of adults especially women at some point. Pathology is unclear. This high powered Finnish trial looked at effectiveness and costs when nearly 400 female office workers with chronic non-specific neck pain were randomly assigned to 12 weeks of dynamic muscle training, relaxation therapy, or ordinary activity.

Neither dynamic muscle training (using dumbbells and stretching techniques) nor relaxation techniques influenced severity of pain, disability, or sick leave over a period of 12 months. Ordinary activity was just as good.

The training groups did report better subjective recovery, and there was a slightly larger range of cervical motion, but this was not clinically relevant.

Cost effectiveness of physiotherapy, manual therapy, and general practitioner care for neck pain: economic evaluation alongside a randomised controlled trial
Korthals-de Bos IBC, Hoving JL, van Tulder MW *et al.*
BMJ, 2003; **326**: 911–914

This Dutch study randomly allocated 183 patients to manual therapy (spinal mobilisation), physiotherapy, or GP care. The manual therapists used slow passive movements up to the limits of the range of motion of the joint. To keep things clear, these techniques were discouraged in the physiotherapy group who used stretching and other postural and relaxation techniques. GPs offered advice on lifestyle as well as on simple exercises along with an educational booklet and

MUSCULOSKELETAL

medication. Manual therapy (gentle active spinal mobilisation) was found to be more effective for treating neck pain than physiotherapy or care by a GP. Active treatment from a manual therapist led to faster recovery in the first 6 months and was cheaper over the year.

Physiotherapy for neck and back pain

Harvey N, Cooper C
BMJ, 2005; **330**: 53–54

This editorial summarises that it is clear that back pain and neck pain share a tendency towards intractability. Biopsychosocial approaches will be necessary to manage this rather than concentrating on physical symptoms alone.

Trials in this area are often hampered by too much diversity – of treatments, of therapists and of approach. Perhaps it is not surprising that they fail to show how one specific intervention improves disability when the psychosocial component to chronicity is so great.

Research into subgroups of patients is needed to tell us who responds best to what. Broad-based public health interventions must work alongside these measures to alter public beliefs about back pain and reduce its medicalisation. Otherwise we might stay in the quagmire we are in at the moment.

MUSCULOSKELETAL

OSTEOPOROSIS

Recent Papers

CASE DETECTION

Quantitative ultrasound and risk factor enquiry as predictors of postmenopausal osteoporosis: comparative study in primary care
Hodson J, Marsh J
BMJ, 2003; **326**: 1250–1251

Use of risk factors is reported to predict osteoporosis poorly so this paper looked at the use of quantitative ultrasound scanning in primary care to predict fracture.

In seven UK general practices, 200 women over 60 years were referred either because of perceived risk or interest. An experienced practice nurse enquired about risk factors and performed a heel ultrasound scan. The GP then referred the patient for DEXA scanning of the hip and lumbar spine.

Risk-factor positive patients were defined as having at least one of the factors in the Royal College of Physicians' 1999 guidelines, e.g. BMI <19 kg/m^2, height loss >2 inches, maternal hip fracture, menopause or hysterectomy <45 years, fracture after age 50, secondary amenorrhoea >1 year.

Risk factor enquiry was a poor predictor – only 19% had osteoporosis and a third of affected women were not identified.

Ultrasound scanning alone had nearly twice the specificity as just using risk factors. Adding ultrasound to risk factor assessment improved sensitivity by 22% and reduced specificity by 4% identifying 90% of the women with osteoporosis.

The improved pick-up rates and predictive values of combining ultrasound with risk factor assessment indicated that more evaluation of this simple, quick approach could be interesting.

TREATMENT

Treatment of postmenopausal osteoporosis
Reginster J-Y
BMJ, 2005; **330**: 859–860

Bisphosphonates account for 70% of the worldwide market of drugs to prevent osteoporosis. There are still no head-to-head trials of alendronate and risendronate, and etidronate now seems outdated. Raloxifene reduces vertebral fractures but evidence on non-vertebral fracture is scant and HRT is off the menu for all but severe climacteric symptoms.

Strontium ranelate is a recent treatment in those with low bone density. Calcium and vitamin D is recommended here as first-line therapy especially where there are deficiencies. As deficiencies are so prevalent and the treatment is so cheap, this author indicates it should be offered to all postmenopausal women over 65.

CALCIUM AND VITAMIN D

Calcium

Calcium did not prevent fractures in elderly women. *Evidence-Based Medicine,* 2006; **11**: 149
The following article is reviewed
Effects of calcium supplementation on clinical fracture and bone structure: results of a 5-year, double-blind, placebo-controlled trial in elderly women
Prince RL, Devine A, Dhaliwal SS *et al.*
Arch Intern Med, 2006; **166**: 869–875

What is the effect of calcium supplementation alone in a population of unselected elderly women?
• Nearly 1500 women over 70 years (average age 75) and not taking any medication were given calcium carbonate 600 mg twice daily, or placebo.

OSTEOPOROSIS

- There were 297 osteoporotic fractures over the 5 years of this Australian study.
- There was no fewer fractures due to calcium based on intention to treat (the preferred method of reporting data such as this, i.e. regardless of compliance).
- The non–ITT analysis showed that in the 57% who were compliant (more than 80% of tablets taken as prescribed), calcium did reduce fractures overall.

The commentary reminds us that non-ITT analysis can undermine the purpose of randomisation. Non-compliant women may be older, weaker and slower.

The study is also uncertain that there were sufficiently high levels of vitamin D in the population for optimum skeletal calcium handling.

However, the trial was large and well-designed and it will remind us to remind our patients on calcium to keep taking the tablets.

Calcium supplementation has a small positive effect on bone mineral density but not fractures in postmenopausal women. *Evidence-Based Medicine,* 2004; **9**: 170
The following research is reviewed
Calcium supplementation on bone loss in postmenopausal women
Shea B, Wells G, Cranney A *et al.*
Cochrane Database Syst Rev, 2004

This meta-analysis of randomised controlled trials in postmenopausal women over 45 years found that calcium supplementation alone has a small positive effect on bone mineral density but does not reduce vertebral fractures. Calcium is cheap and safe and this may add support to increasing intake. Vitamin D also independently reduces risk of fractures in the elderly.

The commentary explains that the cornerstone of fracture prevention in the elderly is the combination of the two, which has been shown to be useful in osteoporosis and in nursing homes. Bisphosphonates may not work as well in those who are deficient in calcium or vitamin D.

Combined calcium and vitamin D

Vitamin D plus calcium, but not vitamin D alone, prevents osteoporotic fractures in older people. *Evidence-Based Medicine,* 2006; **11**: 13
The following article is reviewed
Vitamin D and vitamin D analogues for preventing fractures associated with involutional and post-menopausal osteoporosis
Avenell A, Gillespie WJ, Gillespie LD *et al.*
Cochrane Database Syst Rev, 2005

A review of 38 RCTs trying to clarify the role of calcium and vitamin D came to the following conclusions:
- vitamin D did not reduce hip fractures and the role of vitamin D alone is still somewhat unclear
- vitamin D plus calcium marginally reduced hip fractures (by 19%) – mainly in those in institutionalised care (who may be sunlight deficient). The combination can be recommended for frail older people confined to long-term care institutions
- lack of compliance with medication limits population benefits

OSTEOPOROSIS

Calcium plus vitamin D supplementation and the risk of fractures
Jackson RD, LaCroix AZ, Gass M *et al.*
N Engl J Med, 2006; **354**: 669–683

A report based on 36 282 women enrolled in the Women's Health Initiative also showed the effect of calcium and vitamin D supplements in healthy women between 50 and 79 years based on intention to treat.

It identified:
- increased hip bone density after 7 years of follow up
- no difference in the number of hip or total fractures
- a significant increase in renal calculi

Vitamin D

Effect of four monthly oral vitamin D3 (cholecalciferol) supplementation on fractures and mortality in men and women living in the community: randomised double blind controlled trial
Trivedi DP, Doll R, Khaw KT
BMJ, 2003; **326**: 469–472

This study looked at isolated use of vitamin D in over 2600 people aged 65–85 years living in the community. Unlike most other studies, the group was mainly men and most of the participants were doctors.

They were posted a capsule containing a large dose (100 000 IU) of vitamin D_3 (cholecalciferol) once every 4 months for 5 years and confirmed in a Freepost reply that they had taken it.

Risk of a first fracture was reduced by 22% and findings were similar in men and women.

The results compare with a study of daily combined calcium and vitamin D (800 IU) at similar total doses of vitamin D.

No adverse effects on mortality, cancer or cardiovascular disease were seen.

To prevent one fracture, the number needed to treat would be 250. It's simple, safe and cheap. At less than £1 a year, it is feasible as a population strategy.

Fracture prevention with vitamin D supplementation
Bischoff-Ferrari HA, Willett WC, Wong JB *et al.*
JAMA, 2005; **293**: 2257–2264

This meta-analysis of RCTs attempted to clarify the value of vitamin D supplementation. The majority of patients were women living in the community or in residential care. The results conflict with the study by Porthouse above.
- Oral vitamin D supplementation between 700 and 800 IU/day appeared to reduce the risk of a first hip fracture by 26% (NNT of 50 to prevent one hip fracture in 2 years) versus calcium or placebo.
- First nonvertebral fractures were reduced by 23% (NNT of 28 for one year).
- The dose of cholecalciferol was higher than that usually used so they conclude an oral vitamin D dose of 400 IU/day is not sufficient for fracture prevention.
- The authors argue for high dose vitamin D supplementation in the elderly but cannot say whether calcium is needed to make it work.

Effect of vitamin D on falls: a meta-analysis
Bischoff-Ferrari HA, Dawson-Hughes B, Willett WC *et al.*
JAMA, 2004; **291**: 1999–2006

This meta-analysis of five randomised controlled trials was also reviewed in *Evidence-Based Medicine* (2004; **9**: 169). It concluded that:
- a daily supplement of vitamin D reduced falls in older people by around 20%
- the effect was independent of calcium use
- the number needed to treat was only 15
- benefit has been shown to begin within 2–3 months
- the mechanism is unknown but it may be that vitamin D enhances muscular strength with muscle cell growth
- vitamin D might now be considered for routine use in older people but optimal dose and type of vitamin D is unknown

Recent developments in vitamin D deficiency and muscle weakness among elderly people
Venning G
BMJ, 2005; **330**: 524–526

There are previously unsuspected high levels of prevalence of vitamin D deficiency in elderly people. This is associated with muscle weakness, body sway, and a tendency to falls and fractures.

According to this clinical review, supplementation of 800 IU of vitamin D daily (or an equivalent, such as 100 000 IU every 4 months) is needed to have an effect on falls. Treating elderly housebound people with this should be seriously considered.

Effect of cholecalciferol plus calcium on falling in ambulatory older men and women
Bischoff-Ferrari HA, Orav EJ, Dawson-Hughes B *et al.*
Arch Intern Med, 2006; **166**: 424–430

Does calcium / vitamin D supplementation reduce the risk of falling in the elderly?

This placebo-controlled 3 year randomised controlled trial studied 199 men and 246 women and found the following.
- Combined supplementation reduced the odds of falling in ambulatory older women by 46%.
- Benefit was more evident in less active women with a 65% reduction in falls.
- There was no such benefit recorded in men regardless of their physical activity level.

OSTEOPOROSIS

BISPHOSPHONATES

Bisphosphonates reduce fractures, radiotherapy and hypercalcaemia and increase time to a first skeletal related event. *Evidence-Based Medicine,* 2004; **9**: 83
The following research is reviewed
Systematic review of role of bisphosphonates on skeletal morbidity in metastatic cancer
Ross JR, Saunders Y, Edmonds PM *et al.*
BMJ, 2003; **327**: 469–472

This meta-analysis of 30 trials showed that in metastatic bone disease, bisphosphonates reduce fractures, radiotherapy, hypercalcaemia and increase time to a first skeletal event.

The commentator expresses reservations that the case is not yet won for routine use of these drugs in metastatic cancer. A more important end-point is quality of life which is what really matters to these patients but harder to measure and so less often considered. In addition, meta-analysis is imperfect when high quality data are scant, some studies are not included, some are still in progress and some are unpublished.

Ten years' experience with alendronate for osteoporosis in postmenopausal women
Bone HG, Hosking D, Devogelaer JP *et al.*
N Engl J Med, 2004; **350**: 1189–1199

Long-term studies on the use of bisphosphonates are in short supply. This one looked at 247 postmenopausal women on alendronate.

Treatment with 10 mg of alendronate daily for 10 years increased bone mineral density at the lumbar spine by 14%, at the trochanter by 10% and at the femoral neck by 5%.

Effects of alendronate were sustained, and the drug was well tolerated over a 10-year period. Discontinuation resulted in a gradual loss of effect.

RALOXIFENE

Continuing outcomes relevant to Evista: breast cancer incidence in postmenopausal osteoporotic women in a randomised trial of raloxifene
Martino S, Cauley JA, Barrett-Connor E *et al.*
J Natl Cancer Inst, 2004; **96**: 1751–1761

Raloxifene is a selective oestrogen inhibitor but unlike tamoxifen does not stimulate uterine proliferation. It is indicated for treatment and prevention of postmenopausal osteoporosis.

Four years of raloxifene have been shown by the same researchers to decrease the incidence of invasive breast cancer. There was no change in incidence of oestrogen receptor-negative invasive breast cancer.

This further study was for an extra 4 years and over the 8 years of both trials, the incidences of invasive breast cancer and oestrogen receptor-positive invasive breast cancer were reduced by two-thirds. The trade off was a doubled risk of thromboembolism.

OSTEOPOROSIS

Further studies will be needed to see if the drug has potential in post-menopausal women without osteoporosis who wish to reduce their risk of breast cancer.

The effect of raloxifene after discontinuation of long-term alendronate treatment of postmenopausal osteoporosis

Michalská D, Stepan JJ, Basson BR *et al.*
J Clin Endocrinol Metab, 2006; **91**: 870–877

This randomised study shows that those that have to stop taking alendronate can successfully switch to raloxifene and keep most of the benefit in terms of bone mineral density at the lumbar spine compared with taking a placebo. All of the patients were taking supplemental calcium and vitamin D.

OSTEOPOROSIS

OLDER PEOPLE

What we know already:

- By 2025, almost one-quarter of the population of Europe will be over 65
- By 2050 the overall growth rate of 2.4% per year will result in a threefold increase in the number of people aged 60 or older to 2 billion
- Elderly people at home and in care homes provide an increasing workload for the GP and arrangements for delivering care to the elderly have been haphazard
- Insufficient use of beneficial drugs, overuse of unnecessary drugs and poor monitoring of chronic disease are commonplace
- Assessing five priority domains of unmet need can add 'SPICE' to later life: Senses (vision and hearing); Physical ability (mobility and falls); Incontinence; Cognition; Emotional distress (depression and anxiety)
- Dementia has become a pressing challenge facing healthcare with 5% of those aged over 65 year and 20% of those over 80 years having some degree of dementia
- Inadequate detection, referral and management of dementia has been recognised in primary care and suboptimal psychosocial intervention is widespread
- Between 2001 and 2040, the number of dementia cases is expected to double in developed countries and quadruple in developing countries
- Cholinesterase inhibitors produce small improvements in cognitive and global assessments in Alzheimer's disease
- Falls are a major cause of disability and the associated costs to the NHS are around £1 billion a year
- In the UK approximately 30% of people over 65 years and 50% over 80 years will fall in a given year
- Hip fracture is the commonest reason for admission to an orthopaedic ward, often resulting in death or permanent disability. By 2050, there will be 4.5 million hip fractures in the elderly so prevention will be crucial
- The mean age of hip fracture in women is 81 years. The expected additional life for an 80 year old will be 8.7 years so there is plenty of time to benefit from prophylactic measures
- Diverse risk factors such as balance problems, muscle weakness, use of medication and environmental hazards increase the risk of falls
- Risk factor intervention, muscle strengthening, balance training and withdrawal of psychotropic medications are considered to be likely to be beneficial in falls
- Multifactorial assessment in falls clinics are providing individualised interventions

Guidelines

The National Service Framework for Older People (2001) aims to provide the same levels of care regardless of age. Resources are being targeted towards increased numbers of elderly care specialists and associated nurses and therapists as well as operations such as cataracts and joint replacements.

Since its inception, one-third of older people needing intensive daily help now receive this in their own homes rather than in residential care; delayed discharge from acute beds has reduced by two-thirds; and services for stroke and falls continue to improve.

A New Ambition for Old Age: Next steps in implementing the national service framework. London: Department of Health, 2006 (*www.dh.gov.uk*).

This document emphasises three themes – dignity in care, joined up care, and healthy ageing. Improvements of services in appropriate environments, stronger commissioning arrangements and dealing with any remnants of age discrimination will build on the success of the NSF.

Recent Papers

SCREENING THE ELDERLY

Population-based multidimensional assessment of older people in UK general practice: a cluster-randomised factorial trial
Fletcher AE, Price GM, Ng ES *et al.*
Lancet, 2004; **364**: 1667–1677

This study looked at the controversial area of screening the over 75s in over 100 UK practices. They identified over 43 000 eligible patients and achieved 78% participation.

A brief multidimensional assessment was given to all. A further in-depth assessment with a nurse was given universally to all in one group and only to those targeted by the initial assessment in another group. Referrals as necessary were made according to protocol. Follow up was for 3 years.

No differences in mortality or admission were noted in any of the groups. The improvements found were small enough for the authors to conclude that multidimensional assessment makes no difference to outcomes when the elderly are screened in a manner such as this.

Prevalence of five common clinical abnormalities in very elderly people: population based cross sectional study
de Craen AJM, Gussekloo J, Teng YKO *et al.*
BMJ, 2003; **327**: 131–132

This study looked at the prevalence of five clinical conditions in a group of over 500 people over 85 years.

The number of newly identified patients with anaemia (<13 g/dl in men, <12 g/dl in women) was three times the number previously known and documented.

As a percentage of total cases in the participants, the new cases of:
- diabetes accounted for 10% of all the diabetics
- thyroid dysfunction accounted for 16% of the total
- AF accounted for 42% of the total
- hypertension (>160/95) accounted for 19% of the total

Over 90% of all participants (except for those with previously unidentified AF where it was closer to 80%) had consulted their GP within the previous year.

It is difficult to know what conclusions we should draw about how we should

198

deal with these results but where there is a disease state and opportunity to pick it up, there is food for thought.

RESIDENTIAL CARE

A national census of care home residents
Bowman C, Whistler J, Ellerby M.
Age & Ageing, 2004; **33**: 561–566

This survey of more than 15 000 residents of private nursing homes clarifies the high dependency need of the residents. These data were previously poorly described but essential for commissioning care.

Some 75% were in 'nursing' care and 25% were 'residential', but there was considerable overlap in dependency.

- More than 50% of residents had dementia, stroke or other neurodegenerative disease.
- 78% had at least one form of mental impairment.
- 76% of residents required assistance with their mobility or were immobile.
- 71% were incontinent.
- 27% of the population were immobile, confused and incontinent.

Chronic disease progression and related disability were the principal determinants of the need for residential care in over 90% of residents, rather than the sometimes suggested mix of frailty and social factors.

Case management for elderly people in the community
Black DA
BMJ, 2007; **334**: 3–4
and
Impact of case management (Evercare) on frail elderly patients: controlled before and after analysis of quantitative outcome data
Gravelle H, Dusheiko M, Sheaff R *et al.*
BMJ, 2007; **334**: 31

A UK pilot study looking at case management for frail elderly people, trailblazed a role for the community matron. The Evercare model piloted this in 10 PCTs following US research that nurse practitioners could save money by reducing admissions of long-stay nursing home residents to hospital.

The Department of Health invested enthusiastically, combining elements of nurse-led assessment and intensive case management, only this was in the community not in a nursing home setting.

During the study period there were no significant effects on rates of admission, use of emergency departments or mortality for this high-risk population. Additional services were put in place and people seem to like the extra service but the evidence base for the intervention is weak and the role of nurse practitioners in this area is not supported by evidence. Criticism about failure to produce a properly controlled study before this investment followed. Public funds had largely been spent on travel, consultancy fees and going on courses.

Nurse practitioners seem not to be able to replace a proven intervention such as a comprehensive geriatric assessment as an inpatient, which has been shown to reduce mortality, institutionalisation, and improve function.

Effect of family style mealtimes on quality of life, physical performance, and body weight of nursing home residents: cluster randomised controlled trial
Nijs K, de Graaf C, Kok F *et al.*
BMJ, 2006; **332**: 1180–1184

This Dutch study encouraged family style mealtimes (being served in a group at a dressed dinner table with a choice of food and a member of staff at the table) for nursing home residents, average age 77 years. Although the study was impossible to blind, they found that this simple social interaction maintained quality of life, physical performance and body weight in preference to similar nutritional content eaten from trays. This more convivial approach provides a sense of ambience, structure, security and meaning in a more stimulating environment to ease the psychosocial elements of 'the anorexia of ageing'.

MEDICATION

Sedative hypnotics in older people: meta-analysis of risks and benefits
Glass J, Lanctôt KL, Herrmann N *et al.*
BMJ, 2005; **331**: 1169

More than 10 million prescriptions for hypnotics are dispensed each year in England – 80% are for people over 65 years.

In people over 60, sedative hypnotics do improve the quality of sleep but only in a small way and not enough to outweigh the disadvantages, according to this meta-analysis of 24 RCTs and 2400 participants which looked at any pharmacological agent used for at least five days.

The NNT for improved sleep quality was 13 and the number needed to harm for any adverse event was 6. This ratio indicates that an adverse event is roughly twice as likely as enhanced quality of sleep. Those particularly at risk of falls or who already have cognitive impairment will not get a net benefit. Non-pharmacological therapies such as CBT have been shown to be just as good for insomnia in older people.

DEMENTIA

Improving the management of dementia
England E
BMJ, 2006; **332**: 681–682

This editorial discussed the underdetection and poor management of dementia in the UK.

Unfortunately it rarely presents with clear, well demarcated symptoms. Diagnosis is confusing and there is little training of primary care teams. Tools to aid diagnosis are often not culturally sensitive and community services are often not well coordinated.

The new GMS contract from 2006 highlights dementia with an expectation of improved record keeping, introduction of a dementia register and evidence that patients' needs have been reviewed in the previous 15 months. NICE nevertheless only recommends drug treatment for Alzheimer's in later disease.

Effectiveness of educational interventions in improving detection and management of dementia in primary care: cluster randomised controlled study

Downs M, Turner S, Bryans M *et al.*
BMJ, 2006; **332**: 692–696

Thirty-five UK practices were randomised to new approaches to improved detection of signs of dementia.

Decision support software which is now incorporated into the popular EMIS practice system and is available to 5000 practices in the UK was a simple, practical and successful tool.

Practice-based workshops also significantly improved rates of detection although no intervention led to improvements in management of the cases of dementia.

Cholinesterase inhibitors may be effective in Alzheimer's disease. *Evidence-Based Medicine,* 2006; **11**: 23
The following paper is reviewed
Cholinesterase inhibitors for patients with Alzheimer's disease: systematic review of randomised clinical trials.

Kaduszkiewicz H, Zimmermann T, Beck-Bornholdt HP, *et al.*
BMJ, 2005; **331**: 321–327

NICE sanctions the use of cholinesterase inhibitors in mild to moderate Alzheimer's disease. The consensus at the moment is that they probably have a small beneficial effect on cognition and perhaps behaviour in some patients, but the clinical significance seems arguable. Clinicians often argue that they work in a subset of 10–20% which cannot be identified in advance and so all should be treated.

This systematic review looked at the current evidence surrounding use of cholinesterase inhibitors (donepezil, rivastigmine, or galantamine) in Alzheimer's disease.

The authors found 12 placebo-controlled randomised trials that examined clinical outcomes and identified many areas of poor methodology and possible bias in the published studies. They do nothing to change that consensus.

Good evidence is lacking on treating Alzheimer's disease with these costly drugs. How to identify responders, how long to treat and cost-effectiveness are as elusive as ever.

Non-degenerative mild cognitive impairment in elderly people and use of anticholinergic drugs: longitudinal cohort study

Ancelin ML, Artero S, Portet F *et al.*
BMJ, 2006; **332**: 455–459

This valuable study, in 372 people aged over 60 years in 63 general practices in France, looked at use of anticholinergics and their impact on cognition.

OLDER PEOPLE

As doctors try to spot signs of dementia early, we will need to think how many subtle effects can be explained by drugs.

Polypharmacy is common in the elderly and many drugs have anticholinergic effects including antiemetics, antispasmodics, bronchodilators, antiarrhythmics, antihistamines, analgesics, antihypertensives, antiparkinsonian agents, steroids, ulcer drugs, and psychotropic drugs.

In this study, nearly 10% of subjects used at least one of these drugs for extended periods. Eighty per cent of continuous users were classed as cognitively impaired compared with 35% of non-users. They performed poorly in reaction time, attention, narrative memory, visuospatial construction and language tasks, but not on tasks of reasoning, recall of lists or implicit memory. The patients whose impairment could be explained by the medication were no more likely to deteriorate into dementia.

Some of these, slightly ridiculously, may end up being considered candidates for pro-cholinergic agents.

The ageing brain is easier to poison – the blood–brain barrier is leakier, metabolism is slower and drug elimination is impaired. Use of many non-prescription compounds can further muddy the waters. Doctors need to start associating cognitive dysfunction with anticholinergic toxicity.

PALLIATIVE CARE

Developing primary palliative care
Murray SA, Boyd K, Sheikh A *et al.*
BMJ, 2004; **329**:1056–1057

This editorial argues in favour of the need for coherent services in palliative care within primary care.

Many chronic diseases such as COPD and cardiac failure could benefit from such a structure and doctors might identify those in need of it by asking themselves a simple question – 'Would I be surprised if my patient were to die in the next 12 months?'.

There is uncertainty about the most effective models of care but all agree on a need to target symptoms and maintain quality of life.

GPs with their patient-centred holistic approach in the community and hopefully patient trust are ideally placed to be a part of this. Training GPs with a special interest in palliative care could be one way to enhance collaborative care. Unfortunately out of hours services are even less well set up to facilitate dying at home than they were before.

From April 2006, with the new GMS contract, additional Quality and Outcomes Framework points have been awarded for holding a palliative care register and reviewing those patients on the register at a multidisciplinary team meeting at least three-monthly.

OLDER PEOPLE

Population-based study of place of death of patients with cancer: implications for GPs
Aabom B, Kragstrup J, Vondeling H *et al.*
Br J Gen Pract, 2005; **55**: 684–689

This Danish study showed that the home visits made by GPs and, to a lesser extent, community nurses in the final 3 months of a patient's life were inversely associated with dying in hospital regardless of the nature of the disease.

The GP clearly still has an important role if we wish to facilitate our patients' wishes in their final challenge. However, now that out-of-hours responsibility has changed, it remains to be seen if GPs explore this and if financial backing occurs or whether this may be another role for a specialist nurse with prescribing powers.

Good end-of-life care according to patients and their GPs
Borgsteede SD, Graafland-Riedstra C, Deliens L *et al.*
Br J Gen Pract, 2006; **56**: 20–26

This study interviewed GPs and their patients who had a life expectancy of less than 6 months due to cancer, COPD or heart failure.

Feelings of both doctors and carers were comparable. Areas consistently thought to be important were continuity of care and availability of GPs for home visits outside of traditional hours, as well as professional competence and cooperation with other members of the care team. The more modern, slightly fractured ways of delivering primary care such as part-time jobs and restricted home visits may threaten these valued aspects.

Care of people dying with malignant and cardiorespiratory disease in general practice
McKinley RK, Stokes T, Exley C *et al.*
Br J Gen Pract, 2004: **54**: 909–913

A review of GP records in two UK practices compared care in the last year of life for those with malignant disease to those with cardiorespiratory disease.

The cancer patients were more likely to have had the end of their life identified as such and more likely to have had palliative medication as a result. Both groups otherwise had similar demands in terms of comorbidity and number of consultations. This implies that there may be unmet needs in terms of symptom control in patients who are dying but who have not been identified as terminal.

INFORMAL CARERS

Health of young and elderly informal carers: analysis of UK census data
Doran T, Drever F, Whitehead M
BMJ, 2003; **327**: 1388

This study quantified the burden on informal carers in the UK. For the first time, information from the entire population was gathered on the 2001 census.

Nearly 6 million people are informal carers. Only around half are in good health.

OLDER PEOPLE

- Of children between 5 and 15 years, 114 000 (1.4%) provided informal care.
- Of those over 65 years, more than a million (12%) were informal carers, roughly evenly split between men and women.
- The oldest age group – the over 85s – still contained 44 000 carers, most of whom provided more than 50 hours a week and one third of these rated their health as 'not good'.
- At least 50 hours a week of care were provided by nearly 9000 children and 381 000 over 65s. This is a large burden for children and pensioners. Paid employees would be in violation of the European Working Time Directive.

Training carers of stroke patients: randomised controlled trial
Kalra L, Evans A, Perez I et al.
BMJ, 2004; **328**: 1099

Informal caregivers provide an enormous service to society but receive little training for their role and their needs are often sidelined.

This study looked at the caregivers of 300 stroke patients and found that simple training in basic skills of moving and handling, and simple nursing tasks, reduced the burden of care and improved quality of life in patients and caregivers.

Carers had better psychological outcomes at 3 and 12 months, better 'job' satisfaction and significantly reduced anxiety and depression.

Mortality of patients and number of hospital admissions were similar in both groups but the training markedly reduced costs associated with stroke care. Patients achieved independence at an earlier stage.

FALLS

Preventing falls in elderly people living in hospitals and care homes
Cameron ID, Kurrle S
BMJ, 2007; **334**: 53
and
Strategies to prevent falls and fractures in hospitals and care homes and effect of cognitive impairment: systematic review and meta-analyses
Oliver D, Connelly JB, Victor CR et al.
BMJ, 2007; **334**: 82

This meta-analysis and accompanying editorial describes the certainty and uncertainty surrounding prevention of falls.
- The best outcome of falls to measure is the number of falls prevented rather than reductions in the overall number of fallers.
- Multifaceted interventions in hospital significantly reduce falls but not fallers or fractures.
- Hip protectors significantly reduce hip fractures in care homes but not numbers of falls (there were too few studies on fallers).
- There was no evidence that presence of dementia or cognitive impairment influences the effect of any interventions.
- There is no evidence that effectiveness is improved by adherence.

OLDER PEOPLE

- Evidence was inconclusive for multifaceted interventions in care homes (or any single intervention other than hip protectors including calcium/vitamin D or exercise in care homes).
- Harms such as risks of increased falling with some interventions are not specifically addressed in this review.
- The cornerstones of care remain adequate supervision, encouragement of mobility, individually tailored aids, a safe environment, sensible prescribing, and early treatment of medical complications. Future studies into a standardised multifactorial intervention should involve these elements.

Effectiveness protectors for preventing hip fractures in elderly people: systematic review
Parker MJ, Gillespie WJ, Gillespie LD
BMJ, 2006; **332**: 571–573
and
Hip protectors to prevent femoral fracture
de Rooij SE
BMJ, 2006; **332**: 559–560

This update of a previous systematic review included further studies and ended up revising its original conclusions that hip protectors seem to reduce hip fracture.

Selection bias, publication bias or design and reporting flaws were examined in the context of new evidence. Hip protectors are uncomfortable and unattractive and poor compliance itself also presents huge problems of analysis as well as of interpretation.

Also, different hip protectors may have different effectiveness.

The bottom line is that when people are randomised as individuals rather than in clusters, hip protectors were found to be ineffective for those living at home.

Whether or not they work in institutionalised care is questionable.

The accompanying editorial describes that, in the light of this evidence, these devices should not be widely used until studies show benefit. Hip protectors may yet show some value in specific subgroups of the elderly – perhaps highly motivated people at high risk of fracture where use is backed up by encouragement from nursing staff.

MEDICALLY UNEXPLAINED PHYSICAL SYMPTOMS

What we know already:

- GPs feel that about one-fifth of patients who consult them have physical symptoms not explained by a disease process
- Medically unexplained conditions are poorly understood and thought to represent complex adaptive systems related to biological, psychological, and social factors
- These symptoms generally do not conveniently cluster into well-defined distinct syndromes
- Many patients receive a lot of largely ineffective investigations and treatments in primary care
- Chronic fatigue is severe fatigue causing functional impairment lasting longer than six months
- Chronic fatigue syndrome (CFS) on the other hand is less common and has a more complex definition
- The existence of CFS has been questioned down the years leading to breakdown in communication between doctors and the public
- In a UK survey of 1000 GPs, half did not feel confident with making a diagnosis of CFS/ME and 41% did not feel confident in treatment options
- Parental labelling of children with 'ME' bears no correlation with definitions of CFS
- Treating co-existent anxiety/depression may help alleviate physical symptoms
- Systematic review shows that cognitive behaviour therapy improves pain, disability, and depression in chronic back pain and probably has positive effects in chronic fatigue syndrome

Recent Papers

THE DOCTOR–PATIENT RELATIONSHIP

Managing patients with inexplicable health problems
Fischhoff B, Wessely S
BMJ, 2003; **326**: 595–597

This paper looks at how we go about communicating with patients whose symptoms we cannot explain.

Doctors need to take measures to avoid alienating these patients. The potential for conflict is clear. Patients want explanations and treatments. Doctors want diagnostic certainty. Add in a limited time factor and the potential could be explosive or at least deeply unsatisfactory.

We need to develop trust so we can start to try to comprehend patients' illness beliefs and focus on the facts that most matter to them, e.g. what decisions they are currently facing and which beliefs/misconceptions provide the greatest barriers. If we have information to impart it should be delivered in an organised manner perhaps using a narrative technique that encourages progress. We need to acknowledge uncertainty and avoid certainty where there is none, as loss of trust could send us back to square one. Avoiding the lay label of the hour may seem to reinforce the disability but a strategy of compromise labelling which incorporates and expands on the lay name may lead to better communication. Use of the CFS/ME moniker is such an example. Focusing on symptom relief shows compassion and allows us to avoid the labelling trap.

Do patients with unexplained physical symptoms pressurise general practitioners for somatic treatment? A qualitative study
Ring A, Dowrick C, Humphris G *et al.*
BMJ, 2004; **328**: 1057

This paper examined how patients with unexplained symptoms might pressure their GP for somatic management. Analysing audiotapes of consultations in practices in Merseyside, they found 36 relevant consultations where the doctor agreed that symptoms had existed for at least 3 months, caused significant distress (to the patient) and could not be explained by a recognisable physical disease.
- Abdominal symptoms, headache and limb pain were the most common complaints.
- All but two received somatic treatments.
- Most received a prescription although few asked for one.
- No patient asked for investigation or referral but nearly half received this.
- Reasons for this are usually attributed to pressure from patients.

Patients seem to convey the need for a response while curtailing the doctor's ability to deliver it, putting pressure on GPs in subtle ways by:
- conveying their suffering with graphic and emotive language
- emphasising social effects of symptoms
- describing complex symptom patterns
- negating a doctor's attempts at explanation
- refering to other individuals, e.g. family, as testimony to the severity of symptoms
- using biomedical explanations

The authors state that this research does not support the assumption that patients with unexplained symptoms pressure GPs for symptomatic treatments. This may reflect the need to maintain a long-term relationship. Doctors may respond with symptomatic treatments if they mistake patients' needs, if they lack another solution or if they just feel too helpless.

But if the game is softball in general practice, it is hardball in hospital outpatients. Research in secondary care, where patients may only get one shot at the consultation, shows that treatments are explicitly requested, consequences of the doctor's failure to supply them are trumpeted, and blame is put on doctors for worsening their lot.

Voiced but unheard agendas: qualitative analysis of the psychosocial cues that patients with unexplained symptoms present to general practitioners
Salmon P, Dowrick CF, Ring A et al.
Br J Gen Pract, 2004; **54**: 171–176
and
Normalisation of unexplained symptoms by general practitioners: a functional typology
Dowrick CF, Ring A, Humphris G M et al.
Br J Gen Pract, 2004; **54**: 165–170

This research examined audiotapes of 36 consultations to see whether patients who are considered to have medically unexplained symptoms give opportunities to GPs discuss psychological issues. All but two presented these opportunities. Patients perceived emotional and social problems as symptoms of mood disorder or stress and asked questions about symptoms with explicit concern, cautious reference to more serious possibilities, and even suggestions that disease may be absent.

By missing these cues to tackle elements of their problem with a new perspective, unnecessary symptomatic interventions were used.

Dangers still persist if normalisation – simple empty reassurance – is used without making this relevant to patients' concerns. The patients were much more likely to accept an effective narrative that linked their physical symptoms with psychological factors.

Management of medically unexplained symptoms
Rosendal M, Olesen F, Fink P
BMJ, 2005; **330**: 4–5

This editorial reinforces the need to avoid forcing patients into a biomedical model. Cognitive behaviour therapy is very effective and can be learned and applied by GPs after brief training. Patients accept a combined biological and psychological approach. We know reassuring patients that they are normal is not enough; it is time therefore to adjust our paradigms about the way we communicate, so we can give these patients the same standard of care as we try to for 'medically explainable' symptoms.

CHRONIC FATIGUE

What causes chronic fatigue syndrome?
White PD
BMJ, 2004; **329**: 928–929

Chronic fatigue syndrome, also known as myalgic encephalomyelitis, and increasingly by the shorthand CFS/ME, is an illness of unknown nature and cause, but its existence is generally accepted.

Markers of predisposition for the conditon are being female, having a premorbid mood disorder, and increased use of their GP for up to 15 years prior to diagnosis. Although there may be viral triggers, there is no evidence of ongoing

MEDICALLY UNEXPLAINED PHYSICAL SYMPTOMS

infection. Cortisol levels tend to be low but this may be due to sedentary activity and there is no recognised biological marker for the condition. The heterogeneity of the group makes research tricky.

A paper in the same issue as this editorial (*BMJ*, 2004; **329**: 941) examined the British birth cohort from 1970 and found that 10 year olds whose mothers reported that they 'never or hardly ever' played sport in their spare time had twice the risk of CFS in adulthood.

Other risk factors for children were a limiting long-standing physical condition in childhood and higher social class (remember the term 'yuppie flu'?). However, in contrast to previous studies, there was no associated incidence of CFS/ME with maternal or childhood psychological problems, birth weight, obesity, school absence/ability, and parental illness.

Inactivity increases the perception of effort during exercise – this awareness is a phenomenon called interoception. This can be reprogrammed with graded exercise therapy which along with cognitive behavioural therapy has been shown to be effective.

General practitioners' perceptions of chronic fatigue syndrome and beliefs about its management, compared with irritable bowel syndrome: qualitative study
Raine R, Carter S, Sensky T *et al.*
BMJ, 2004; **328**: 1354–1357

GPs tend to negatively stereotype patients with CFS but not patients with irritable bowel syndrome.

Discussions with a random sample of 46 UK doctors identified these reasons for antipathy towards CFS cases:
- lack of a precise bodily location which would allow a plausible pathological mechanism
- reclassification and relabelling of the condition over time
- patients can be seen as using the sick role to flout the work ethic
- conflict between doctor and patient over causes and management

These barriers to effective clinical management explain why doctors feel less comfortable and more hopeless dealing with CFS rather than irritable bowel syndrome.

Referral for mental health interventions, which have been proven to be useful, was unlikely as many doctors were not familiar with the interventions or thought them unavailable or unnecessary.

The management of children with chronic fatigue syndrome-like illness in primary care: a cross-sectional study
Saidi G, Haines L
Br J Gen Pract, 2006; **56**: 43–47

Little is known about the characteristics of children with CFS/ME who present to primary care. This survey identified around 100 patients from 62 practices aged 5–19 years who consulted their GP with severe fatigue lasting over 3 months and who filled in questionnaires which were considered by a clinical panel to meet CFS criteria.
- 73% were girls, 94% were white, mean age was 12.9 years, and median illness duration was 3.3 years.

- GPs had principal responsibility for 62%.
- A diagnosis of CFS/ME was made in 55%, one-third of these within 6 months.
- Half had illness of moderate severity.
- Paediatric referrals were made in 82% and psychiatric referrals in 46% (median time of 2 and 13 months respectively).
- Advice was given on setting activity goals, pacing, rest and graded exercise.

GPs look after the majority of these patients and seem to be successful in fairly rapid diagnosis and appropriate interventions. Cases were milder than in tertiary care but similar in characteristics.

IRRITABLE BOWEL SYNDROME

Prevalence of irritable bowel syndrome: a community survey
Wilson S, Roberts L, Roalfe A et al.
Br J Gen Pract, 2004; **54**: 495–502

This postal survey from Birmingham set out to find a true prevalence for irritable bowel syndrome (IBS).

A follow up survey went to patients with positive symptoms and, with a return of 57%, they found that:
- prevalence of IBS was 10.5% – 7% of men and 14% of women
- reduced quality of life was marked with symptom profiles characterised by diarrhoea (25%), constipation (24%) and alternating symptoms (47%)
- over half had consulted their GP within the previous 6 months and 16% had been referred to hospital
- the majority self-medicated with over-the-counter medication and alternative therapies
- less than half of those reporting symptoms of IBS according to the well-validated Rome II criteria had received a diagnosis of IBS

A randomised controlled trial of self-help interventions in patients with a primary care diagnosis of irritable bowel syndrome
Robinson A, Lee V, Kennedy A et al.
Gut, 2006; **55**: 643–648

A self-help book incorporating best evidence on lifestyle, diet, drugs and alternative treatments for IBS was studied in a randomised trial over a year.

Based on intention to treat, there were an average of 1.5 fewer primary care consultations and 0.22 fewer hospital consultations from those who received the book. This group reported slightly greater global improvement in illness even though there was no specific effect on symptoms or quality of life.

An additional self-help group session had no discernable impact, but the book seemed to make a measurable difference.

MEDICALLY UNEXPLAINED PHYSICAL SYMPTOMS

Cognitive behaviour therapy in addition to antispasmodic treatment for irritable bowel syndrome in primary care: randomised controlled trial
Kennedy T, Jones R, Darnley S
BMJ, 2005; **331**: 435–437

Of 149 patients with moderate or severe IBS who were all taking but were resistant to mebeverine, half were randomised to additional CBT given by primary care nurses. Additional benefit on the severity of symptoms was shown at 6 months and this may be a useful intervention for some that can be performed in primary care. The effect was wearing off by the end of the year however.

MEDICALLY UNEXPLAINED PHYSICAL SYMPTOMS

DEPRESSION

What we know already:

- Depressive disorder is a major health problem in primary care. Costs reach around £9 billion in England each year and reductions in quality of life are comparable to those seen in major chronic physical diseases
- Depressive disorders accompany many chronically morbid physical disorders
- Nine out of ten depressed patients are treated only in primary care
- Only 40% of patients are diagnosed on the first consultation but review increases pick-up rates. Up to half of these disorders remain undetected including one in six who has severe symptoms of depression
- Screening is not improved by routinely administered questionnaires prior to consultation
- About half of these disorders remain undetected including one in six who have severe symptoms of depression
- Half resolve without treatment. The danger of missing depression in the past may therefore have been overstated but undertreatment is still identified as a major problem
- Effective treatments include medication, psychological techniques, exercise and self-help materials
- There is no significant difference in efficacy between SSRIs and tricyclics but withdrawal from treatment is more common with tricyclics
- Depression in primary care may have a different aetiology and natural history from cases in secondary care. Research on these milder levels of depression and dysthymia is sparse
- Outcomes improve with enhanced follow-up by telephone or direct contact with primary care and mental health workers. Some psychotherapies may simply have a compliance-enhancing effect
- The Hampshire Depression Project educated GPs on use of a clinical practice guideline. It failed to increase diagnosis or treatment of depression, implying that the problem is more complex than researchers may have thought
- GPs can be effective in cognitive behaviour therapy (CBT) after an extensive instruction programme. However, brief training for GPs does not improve patient outcomes but does increase referral rates
- Suicide rates are higher in those who have a history of parasuicide by a factor of at least 40 – an effect that persists for at least 2 years
- The idea that parasuicide and suicide involves different populations has turned out to be untrue
- Women have higher rates of deliberate self-harm and parasuicide than men
- Up to 15% of those with unipolar depression eventually commit suicide
- About one in six people repeat self-harm within a year of an episode
- 3–5% of those who self-harm commit suicide with 10 years
- Physical conditions such as visual impairment, malignancy and neurological illness are strongly linked with suicide in the elderly

Guidelines

The National Service Framework (NSF) for mental health was released in September 1999 to improve quality and structure of mental health services. It has seven standards focusing on mental health promotion and addresses standards for primary care, prevention of suicides and the problems of carers.

Depression: management of depression in primary and secondary care. *NICE*, December 2004

The short-term physical and psychological management and secondary prevention of self-harm in primary and secondary care. *NICE*, 2004.

Recent Papers

GENERAL

NICE guidelines for the management of depression
Middleton H, Shaw I, Hull S et al.
BMJ, 2005; **330**: 267–268

The NICE guidelines advocate a stepped care approach, clarifying guidance on treatment of moderate to severe depression with SSRIs as the first choice of medication. They support the use of CBT but no other psychodynamic psychotherapies.

The advice for mild depression will not be much help in uncertain decisions when a particular case may or may not benefit from medication, but this reflects the evidence available.

These milder presentations may be subthreshold disorders where doctors allow the medicalisation of unhappiness in order to legitimise the engagement, when all that people may really need in these times of growing social isolation is some support.

DETECTING DEPRESSION

Should we screen for depression?
Gilbody S, Sheldon T, Wessely S
BMJ, 2006; **332**: 1027–1030

GPs are increasingly being required to screen patients for depression as part of their enhanced services.

NICE recommends targeting those at high risk but screening programmes need to ensure they do more good than harm and in the case of depression this is far from clear.

A variety of screening questionnaires have been used but practices rarely keep using them once the trial is over. A prevalence of under 10% makes even a test with good sensitivity and specificity have a positive predictive value of under 50%, leading to a lot of unnecessary follow-up. In addition, there is little to suggest that patients appreciate this sort of screening very much.

Although drugs and psychological interventions are effective, they are less so in cases of mild depression – perhaps the very depression that GPs see most often. Even prescribing of drugs can be somewhat *ad hoc*, with drugs not continued for as long as they should be.

Evidence is therefore scant that screening improves outcomes.

It would seem to be a 'no-brainer' to screen those at high risk such as those with physical illnesses or alcohol problems, but there are no studies that evaluated this strategy. With a lack of randomised data on the harms of screening (stigma, medicalisation, discrimination by insurance companies, etc.), the authors do not recommend even this approach.

Screening has a role when good collaborative care systems are in place, for example, in diabetics already attending a review process on a regular basis.

Population strategies will only be effective when our efforts minimise the chronic long-term effects of this relapsing condition rather than uncover more minor morbidity that may have got better without interference.

Although screening for depression does not yet meet the criteria of the National Screening Committee, this fact seems to have been bypassed by the enormous size of the problem and the availability of antidepressants.

Managing depression in primary care
Tylee A, Jones R
BMJ, 2005; **330**: 800–801

Primary care is still the 'right place' for most depression to be treated but it is easy to criticise primary care for its role in depression and the concerns over SSRIs has not helped. There are many reasons why we fail to pick up the diagnosis:
- patients may attribute symptoms wrongly
- patients insufficiently active in seeking care, feeling undeserving of the doctor's time and uncertain whether the problems were legitimate
- presentation of physical rather than psychological symptoms
- patients may attend too infrequently
- GPs may have negative attitudes towards mental health problems and may lack time or consulting skills

Screening for depression in primary care with two verbally asked questions: cross sectional study
Arroll B, Khin N, Kerse N
BMJ, 2003; **327**: 1144–1146

This New Zealand study validated a two-question tool for screening for depression.

Screening tests are usually in written form but importantly here the questions were asked verbally. They were:
- during the last month have you often been bothered by feeling down, depressed, or hopeless?
- during the past month have you often been bothered by little interest or pleasure doing things?

A positive screen occurred when either question was positive and prompted further assessment.

They picked up most of the cases of depression with a sensitivity of 97% and a reasonable specificity of 67% – acceptable for screening in a 'low prevalence' setting. After asking the two questions, the GP diagnosis had a sensitivity of 77%, a specificity of 86%, a positive likelihood ratio of 5.4, and a negative likelihood ratio of 0.27 (the PPV was 27% and the NPV 98.2%).

DEPRESSION

The intervention is pleasingly brief, has reasonable statistics and avoids the use of more cumbersome questionnaires.

Effect of the addition of a 'help' question to two screening questions on specificity for diagnosis of depression in general practice: diagnostic validity study
Arroll B, Goodyear-Smith F, Kerse N *et al.*
BMJ, 2005; **331**: 884

An extension to this system added a third question
  • 'is this something with which you would like help?'
The three possible responses are 'no,' 'yes, but not today,' or 'yes'.

The help question alone had a sensitivity of 75% and a specificity of 94%. It improved the GP diagnosis to a specificity of 94% without changing sensitivity, making it a good way to avoid false negatives.

The study was carried out in a community setting by GPs, in consecutive patients, excluding those on psychotropic drugs. The authors suggest using these questions on all new patients who have not been to see their GP for about 2 years.

How many conditions can a GP screen for?
Del Mar C, Glasziou P
BMJ, 2003; **327**: 1117

This editorial accompanies the paper above with a review of our changing practices. It is an interesting article which casts doubt on our way of detecting disease. It challenges the role of taking a thorough history as an 'unhelpful' approach. The era of doctors formulating their plans from a muddle of questions may be ending. Its effectiveness is after all unproven and largely based on habit and ritual.

Clinical prediction rules may help us separate the 'wheat from the chaff' in future. The Mini-Cog, for example, shows promise for detecting dementia but more such tools are needed as we are at the dawn of the 'diagnostic age'. Our rituals will be exposed and the useless habits discarded. Not without a fight of course; we will not give up our old-fashioned clothing easily. The authors predict a deeper impact on our daily work from this concentrated approach to evidence-based diagnostics than we have seen so far for evidence-based interventions.

ANTIDEPRESSANTS

A qualitative study exploring how GPs decide to prescribe antidepressants
Hyde J, Calnan M, Prior L *et al.*
Br J Gen Pract, 2005; **55**: 755–762

A qualitative study of 27 Bristol GPs found that:
  • GPs balance clinical and social criteria in the decision to employ antidepressants
  • the preferred strategy is 'wait and see', but antidepressants are used appropriately earlier in illness that is perceived as severe, classic or persisting
  • decisions depend on time constraints, lack of alternative psychological services options, cost of prescribing, and perceived attitude of patients
  • this suggests the 'watchful waiting' guidance of NICE will be well received

Efficacy of antidepressants in adults
Moncrieff J, Kirsch I
BMJ, 2005; **331**: 155–157

> This controversial but fascinating paper suggests that, after all, antidepressants have no clinically meaningful benefit.
>
> The NICE meta-analysis of placebo-controlled trials, they argue, identifies differences in symptoms so small as to be unlikely to be clinical important. This is consistent with other meta-analyses performed.
>
> Lack of consensus on what an important difference is does not help. Statistical aberrations such as publication bias and methodological aberrations such as poor blinding may explain the small levels of apparent superiority seen.
>
> In addition they argue that the claim that antidepressants work better for severe rather than mild depression is far from proven.
>
> The paper calls for a re-evaluation of our entire approach to treating depression and a need to address the now raised expectations of society.

Efficacy and safety of second-generation antidepressants in the treatment of major depressive disorder
Hansen RA, Gartlehner G, Lohr KN et al.
Ann Intern Med, 2005; **143**: 415–426

> Reviewing 46 head-to-head randomised, controlled trials comparing one second-generation antidepressant with another, this systematic review found no major differences in the numbers of adults with major depression who responded to any particular drug. Adverse events varied in nature but not incidence.
>
> Almost all (96%) of these trials were sponsored by the pharmaceutical industry or had financial ties to the industry. Sponsorship was associated with a 5% advantage for the sponsor's drug over the comparator drug, and publication bias obscured the evidence even further.

PSYCHOTHERAPY

The future of psychotherapy in the NHS
Goldbeck-Wood S
BMJ, 2004; **329**: 245–246

> This editorial provides a nice review of the controversial role of and evidence in favour of psychotherapy.
>
> Demand for services is great but its legitimacy has never been more in question. The government is in favour of patient choice but evidence on cost-effectiveness is patchy at best.
>
> Neither is psychotherapy formally recognised as a profession. Regulation is voluntary and treatments delivered behind the closed doors of the therapist are a lottery for patients. Attitudes of some have not helped open the door to government money and interventions are in danger of appearing to be a private luxury for the wealthy.
>
> The therapist may be the most important factor in treatment rather than the type

DEPRESSION

of therapy chosen but relapse rates still look high. Someone needs to get off their couch and produce some serious evidence.

COGNITIVE BEHAVIOURAL THERAPY

Cognitive behaviour therapy reduced relapses in recurrent major depressive disorder. *Evidence-Based Medicine,* 2005; **10**: 82
The following paper is reviewed
Six-year outcome of cognitive behavior therapy for prevention of recurrent depression
Fava GA, Ruini C, Rafanelli C *et al.*
Am J Psychiatry, 2004; **161**: 1872–1876

This small study of 45 patients with three or more episodes of depression used 30-minute sessions of CBT once a fortnight while antidepressants were tapered off. Relapse rates were only 25% compared with 80% on usual treatment. The low relapse rate was maintained over 4 years, at which point it was 40% (compared to 80% with usual care).

The study is interesting if not generalisable. All the interventions were performed by the same psychiatrist who achieved a 100% follow up in his loyal patients.

A further study summarised in *BMJ* (2005; **331** – 5 Nov) randomised over 170 people to an 8 week course of CBT. Those at highest risk (with five or more episodes of major depression in the past) had an absolute risk reduction of 26% with CBT (NNT of only 4). The benefits lasted for the duration of the trial. Extraordinarily, it did not prevent relapses for those with fewer episodes of depression, but seemed to prolong remission only for those at highest risk.

Opportunity cost of antidepressant prescribing in England: analysis of routine data
Hollinghurst S, Kessler D, Peters TJ *et al.*
BMJ, 2005; **330**: 999–1000

Resources associated with threefold increases in levels of NHS antidepressant prescribing in England between 1991 and 2002 could have employed 7700 therapists (26 per PCT) to deliver six sessions of CBT to 1.5 million patients – more than one-third of adults with depression or mixed anxiety depression.

Although not a perfect cost analysis, this study gives us an idea that this alternative to antidepressants may actually float.

POSTNATAL DEPRESSION

Psychosocial and psychological interventions for prevention of postnatal depression: systematic review
Dennis C
BMJ, 2005; **331**: 15

Postnatal depression is a major health issue. Sufferers are likely to experience future depression and endure impaired maternal–infant interactions. Psychological and psychosocial risk factors such as life stress, marital conflict, self esteem, and lack of social support have been identified.

This systematic review of 15 trials, however, did not find that any diverse interventions in these areas in the form of classes, debriefings and interpersonal psychotherapy, reduced the number who went on to develop postnatal depression. Targeting of at-risk women may be more effective.

MANAGEMENT PROGRAMMES

Long term outcomes from the IMPACT randomised trial for depressed elderly patients in primary care
Hunkeler EM, Katon W, Tang L et al.
BMJ, 2006; **332**: 259–263

Few studies deal specifically with the needs of elderly depressed patients.

The IMPACT trial – Improving Mood Promoting Access to Collaborative Treatment – involved 1801 patients, mean age 71 years, who met the DSM-IV criteria for major depression or dysthymia. The trial has already reported benefits in outcome over a year with a management programme involving a depression care manager (a nurse or psychologist), who personalises and supports a treatment plan which may use drugs and psychological modalities in liaison with a psychiatrist and a primary care physician.

The intervention group used more drugs and more psychotherapy, raising the suggestion that the case worker may just have removed some barriers to accessing care.

However, this further study extends the original findings.

One year after IMPACT resources were withdrawn, the active engagement of these elderly and often reluctant patients was still paying dividends in terms of less depression, healthier lives and better physical functioning.

The particular care manager may be an important factor as it was still not possible to determine which part of the package led to the enduring benefits.

Collaborative care for depression
Simon G
BMJ, 2006; **332**: 249–250
and
Depression should be managed like a chronic disease
Scott J
BMJ, 2006; **332**: 985–986

Undertreatment has resulted from doctors failing to prescribe effectively and from patients failing to take their drugs. Non-specific counselling is not going to solve the problems of case management and even CBT is not for everybody.

Collabarative care models, however, have successfully used structured collaboration between patient, specialist and primary carers combined with evidence-based protocols to actively monitor adherence to treatment and clinical outcomes. These two editorials note that evidence has consistently shown the value and the acceptability of this strategy. IMPACT used such an approach with brief monthly

DEPRESSION

follow-up telephone calls documenting persisting benefit after 2 years – valuable evidence of a successful intervention for such a relapsing and remitting chronic disease.

The research is clear. Now it is time to disseminate the message and graduate from the *ad hoc* management of isolated acute episodes of depression and attend to the maintenance and continuation phases. These chronic disease management models can be as effective in depression as they have been in asthma and hypertension.

Patient involvement in primary care mental health: a focus group study
Lester H, Tait L, England E *et al.*
Br J Gen Pract, 2006; **56**: 415–422

The personal experience of psychiatric patients can enhance the care of others. Patients with serious mental illness in this survey felt that early contact with someone who had been in their shoes would have given them valuable insight into their new diagnosis and the issues they would be facing. The survey of 39 GPs and 45 patients also failed to yield examples of a shared-decision making approach to the consultation. Patients felt that decisions were made by the health professional and felt unable to challenge this due to a lack of information about alternatives.

Daily practicalities such as resource limitations impact on the ability to provide a better service but this may be an excellent area for voluntary patient groups to help out.

Delivering interventions for depression by using the internet: randomised controlled trial
Christensen H, Griffiths KM, Jorm AF
BMJ, 2004; **328**: 265

This Australian paper compared internet interventions for dealing with depression in the community, obtaining its recruits by sending questionnaires randomly to names on an electoral role.

One approach was a psychoeducation website called BluePages offering information, and the other, called MoodGYM, offered interactive CBT. Lay interviewers contacted all participants weekly to direct the use of the websites. An 'attention placebo' consisted of weekly contact with an interviewer to discuss lifestyle factors such as exercise patterns.

Both interventions were effective in reducing symptoms of depression by week six. MoodGYM was also good for reducing dysfunctional thinking.

This shows the internet to be a feasible and powerful tool, highly acceptable to patients in the community with low dropout rates.

DEPRESSION

Most selective serotonin reuptake inhibitors lead to adverse events that appear to outweigh the benefits in children. *Evidence-Based Medicine,* 2004; **9**: 181
The following paper is reviewed
Selective serotonin reuptake inhibitors in childhood depression: systematic review of published versus unpublished data
Whittington CJ, Kendall T, Fonagy P *et al.*
Lancet, 2004; **363**: 1341–1345

This review of six published and six unpublished trials on the safety and effectiveness of SSRIs for treating depression in children made the following conclusions:
- fluoxetine improves symptoms with no increase in adverse events
- paroxetine, sertraline, venlafaxine and citaloporam probably do more harm than good
- assumptions of efficacy should not be extrapolated to children based on adult studies
- the placebo response and adverse effects are enhanced in children
- caution should be taken when interpreting marginally positive results as on reanalysis benefits can evaporate
- access to unpublished data is critical to avoid 'evidence-biased medicine'

Treatment of major depressive disorder in children and adolescents
Ramchandani P
BMJ, 2004; **328**: 3–4

This editorial refers to advice in 2003 that most SSRI antidepressants are no longer to be used in treating major depressive disorder in children due to increased risk of suicidal thoughts and self-harm. Only fluoxetine has a favourable risk-benefit balance as things stand and even that will only be of use to around one in ten cases.

Unfortunately they have been widely used – around half the 40 000 under eighteens using antidepressants have been on one of these 'contraindicated' medications.

How should we treat them now? We know depressive symptoms in adolescents are common and often transient. For less severe symptoms, psychological treatments should be opted for, particularly in younger patients, but drugs may be necessary for more severe depression. Fluoxetine is probably first line as evidence for the effectiveness of tricylics is sparse and their toxic effects are well-known, particularly in overdose. Guidance has had to be based on only a few trials as high-quality unbiased evidence in is short supply in this area.

DEPRESSION

Fluoxetine plus cognitive behavioural therapy was most effective for adolescents with major depressive disorder. *Evidence-Based Medicine,* 2005; **10**: 46
The following paper is reviewed
Fluoxetine, cognitive-behavioral therapy, and their combination for adolescents with depression: treatment for Adolescents with Depression Study (TADS) randomized controlled trial
March J, Silva S, Petrycki S *et al.*
JAMA, 2004; **292**: 807–820

The largest independent treatment trial for adolescent depression found that combined CBT and fluoxetine was the best option for moderate to severe depression in adolescents. There were concerns over fluoxetine related to trends towards adverse events and suicide, but not enough to reach statistical significance. With CBT having limited availability, fluoxetine is still the next treatment of choice in adolescents with significant depression, although a small number may experience harm-related events and need close monitoring.

SUICIDE

Factors influencing help seeking in mentally distressed young adults: a cross-sectional survey
Biddle L, Gunnell D, Sharp D *et al.*
Br J Gen Pract, 2004; **54:** 248–253

Half of over 3000 young adults (aged 16–24 years) in this UK study replied to a standard validated questionnaire designed to identify mental disorder.
- Suicidal thoughts occurred at similar levels in males and females (around 13–15%) but less than one in five had been to their GP about this.
- Twice as many women as men had sought help for a psychological problem from friends or family.
- Men appear to need higher levels of morbidity in order to seek help or confide in someone. This may increase their risk of crisis and suicide.

Primary care services may need to refocus on the removal of the barriers that prevent consultations prior to suicide. One is certainly the stigma that mental health disorders still attract.

A qualitative study of help seeking and primary care consultation prior to suicide
Owens C, Lambert H, Donovan J *et al.*
Br J Gen Pract, 2005; **55**: 503–509

A qualitative study found that relatives and friends often played a key role in determining whether or not suicidal individuals sought medical help.

Half the suicides in the study had consulted in the final month of their life and many were persuaded to do so by a relative or friend. Of the others, some had not suggested going to the GP because no-one was aware how serious the situation was.

More attention paid to these lay networks to combine medical and non-medical strategies might prevent suicides.

DEPRESSION

General practitioner contacts with patients before and after deliberate self-harm
Houston K, Haw C, Townsend E *et al.*
Br J Gen Pract, 2004: **53**: 365–370

Interviews were held with 139 deliberate self-harm patients presenting to a general hospital to help clarify the role of the GP in these patients.

They found the following:
- 91% had a psychiatric disorder and 28% were under psychiatric services
- two-thirds had contacted their GP in the month before self-harming, but only 13% expressed suicidal thoughts at this consultation
- 41% consulted their GP in the week after the harming episode, and over half discussed their reasons for it
- two-thirds of people were happy with their follow up consultation

The authors find the main role of the GP in preventing suicidal behaviour is in detecting and treating depression and in the aftercare of deliberate self-harm episodes.

SSRIs AND SUICIDE

Association between suicide attempts and selective serotonin reuptake inhibitors: systematic review of randomised controlled trials
Fergusson D, Doucette S, Glass KC *et al.*
BMJ, 2005; **330**: 396

This systematic review of 702 published RCTs with 87 650 patients compared SSRIs with either placebo or other active treatments in patients with depression and other clinical conditions.
- There was an almost twofold increase in suicidal attempts in users of SSRIs compared with placebo or other therapeutic interventions other than tricyclics.
- NNT for harm for SSRIs was 684.
- Users of SSRIs had no increase in fatal suicidal attempts compared to placebo.
- No differences were observed when overall suicide attempts were compared between users of SSRIs and tricyclic antidepressants. This conclusion was shared by case-control analysis on nearly 150 000 primary care records with a first prescription of an antidepressant (*BMJ*, 2005; **330**: 389).

Suicide, depression, and antidepressants
Cipriani A, Barbui C, Geddes JR
BMJ, 2005; **330**: 373–374

This editorial gives us some help on the SSRI debate by reminding us that study designs influence the conclusions we can make. These are the insights the authors summarise:
- SSRIs and tricyclics may induce and worsen suicidal ideation and suicide attempts in the early phase of treatment possibly due to agitation and activation
- at this time close follow up and family involvement should be considered
- patients should be advised to avoid sudden discontinuation of therapy
- evidence in favour of antidepressants cannot necessarily be extrapolated to mild depression

DEPRESSION

- in children and adolescents on SSRIs and other antidepressants, evidence of suicidal behaviour and lack of long-term data should discourage routine prescribing

---

The risk of suicide with selective serotonin reuptake inhibitors in the elderly
Juurlink DN, Mamdami MM, Kopp A *et al.*
Am J Psychiatry, 2006; **163**: 813–821

This case control study in 1138 cases in Ontario, also reviewed in the *BMJ* (2006; **332** – 20 May), revisits the question of suicide and SSRIs.

They concluded starting treatment with SSRIs – fluoxetine, fluvoxamine, paroxetine, sertraline and citalopram (venlafaxine was not included) – was associated with a risk of suicide five times higher than any other class of antidepressant. This was predominantly related to violent suicide in young men but only apparent in the first month of treatment.

The absolute risk was still low – estimated as 1 in 3300 for SSRIs and 1 in 16 000 for those on other antidepressants.

Because of the way they matched the cases to controls, the authors feel this is unlikely to be due to doctors giving SSRIs to those more prone to suicide.

The risk of undertreatment is still likely to be much worse than these observations.

Further research

- A Swedish study in nearly a million 18 year old men has shown a strong inverse association between intelligence test scores and risk of suicide with twofold to threefold higher risks in those with lowest and highest scores. This may reflect the importance of cognitive and problem-solving ability to work through life's crisis points. *BMJ*, 2005; **330**: 167.
- Giving CBT to people who attempted suicide reduces the recurrence rate by 50% according to a randomised trial of 10 sessions per patient with follow up at 18 months. Interestingly there was no difference in suicidal ideation, just presumably the ability to deal with it and ride out the crisis points. *JAMA*, 2005; **294**: 563–570.
- A US study looked into worries that asking about suicidal ideation or behaviour in teenagers (average age 15 years) during a screening program might create distress or increases suicidal ideation. Reassuringly, they found no evidence to support this and the questions seemed to be beneficial in high-risk groups. *JAMA*, 2005; **293**: 1635–1643.

DOMESTIC VIOLENCE

What we know already:

- Domestic violence (a.k.a. intimate partner abuse) includes emotional, sexual, and economic intimidation as well as physical violence. It is a major public health problem
- Consequences include injury in the short term and chronic health problems, sexually transmitted disease and mental illness in the long term
- A minority of health professionals are in favour of screening for domestic violence. Most feel ill-equipped to screen, are afraid of annoying or endangering patients, and do not know what to do with a positive screen
- Systematic review suggests that there is insufficient evidence to justify screening. The most important factor against it is the lack of proof that interventions are successful and not harmful
- One-quarter of women in the UK report being assaulted by an intimate partner and many do not know how to get help
- One in seven men experience physical assault by a current or former partner but incidents in men are likely to involve less fear and injury
- Children growing up with domestic violence are 30–60% more likely to develop emotional, behavioural, educational and health problems
- Children are more likely to repeat these patterns as an adult
- There is limited research of GP management of partner abuse and studies on interventions are rare

Guidelines

Domestic violence: the general practitioner's role. *RCGP*, 1998.

Domestic violence: a resource manual for health care professionals. *Dept of Health*, 2000.

The WHO multi-country study on women's health and domestic violence against women. *World Health Organization*, 2003.

Recent Papers

PREVALENCE

Association between depression and abuse by partners of women attending general practice: descriptive, cross sectional survey
Hegarty K, Gunn J, Chondros P *et al.*
BMJ, 2004; **328**: 621–624

> This study showed that physical, emotional, and sexual abuse were strongly associated with depression in 1257 women attending Australian general practice.

DOMESTIC VIOLENCE

There was an 18% prevalence of current depression and a 24% prevalence of intimate partner abuse in the previous year.

Overall, one-third of the women had experienced some form of abuse but only one-third of those had ever told a doctor. Few had ever been asked.

Although the study was not designed to infer causation, the association remained after adjusting for other significant socio-demographic factors such as poor education, low income, unemployment and being abused as a child.

Doctors should be alert to the possibility of abuse in their depressed patients.

CASE IDENTIFICATION

The acceptability of routine inquiry about domestic violence towards women: a survey in three healthcare settings
Boyle A, Jones P
Br J Gen Pract, 2006; **56**: 258–261

This study took place in three general practices, one emergency department and an antenatal clinic. Questionnaires were used to determine the characteristic of women who found inquiry concerning domestic violence unacceptable. Of 2300 women, 63% responded:
- 8.4% of those that responded found inquiry unacceptable
- abuse within a year was strongly associated with finding inquiry unacceptable
- lifetime abuse was not associated with finding inquiry unacceptable

The authors conclude that screening for domestic abuse in this way is acceptable to most women particularly if they have recently been free from abuse.

Routinely asking women about domestic violence in health settings
Taket A, Nurse J, Smith K et al.
BMJ, 2003; **327**: 673–676

This is an excellent review arguing that the health sector can no longer avoid its responsibility in tackling domestic violence or as the authors prefer 'partner abuse'. They argue strongly in favour of 'routine enquiry' as opposed to screening.
- The rates of disclosure of abuse without direct questioning are known to be poor and routine enquiry may be the only pragmatic way of getting to the truth.
- It has a high level of acceptability although a minority of women do not like the idea.
- Health services are familiar with uncovering problems and, with their frequent opportunities for contact, are the best place for such enquiry.
- Women experiencing domestic violence have three times the usual consultation rate.
- The presence of depression may heighten awareness to possible partner abuse and encourage enquiry.
- Some studies show positive outcomes from outreach services in terms of reduced violence over time and leaving abusive relationships.
- Training for health professionals is urgently needed. Reform at a structural and policy level needs local leaders to coordinate training and support.

Protocols that prioritise safety are essential to alleviate concerns from health professionals about 'opening a can of worms'. This will also ease their ambivalence, frustration and worry at dealing with issues of child protection, legalities, and pressure of time.

MANAGEMENT

Intimate partner violence
Ferris L
BMJ, 2004; **328**: 595–596

That intimate partner violence affects entire families including children makes its impact even more shocking. Unfortunately, the lack of proven interventions in both the developed and developing world creates difficulties for doctors.

Is there sufficient evidence of lack of harm from our efforts to warrant going ahead? There is a consensus on casting a wide net for the problem but following up on specific presenting clues is the usual way of identifying cases of abuse until more evidence shows us another path. We should screen for depression at the same time as plenty of research has shown us that our time is well spent doing this.

Pathways of referral need to be defined. Victim support interventions seem to be a good place to start. Emergency shelter and legal advice might be useful. A structured programme would be nice but in the meantime doctors must recognise and acknowledge the situation non-judgementally then respond with referral to one or more interventions.

General practitioner management of intimate partner abuse and the whole family: qualitative study
Taft A, Broom DH, Legge D
BMJ, 2004; **328**: 618

This study of 28 Australian GPs found that their own stress and difficulty in resolving tensions led to neglect of risks to children, contraindicated practices, unsuccessful attempts at counselling and breaks in confidentiality between the couple.

It illustrated how poor Australian doctors were at their attempts to resolve partner abuse issues. They were confused about when normal conflict became abnormal and seemed to underestimate the number of cases on their books.

The empathetic GPs suffered with non-compliant patients and lack of positive feedback. Feelings of despair and helplessness were common and female GPs got the brunt of it. The GPs on the other end of the spectrum were concerned how much money they were losing due to long consultations.

Responses to the male partners – the abusers coming in for treatment for their depression, pain and alcohol problems – could be hostile. Some entered into raising the issues in a watered down version of amateur counselling despite this model being contraindicated due to the associated risks.

Some, of course, just ignored the problem and most doctors overlooked the impact on children despite the powerful catalyst this can be for change. They did not feel equipped to help and were distrusting of child protection services.

CLINICAL ISSUES

DOMESTIC VIOLENCE

Unfortunately there were few agencies to which to refer patients and little information on whether intervention is beneficial.

Intimate partner abuse cannot be solved by general practice alone but identification and referral plays a critical role in the process.

This study reinforces the need for guidelines for managing the whole family, acting on behalf of children and the need to refer to specialist agencies. Training, supervision and support for the health professionals is needed to cope with the stress of this difficult work.

DOMESTIC VIOLENCE

SCREENING CONCEPTS

Recent Papers

Health professionals' and service users' interpretation of screening test results: experimental study
Bramwell R, West H, Salmon P
BMJ, 2006; **333**: 284

Different groups of people draw differently incorrect conclusions when presented with results of screening.

This study looked at the interpretations of people involved in antenatal care – midwives, obstetricians and pregnant women and their companions.

The data were related to the blood test for Down syndrome that is offered to all pregnant women and actually predicted a 50% probability of Down syndrome.

- 86% of the responses were incorrect.
- The incorrect answers given were mostly very high or very low.
- Obstetricians gave more correct answers but still were right only 43% of the time.
- Pregnant women interpreted correctly in 9%.
- Midwives – the major provider of information - interpreted correctly in 0% of cases.
- Many health professionals were confident in their incorrect answers, displaying a lack of insight into the meaning of crucial information.
- Presentation of the information as frequencies (which is presumed to promote a more natural style of reasoning) rather than percentages improved interpretation but only in obstetricians – to 65%. Almost all the others were still wrong.
- Participation was voluntary so things could be even worse in reality.

Ways of conveying information sorely need updating, with visual aids, for example. They need to be relevant to the academic ability and level of education of patients and others interpreting them.

More and more screening technologies are becoming available and we are making more use of probabilistic information. It is crucial to draw correct conclusions from the information we gather. If we do not, the concept of screening is damaged.

Screening without evidence of efficacy
Law M
BMJ, 2004; **328**: 301–302

Screening has intuitive appeal to doctors and patients. The idea that early diagnosis means definitive gain is seductive and has led to procedures that have side-stepped the usually necessary gold standard of a randomised controlled trial or two.

Law mentions the example of the prostate where one-third of healthy American males over fifty have had their PSA measured compared to 5% in Britain.

SCREENING

Available evidence indicates that the British are right to reject the test. High levels indicate advanced disease that may present too late to affect mortality. A study using a threshold of 10 µg/l put false positives in men over 70 at 4% and discovered that 15 out of 16 cases detected already has advanced extra-prostatic tumour. At the more common cut off of 4 µg/l, 22 of 33 had such spread and the false positives in the vulnerable over 70s (who have 84% share of the mortality of prostatic cancer) reached an unacceptable 18%. The test has poor specificity and the only thing we do know for a fact is that it causes harm through unnecessary investigation and treatment.

Studies have shown that screening can reveal cancers that would never have presented clinically. One randomised trial looking for lung cancers failed to show improved outcomes from earlier detection over a period of 11 years. Overdiagnosis of indolent cancers in asymptomatic patients is an unresolved problem.

Breast self-examination and testicular self-examination have failed due to lack of scientific rigour. Both had been advocated on the assumption that they could do no harm. They do. More biopsies and more anxiety. Same deaths. Law argues public health bodies need to avoid promoting unproven screening procedures when health resources are limited.

EDITOR'S CHOICE: The screening industry
Smith R
BMJ, 2003; **326**: 26 April

This piece starts with a look at the flavour of the month – whole body CT scanning. Intensely marketed in the US, it highlights medicine's failure to define 'normal'. Our usual method of taking two standard deviations from the mean fails us when there are thousands of measurements. Many will cross into the 'abnormal' 5% threshold and the only question becomes exactly how abnormal each of us is! Not terribly helpful some may argue. The 'devil of false positives' is on our shoulder and highlights our limited understanding of the natural history of disease. Which abnormalities signify significant conditions? Of course, it may be profitable for the screening industry for none of us to be normal. Smith refers to a concept of 'rational ignorance' which may still be bliss.

Screening for cancer with computed tomography
Swensen SJ
BMJ, 2003; **326**: 894–895

Swensen quotes his own work on chest screening with CT and its success in detecting smaller (down to 3 mm) lung cancers at earlier treatable stages with improved detection over chest radiography.

However, there are caveats:
- some lung cancers may progress too rapidly for this process to be useful. We do not know how early metastasis occurs
- others may progress too slowly and not pose a threat to the patients
- if we found incidence was the same in smokers and non-smokers, it may be a case of 'dying with' rather than 'dying from'
- false positives from CT scans may be too high (over 70% in Swensen's series)

SCREENING

- mortality from investigative surgery such as wedge resections may be too high
- radiation from follow-up may cause more cancer deaths than it saves
- cost per life year gained may be too high

Whole body CT magnifies the concerns that result from localised CT. In his own research, Swensen found 700 ancillary findings including four renal cell carcinomas, three breast cancers, two lymphomas, two gastric tumours, and 114 abdominal aortic aneurysms. However, most were false positives and led to unnecessary investigations and interventional procedures which 'adversely affected quality of life'.

The question of whether we can affect outcome remains. Does it do more good than harm and will market forces wait for the answer? Doctors disagree with each other and ethicists refer to this conflict as equipoise. Randomised trials are awaited but it could take a decade.

In the meantime? Informed consent requires doctors to be clear that such screening has no proven benefit and if benefit exists it could be outweighed by life-threatening risk.

SCREENING

COLORECTAL CANCER

What we know already:

- Bowel cancer is second only to lung cancer as a cause of cancer deaths in the UK. Five year survival rates remain below 50%
- In 2004, the number of deaths exceeded that from breast and cervical cancer combined – both of which have effective screening programmes
- Colorectal cancer evolves slowly from premalignant polyps providing a large window of opportunity for screening
- The government first announced its aim to introduce bowel cancer screening in the NHS Plan in 2000
- Contenders for screening are immunochemical FOB test, flexible sigmoidoscopy, colonoscopy, virtual colonoscopy and faecal DNA tests, but evidence is strongest for guaiac FOB testing
- Virtual colonoscopy where the bowel is pumped up creating a pneumocolon prior to CT scanning is not yet a consistent enough technique to recommend
- Pilot trials have shown that screening with guaiac-based testing of faecal occult blood (FOB) is the only method yet shown to cut the death rate from colorectal cancer (by around 15–18%)
- Studies showed that FOB testing would detect one or two bowel cancers for every 1000 people screened. An additional three or four people would have pre-cancerous lesions removed
- The US has recommended FOB testing from the age of 50 years since the 1980s – around 40% of the population complies with this advice but their more unregulated approach often uses colonoscopy in favour of faecal testing
- Colonoscopy is increasingly popular and yet we cannot say for certain whether it saves lives. It may not be cost-effective and a decent randomised trial is needed
- Rectal bleeding occurs in 40% of patients with colorectal cancer
- The high prevalence and resulting low predictive value of symptoms such as rectal bleeding, changes in bowel habit, and abdominal pain means that most affected patients have a very low chance of cancer
- Aspirin may have a role as a reasonably effective treatment to prevent adenomas in high risk patients

Guidelines

Referral guidelines for suspected cancer. *NICE*, 2005.

Recent Papers

SCREENING METHODS

Results of the first round of a demonstration pilot of screening for colorectal cancer in the United Kingdom
UK Colorectal Cancer Screening Pilot Group
BMJ, 2004; **329**: 133

This research set out to see whether the extension of the success of FOB testing could work at a population level within the NHS.

Nearly half a million people aged 50–69 years living in England and Scotland were invited to take part. Patients were sent a testing kit through the post and smeared a small sample of stool onto a piece of card and send the card back to the testing centre. Those testing positive for blood were investigated with colonoscopy. Results were as follows:

- uptake was 57% showing high levels of acceptance which might be further increased by invitations direct from the patient's own practice
- women were more likely to comply than men possibly because they have more exposure to screening
- there was a positive test result in nearly 2 in 100 with cancer detected at 1.62 per 1000 people screened
- the uptake of colonoscopy among positives was 81.5%. Of these, 0.56% required brief hospitalisation for bleeding or abdominal pain. Two people had perforations (0.05%)
- the positive predictive values of a positive test result were 11% for invasive cancer and 35% for adenoma
- the cost of screening was about £5900 per life year saved

FOB testing is not perfect as the test may only be about 50% sensitive in a screening context, but evidence clearly now shows it can have a major impact on mortality from colorectal cancer. Screening with this method has been shown to be feasible within the context of the United Kingdom's NHS. An increase in provision of endoscopy services will be needed promptly.

Impending or pending? The national bowel cancer screening programme
Atkin WS
BMJ, 2006; **332**: 742
and
Colorectal cancer in primary care
Weller D
BMJ, 2006; **333**: 54–55

These editorials discuss the considerable challenges for primary care in trying to recognise potential cases of colorectal cancer while avoiding unnecessary investigations.

We certainly need to reduce the burden of disease and reverse our low ranking of survival rates. This means diagnosis must be made at an earlier stage – preferably when asymptomatic.

England is introducing bowel cancer screening based on the strong evidence of

SCREENING

effectiveness and acceptability of FOB testing, but the rollout has been slower than expected. Although some funding was in place in 2004, a phased rollout is not expected to cover the country until 2010, screening 60–69 year olds – around 3 years later than in France (who currently target those aged 50–74 years).

The reasons are clear. Without enough accredited endoscopists in place for the estimated 30 000 colonoscopies needed, people may wait too long or even end up getting priority over those who already have symptoms.

Recruitment for the screening programme and follow up is to be organised centrally but some of the workload will spill over to primary care and inevitably patients outside of the nominated age group will request screening.

In the future, diagnostic algorithms based on symptoms scores could help us prioritise referral decisions as we learn more about the predictive values of different symptoms in primary care populations. Perhaps even risk tables, like those used to evaluate cardiovascular risk, might turn out to be useful.

Does a negative screening colonoscopy ever need to be repeated?
Brenner H, Chang-Claude J, Seiler CM *et al.*
Gut, 2006; **55**: 1145–1150

Colonoscopy is traditionally repeated every 10 years after an initial negative result.

This research suggests that it need not be repeated for 20 years if at all.

This population-based case-control study was adjusted for confounders and found that a previous negative colonoscopy reduces the risk of a positive finding in the future for at least 20 years, particularly if performed after the age of 55 years.

Increased time interval between colonoscopies increases safety by diminishing complications and the cost-effectiveness of screening.

Positive predictive value of fecal occult blood testing in persons taking warfarin
Bini EJ, Rajapaksa RC, Weinshel EH
Am J Gastroenterol, 2005; **100**: 1586–1592

A useful prospective study over a 5 year period that looked at concerns related to warfarin use during FOB testing concluded:
- warfarin use did not decrease the positive predictive value of FOB testing
- there is therefore no need to discontinue warfarin prior to FOB testing
- positive FOB in patients taking warfarin must not dismissed as a false positive

---

Colonoscopic screening of average-risk women for colorectal neoplasia
Schoenfeld P, CONCeRN Study Investigators
N Engl J Med, 2005: **352**: 2061–2068

When used for colorectal cancer screening in asymptomatic women, flexible sigmoidoscopy would have picked up only 35% of malignant or potentially malignant lesions, much less than the 66% found in a related study for men.

In the Colorectal Neoplasia Screening with Colonoscopy in Average-Risk Women at Regional Naval Medical Centers (CONCeRN) study, 15% of women had a family history of bowel cancer and as a group they were average risk.

The investigators conclude that colonoscopy is the preferred method of colorectal cancer screening in average risk, asymptomatic women. In the US where this study was done, it is widely use anyway.

RISK ASSESSMENT

Risk in primary care of colorectal cancer from new onset rectal bleeding: 10 year prospective study
du Toit J, Hamilton W, Barraclough K
BMJ, 2006; **333**: 69–70

This was a study in one general practice of patients aged over 45 years who bled rectally and where one of the GPs was familiar with sigmoidoscopy. Some patients received further investigation with barium enemas or colonoscopy.
- The annual rate of new rectal bleeding in this UK general practice population was 9/1000.
- Only two of the patients with cancer had diarrhoea, showing how negatively predictive it is.
- Over a decade, 265 reported rectal bleeding of which 1 in 10 had colonic neoplasia (5.7% had colorectal cancer and 4.9% had colonic adenoma).
The authors state that this incidence means that regardless of other symptoms, rectal bleeding warrants urgent referral in those over 45.

Predicting colorectal cancer risk in patients with rectal bleeding
Robertson R, Campbell C, Weller D et al.
Br J Gen Pract, 2006; **56**: 763–767

This observational study of over 600 patients with rectal bleeding looked at symptoms predictive of colorectal cancer.

Significant predictors included blood mixed with the stool, which had a likelihood ratio of 1.5, and age, particularly if over 70 years. In patients with bleeding not mixed with stool and who had haemorrhoids, a cancer, although less likely, was still present in 2%.

These authors conclude that rectal bleeding in isolation had insufficient diagnostic value to be useful in general practice.

Factors identifying higher risk rectal bleeding in general practice
Ellis BG, Thompson M
Br J Gen Pract, 2005; **55**: 949–955

This study also looked at the predictive and diagnostic value of factors in bowel cancer. Some 319 consecutive patients aged 34 years were studied. A questionnaire asked about symptoms and further investigation was with flexible sigmoidoscopy, followed by review at 18 months.
- 3.4% of this age group had colorectal cancer.
- This increased to 9.2% when rectal bleeding was associated with a change in bowel habit and to 11.1% when peri-anal symptoms were absent.
- 36% of cancer patients had a palpable rectal mass.

Iron deficiency anaemia in general practice: clinical outcomes over three years and factors influencing diagnostic investigations
Yates JM, Logan ECM, Stewart RM
Postgrad Med J, 2004; **80**: 405–410

Studies in patients referred to hospital for anaemia have shown that 5–15% have a gastrointestinal cancer. What happens to patients with anaemia in general practice?
   In this study of patients with iron deficiency anaemia presenting to their GPs:

- 43% of patients had investigations within 3 months and serious pathology was found in 30% of these
- 21% of patients were either considered unfit or refused to have further investigation. Independent predictors of non-investigation were mild anaemia, being female, previous history of anaemia, and age under 65
- during the entire study period gastrointestinal cancers, principally colorectal, were diagnosed in 11%

The authors conclude that there is a risk of delayed diagnosis of gastrointestinal cancer in patients presenting to primary care, as prevalence of serious underlying pathology is similar to cases referred to secondary care.

ROLE OF ASPIRIN

Long-term use of aspirin and nonsteroidal anti-inflammatory drugs and risk of colorectal cancer
Chan AT, Giovannucci EL,. Meyerhardt JA *et al.*
JAMA, 2005; **294**: 914–923

The Nurses Health Study has been collecting data every 2 years since 1976. This study showed that when used for primary prevention, aspirin did indeed reduce incidence of colorectal cancer, but the effect only becomes significant after 10 years and seems to need high doses up to 325 mg. Wider study is indicated but the trade-off in gastric bleeding will surely be damning.

SCREENING

PROSTATE CANCER

What we know already:

- There are 27 000 new cases of prostate cancer a year in the UK making it the second most common cancer in men causing almost 10 000 deaths a year
- Screening has been a controversial area due to a lack of evidence that intervention affects mortality, enormous scope for over-diagnosis and a lack on consensus on treatment
- Serum prostate-specific antigen (PSA) has been adopted for case finding among asymptomatic men and has substantially increased the detection of prostate cancer
- The main cause of elevated serum PSA concentration is benign prostatic hyperplasia
- In men under 60, PSA (at a cut off of 4 µg/l) fails to identify 8 out of every 10 men who later have prostate cancer. In older men 65% of cancers would be missed
- Radical prostatectomy may reduce deaths from prostate cancer and reduce local and distant progression. However, there is no evidence of an overall reduction in mortality compared to watchful waiting
- More trials are needed for the full picture and any benefits that might be shown would have to be balanced with the adverse effects of surgery such as urinary and erectile dysfunction
- Poor communication of the risks of screening means men have been shown to want wider access to PSA testing
- In the future, new tests could identify genes such as E2F3 which help to predict aggressiveness of prostate cancer

Recent Papers

PROSTATE SPECIFIC ANTIGEN

The prostate specific antigen era in the United States is over for prostate cancer: What happened in the last 20 years?
Stamey TA, Caldwell M, McNeal JE et al.
J Urol, 2004; **172**: 1297–1301

Looking at over 1300 radical prostatectomies over 20 years up to 2003, the authors found that many variables decreased linearly during that period, including:

- palpable nodules on digital rectal examination from 91% to 17%
- average age of prostatectomy from 64 to 59 years
- average PSA levels from 25 to 8 µg/l
- average volume of the largest cancer from 5.3 to 2.4 cm^3

Although serum PSA was related to prostate cancer 20 years ago, in the last 5 years PSA has only been related to prostate size and therefore is a guide for benign prostatic hyperplasia. This is worth repeating, the only trend relating to PSA value was prostatic weight.

They add:

- prostate cancer is being overenthusiastically treated
- better markers are needed that reflect the size and grade of prostate cancer.

SCREENING

- improved practice of clinical examination would help as palpable cancers usually require intervention

The author of this paper developed PSA testing and is consigning it to the rubbish bin as a detector of cancer. Unfortunately the prostate screening industry is a juggernaut and it will take time to make a change.

According to Stamey, however, the 'PSA era is over'.

Operating characteristics of prostate-specific antigen in men with an initial PSA level of 3.0 ng/ml or lower
Thompson IM, Ankerst DP, Chi C *et al.*
JAMA, 2005; **294**: 66–70

Three-quarters of US men older than 50 years have been screened for PSA for prostate cancer. This study of nearly 19 000 healthy men found there was no cut-off point of PSA with simultaneous high sensitivity and high specificity for screening healthy men for prostate cancer. Rather there was a continuum of prostate cancer risk at all values of PSA. The patient will have to weigh the final decision.

The effectiveness of screening for prostate cancer
Concato J, Wells CK, Horwitz RI *et al.*
Arch Intern Med, 2006; **166**: 38–43

In this case-control study, no mortality benefit was found from prostate screening with PSA, with or without digital rectal examination. The authors say that routine testing should not be endorsed and the focus should be on fully informing the patients about the uncertainty of screening. The risks of unnecessary biopsies, overdiagnosis, sexual dysfunction and urinary incontinence all need to be taken into account. Reductions in overall prostate cancer mortality rates in the US mirror those in countries which have no claim that they routinely screen.

NATURAL HISTORY

Natural history of early, localized prostate cancer
Johansson JE, Andren O, Andersson SO *et al.*
JAMA, 2004; **291**: 2713–2719

The word 'indolent' is often used to describe the progress of early-stage prostate cancer. This population-based cohort study looked at the natural history of the disease further into the long-term and came up with some interesting conclusions.

They observed 223 men with early prostate cancer and no initial treatment for an average of 21 years. The indolent course ran for 10–15 years. After this there was a substantial drop in survival from prostate cancer as well as in survival without metastases. The prostate cancer mortality rate tripled from 15 per 1000 person-years during the first 15 years to 44 per 1000 person-years afterwards.

They conclude that because aggressive progression locally and metastatically may develop in the long term, we should consider early radical treatment among patients expected to live more than 15 years.

Clinical features of prostate cancer before diagnosis: a population-based, case-control study
Hamilton W, Sharp DJ, Peters TJ *et al.*
Br J Gen Pract, 2006; **56**: 756–762

Predictive features of prostate cancer are largely unknown. This study looked at the medical records of over 200 patients relating to the 2 years prior to diagnosis of prostate cancer. They found eight features which were predictive of prostate cancer.

Coming in with positive predictive values at around 3% were urinary retention, impotence and hesitancy. At around 2% were nocturia and frequency. Abnormal rectal examination deemed benign around 3%, and if deemed malignant 12%. More mildly positive associations were haematuria and weight loss. The authors conclude that most men with prostate cancer present with these symptoms and they offer the data to help guide triage for referral.

MANAGEMENT

20-year outcomes following conservative management of clinically localized prostate cancer
Albertsen PC, Hanley JA, Fine J
JAMA, 2005; **293**: 2095–2101

This retrospective cohort study used registry data along with histology and hospital records to review the progress of 767 men aged 55–74 years with clinically localized prostate cancer.

They found that men with low-grade prostate cancers have a very small risk of dying from prostate cancer during 20 years of follow-up and that the annual mortality rate from prostate cancer appears to remain stable even 15–20 years from diagnosis. Aggressive treatment for localized low-grade prostate cancer was therefore thought to be inappropriate.

Further Research

- Widespread testing of PSA leads to overdiagnosis of prostate cancer. A study from East Anglia estimated that around half the prostate cancers were over-diagnosed and would not have come to light in the patient's lifetime in the absence of screening. Those who would promote population testing are on ever shakier ground. *Br J Cancer,* 2006; **95**: 401–405.

- When prostate cancers are diagnosed despite a low PSA level of <4.0 µg/l, they are no less clinically significant. Research shows that many of these tumours are high-grade, high-volume and extraprostatic. *BJU Int,* 2004; **93**: 499–502.

- A study of nearly 3000 men over 62 years who never had a PSA level of more than 4.0 µg/l nor an abnormal digital rectal examination, confirmed that prostate cancers detected on biopsy, including high-grade cancers, are not rare among such men. Prevalence of cancer increased as PSA increased, reaching over a quarter of those with PSA values of 3.1–4.0 µg/l. Overall, when biopsied after 7 years in the study, 15% of men had prostate cancer. *N Engl J Med,* 2004; **350**: 2239–2246.

SCREENING

AORTIC ANEURYSM

> ## What we know already:
>
> - Every year about 6000 men die from a ruptured abdominal aortic aneurysm in England and Wales. Death rates are around 50%
> - This is only about 2% of all deaths in men but the condition is largely preventable
> - Prevalence seems to be increasing although deaths from other atherosclerotic conditions are reducing
> - Aortic aneurysms can be detected with a simple ultrasound examination
> - Ultrasound screening for aortic aneurysm has been shown to be of value in older men fit enough for surgery and who would choose to have it if an aneurysm of more than 5.5 cm was found
>
> ## Key trial
>
> ### The Multicentre Aneurysm Screening Study, 2002
> This large UK randomised 'MASS' study looked into the effect of screening for abdominal aortic aneurysm with ultrasound and showed that it reduced mortality in men between 65 and 74 years of age by 42%.
>
> Uptake was high at 80% and, over the 4 year study period, the scanned group had less aneurysm-related mortality and fewer ruptured aneurysms.
>
> The mean cost of screening a patient was £63. Cost for elective aneurysm repair was nearly £7000 and for emergency surgery just over £11 000. Screening 710 subjects prevents one death. The estimated cost after 10 years was £8000 per life year gained, which is well within desired NHS margins and as effective as other screening programmes.
>
> However, there were a few caveats. Results cannot be generalised to women, or to men outside the 65–74 year age group. In older patients, other co-morbid conditions influence surgical outcomes and therefore the benefits for life expectancy.
>
> Surgical intervention is high-risk, very resource intensive and not many lives will be saved. It is estimated that screening could prevent 14 aneurysm-related deaths in 10 000 patients over 4 years. Follow up scans may need to be large in number for those with moderate-sized aneurysms.

Recent Papers

Screening for abdominal aortic aneurysms: single centre randomised controlled trial
Lindholt JS, Juul S, Fasting H et al.
BMJ, 2005; **330**: 750

The findings of the MASS trial were reproduced in a group of 12 639 Danish men aged 64–73 years (mean age 68 years), as follows:
- more than three-quarters of the group accepted the invite
- 4% of those screened had abdominal aortic aneurysms

- screening reduced deaths specifically due to abdominal aortic aneurysm (not overall mortality), averting 3 deaths for every 1000 screened (NNT to save one life = 352)
- screening reduced the rate of emergency surgery by 75%
- this was offset by a 3–4-fold increase in the total number of aneurysm operations
- screening a population with high prevalence will be most cost effective

Clearly, screening is effective in a population of men 64–73 years of age. The most effective strategy and benefits of the less traumatic intervention of endovascular aneurysm repair merit more research (*Evidence-Based Medicine*, 2005; **10**: 142).

Screening for abdominal aortic aneurysms in men
Earnshaw JJ, Shaw E, Whyman MR *et al.*
BMJ, 2004; **328**: 1122–1124

The Gloucestershire aneurysm screening project has been running since 1990. They invite 65 year old men to an ultrasound at their local practice and screen 3000 men a year. A nurse coordinator runs the show and sonographers are paid on a sessional basis. Ten men are examined in an hour and get their results immediately. Men with an aorta > 40 mm in diameter are referred to a vascular surgeon. They are scanned every 6 months and elective repair is considered at 55 mm. Annual recalls with the current year's 65 year old men are offered to those with an aortal diameter of 26–29 mm. The rest are discharged.

After 13 years, mortality and incidence of rupture have fallen. Elective surgery has increased and emergency surgery has reduced. Operative mortality for elective repair has reduced from 6.5 to 4.4%.

The scheme misses the 10% that die from ruptured aneurysms before reaching 65 years but aims to be a cost-effective programme. Costs would increase markedly if an extra scan was given before hitting 65 years but they propose targeting those at high risk, i.e. smokers or those with a family history, hypertension or arterial disease.

Starting a widespread scheme could overwhelm vascular services and would need to be sensitively co-ordinated. But it could also lead to additional opportunities to target men at high cardiovascular risk for disease modifying interventions.

Population based randomised controlled trial on impact of screening on mortality from abdominal aortic aneurysm
Norman PE, Jamrozik K, Lawrence-Brown MM *et al.*
BMJ, 2004; **329**: 1259

This Australian study was not able to show a benefit when the invited age range was extended to 65–83 year olds. Population screening did not significantly reduce death rates in this age group because so many failed to attend. There was substantial benefit for those who did attend (mainly in the 65–75 year age group) but this was diluted in the final analysis. They failed to exclude men who were unlikely to attend and those would have been ineligible for surgery had they attended.

They also thought that methods of recruitment were important, as patients may be more likely to attend when asked by their GP as opposed to a research group.

SCREENING

They verified that identifying a clear target group is a crucial part of a screening initiative.

National screening programme for aortic aneurysm

Greenhalgh RM
BMJ, 2004; **328**: 1087–1088

The call for a national screening programme has had a good reception on the back of the research above. Critics, however, point to the lack of evidence of either overall survival benefit or that benefits outweigh the physical and psychological harms.

It has been shown that we have a good simple test: it is possible to measure aortic aneurysm with a repeatability of as little as 2–3 mm. But there is a real risk of overwhelming vascular services.

Screening of US patients with peripheral arterial disease ('Legs for Life') showed that 25% were at risk from ruptured abdominal aortic aneurysm and suggested that targeting high risk atherosclerotic patients would be more cost effective. Leaving out women may also be difficult politically (aneurysms are not as common in women but rupture is more frequent and occurs at a smaller diameter). But if we go ahead with a programme, death from a ruptured abdominal aortic aneurysm could become a rarity. The middle of the night drama could be a thing of the past. Hospital resources will be saved and antisocial hours will be spared. The infrastructure of the NHS means that Britain could lead the way.

SCREENING

BREAST CANCER

What we know already:

- The risk–benefit of mammography is still uncertain. More work is needed on whether the number of cancer patients created by screening allows a net benefit
- Studies have shown rates of breast cancer mortality falling by 28–65% (median 46%) in recent years
- Breast screening saves lives and is cost effective. Screening with mammography saves 1400 lives per year in England at a cost of £3000 per year of life saved
- Mammography is not going to prevent most breast cancer deaths. But for every 400 women screened over a 10 year period, one less woman dies from breast cancer as a result of the NHS screening programme in England
- Doubts over the risk–benefit profile of mammography are being dispelled. Agreement is wider than ever that mammography saves lives but concerns such as over-diagnosis linger
- Evidence of benefit in the 40–49 year age group is weak and non-existent in those under 40 where false positives are higher and there is increased potential for radiation carcinogenesis
- Regular breast examination does not reduce breast cancer mortality but may increase harm such as the number of women who have biopsies with benign results.

Guidelines

Screening for breast cancer in England: past and future. *Advisory Committee on Breast Cancer Screening.* February 2006 (www.cancerscreening.org.uk/breastscreen).

Recent Papers

REFERRAL

The '2-week rule' for suspected breast carcinoma: a qualitative study of the views of patients and professionals
Cornford CS, Harley J, Oswald N
Br J Gen Pract, 2004; **54**: 584–588

This qualitative study using semi-structured interviews looked at the impact of the 2-week rule for referring women with suspected breast cancer from the perspective of the patients and of healthcare professionals.
- All women experienced considerable worries in the time leading up to diagnosis.
- Personal fears included images of death and mutilating surgery.
- This affects relationships with others, and they use 'selective telling' to help control overanxiety and prevent anxiety in friends and family.
- Women recognised that GPs may not be able to tell them exactly what is wrong but did not mind as long as something was to be done.

SCREENING

- Doctors and patients wanted quick referral to reassure patients that they did not have cancer.
- Patients need improved information about breast symptoms and the referral process.
- Patients place great value on good communication but there was an absence of such concerns in the accounts of the professionals.
- GPs and specialists felt that the 2-week rule was good for reducing anxiety, but thought it might cause longer waits for other patients and increase pressure on hospital services.
- GPs were concerned about missing diagnoses in patients statistically unlikely to have carcinomas.

BREAST SELF EXAMINATION

Breast self examination
Austoker J
BMJ, 2003; **326**: 1–2

This author refers to the Shanghai trial as a high quality trial and describes its conclusions as the last word on the subject and a full stop to a decade of controversy and confusion. Cancers detected in the trial were the same in number and in stage as the control group.

Breast self examination had been recommended for 70 years without compelling proof of efficacy. In fact only a small proportion of women ever did it – one study reported only around 20% of female doctors examined their breasts regularly. The anxiety that went with the investigation of all the benign lesions found could have led to delay in finding a further possibly malignant lump. There was never even a consensus on how to do it and the frequency was arbitrarily chosen.

The policy of breast awareness has probably added to the confusion but is still very important to avoid delay in presentation of new symptoms.

MAMMOGRAPHY

Screening for breast cancer
Dixon JM
BMJ, 2006; **332**: 499–500

This editorial claims that the controversy over whether or not breast screening with mammography saves lives should be at an end.

Criticisms resulted for early data which now seem to be methodologically inferior.

Previous trials which found no reduction in mortality have been noted by the Advisory Committee on Breast Cancer Screening as having poor methodology, for example, randomising groups rather than individuals. The report also notes the following.

- Criticism that some women receive mastectomy for disease that would never have presented anyway is a red herring. Saving lives with earlier diagnosis mean that women inevitably have the opportunity to die of something other than breast cancer.

- One in eight women who have cancer on screening would never have had their cancer diagnosed but the mastectomy rate is lower than in those who present with symptoms.
- The report estimates that screening actually spares 1 in 8 breast cancer sufferers from mastectomy through earlier diagnosis. This should help to allay the fears of the sceptics of breast screening.
- False positives will always happen and quality assurance measures need to continue to minimise the anxiety and costs that these cause. Digital mammography may help to reduce the figures.
- During the 17 years of the UK breast screening programme, improvements have been made in terms of improved resolution with higher quality equipment, more views and double reading.
- Interval cancers – those that present between mammograms – need better quality data to ensure that all units are delivering a high quality service.

Rate of over-diagnosis of breast cancer 15 years after end of Malmö mammographic screening trial: follow-up study
Zackrisson S, Andersson I, Janzon L et al.
BMJ, 2006; **332**: 689–692

Estimates of the rate of over-diagnosis of breast cancer as a result of mammography have varied from 5 to 50%. A long follow up is necessary to estimate the real magnitude of the effect and the Malmö study had this.

This was a Swedish study that randomised 42 000 individual women aged 45–69. The first cohort was born as early as 1908 and the control groups were never invited for screening.

Fifteen years after the trial ended, they measured a 10% rate of over-diagnosis – detection of cases that would never have come to clinical attention without screening with mammography.

Impact of use of hormone replacement therapy on false positive recall in the NHS breast screening programme: results from the Million Women Study
Banks E, Reeves G, Beral V et al.
BMJ, 2004; **328**: 1291–1292

Previous studies have reported that use of hormone replacement therapy (HRT) increases the risk of being recalled after mammography for further assessment, without eventual diagnosis of breast cancer – 'false positive recall'.

The Million Women Study included 88 000 postmenopausal women from 50 to 64 years between 1996 and 1998. Breast cancer was diagnosed in 0.5%, and 3% had false positive recall.

False positive recall was significantly increased in current users (with an increase of 64%) and past users of HRT. The effect decreased with time but was still significant 5 years after stopping HRT.

Use of HRT was estimated to have been responsible for around 20% of the false positive recall in the NHS breast screening programme, or around 14 000 cases per year.

SCREENING

Effects of conjugated equine estrogens on breast cancer and mammography screening in postmenopausal women with hysterectomy
Stefanick ML, Anderson GL, Margolis KL *et al.*
JAMA, 2006; **295**: 1647–1657

The oestrogen-only arm of the Women's Health Initiative found a possible protective effect of conjugated oestrogens against breast cancer – reassuring for those women with prior hysterectomy who are appropriate for this therapy. Compared to those on placebo, the oestrogen group had a hazard ratio of 0.67.

In this high quality study, all the women underwent routine mammography at the start of the study, then annually. The oestrogen group required more follow up in terms of more mammograms at shorter intervals. More abnormal mammograms led to more need for biopsies. However, ultimately the good news was that there was no sign of an increase in the incidence of breast cancer over the 7 years of study.

Influence of personal characteristics of individual women on sensitivity and specificity of mammography in the Million Women Study: cohort study
Banks E, Reeves G, Beral V *et al.*
BMJ, 2004; **329**: 477–479

This further research from the Million Women Study examines how lifestyle, hormonal, and other factors influence the value of mammography.

In addition to the influence of HRT (which increased recall), they found two other factors had a negative effect on efficiency, and possibly effectiveness of mammography: previous breast surgery and being thin (body mass index <25). All three factors are associated with increased mammographic density, which the authors offer as a plausible explanation for the findings. There was no such effect from past oral contraceptive use, family history, parity, smoking, or alcohol consumption.

Presentation on websites of possible benefits and harms from screening for breast cancer: cross sectional study
Jørgensen KJ, Gøtzsche PC
BMJ, 2004; **328**: 148

This paper looked at how information is presented on the internet and compared information from advocacy groups, government institutions and consumer organisations.

In the European Union an average of 23% of the population use the internet to find information about health issues. This will surely only increase with time and yet the information available is very mixed.

The authors found that in their searches:

- advocacy groups and governmental organisations chose information that shed a positive light on screening probably because screening programmes depend on high participation rates
- there were potential conflicts of interests. For example, all the advocacy groups accepted industry funding whereas the three consumer organisations acknowledged the risk of bias related to industry funding, and two of them did not accept such funding at all

- research quoted was selective rather than representative and there was wide-spread omission of adverse effects
- overdiagnosis (around 30% of cases) and overtreatment, the major harms of screening, were under-reported except by the consumer organisations. Only 18% of publications mention false positives and false negatives
- few people appreciate that screening contributes to the rise in incidence of breast cancer
- serious consequences of increased use of unnecessary radiotherapy were infrequently mentioned and even then usually downgraded
- inflated claims of saved mastectomies were not uncommon (the opposite – an increase in mastectomy – seems to occur)
- information was often misleading – women are not told the numbers needed to screen to prevent one death – or erroneous, not reflecting recent findings. The exception again was the consumer sites, which were much more balanced and comprehensive
- positive spin was commonplace – terms like 'psychological distress' are abandoned for the more friendly and less threatening 'anxiety'
- in one study half of those who failed to attend for a second mammogram said it was due to pain experienced previously, despite the process often being said to be painless
- only the consumer sites reliably mentioned that detected cancers may never progress

They concluded that material provided by professional advocacy groups and governmental organisations is 'severely biased in favour of screening' and that few websites live up to accepted GMC standards for informed consent. Requirements for consent need to be particularly strict when dealing with a healthy population. Are we in danger of sacrificing our role as informers in order to be paternalistic and push the NHS agenda?

MRI

Efficacy of MRI and mammography for breast-cancer screening in women with a familial or genetic predisposition
Kriege M, Brekelmans CT, Boetes C *et al.*
N Engl J Med, 2004; **351**: 427–437

Nearly 2000 Dutch women with at least a 15% lifetime risk of breast cancer underwent clinical examination six monthly and were screened annually by MRI and mammography.

MRI appears to be around twice as sensitive as mammography in detecting tumours in high risk women with an inherited susceptibility to breast cancer, i.e. it is good at ruling out breast cancer. But it was a little less specific, meaning more false positives and unnecessary follow-ups and biopsies.

It is not so good for low or average risk women. Further studies are needed to identify who will benefit most as it is expensive and in this study 5% were lost to follow up (mainly due to claustrophobia).

SCREENING

Screening with magnetic resonance imaging and mammography of a UK population at high familial risk of breast cancer: a prospective multicentre cohort study (MARIBS)
Leach MO, Boggis CR, Dixon AK *et al.*
Lancet, 2005; **365**: 1769–1778

Another study supports the increased sensitivity of MRI for detecting breast cancer in young women aged 35–49 years with a strong family history or a proven genetic predisposition. Of the 35 cancers found, 77% were detected by MRI and 40% by mammography.

MRI was more sensitive, mammography slightly more specific. So MRI will have more false positives at further increased cost and it is still unclear whether this saves lives.

Combining the two procedures may be the most effective method.

Further Research

- Contrary to popular belief, cancer does not run a more benign course in the elderly. A study that looked at the likelihood of metastases found no differences in the over 70s that were attributable to age. The disease behaved as a function of its stage rather than the age of its host. The authors vote for the same treatment and the same screening options regardless of age. *Cancer*, 2004; **100**: 1807–1813.

- Obesity lowers the specificity of mammography typically increasing risks of a false positive by 20% according to this study. Sensitivity was unchanged. Poor image clarity seems to be taking the blame. Prewarning during informed consent will help to reduce the burden of distress that will accompany the additional imaging required. *Arch Intern Med*, 2004; **164**: 1140–1147.

CERVICAL CANCER

What we know already:

- Worldwide 400 000 women contract cervical cancer annually – the second most common malignancy in women after breast cancer
- Screening began in 1964 and was relaunched in 1988 with a more efficient recall system
- Controversies over screening intervals, methods of cytology and HPV testing continue to be debated
- Cytology remains the gold standard for cervical cancer detection in Europe and the US but relies on subjective interpretation. Optimum screening intervals are still hotly debated
- The NHS programme has led to a 42% drop in the incidence of cervical cancer in England and Wales between 1988 and 1997
- To prevent one death, around 1000 women need to be screened for 35 years, 150 women have an abnormal result, over 80 are referred for investigation, and over 50 have treatment
- Estimates of the need for retesting due to inadequate smears reach 300 000 women per year. Many women have to be screened and treated to prevent a single cancer
- A range of screening strategies are possible. They involve combinations of liquid based cytology, earlier referral of those with mild dyskaryosis for colposcopy, stratifying referral with HPV testing, or screening primarily with HPV testing
- HPV is present in virtually all cases of cervical cancer and prevalence in precancerous lesions varies from 80 to 95%
- Continuing research has so far shown HPV vaccines to be safe and highly effective in the medium term and widespread programmes for vaccination are being developed

The screening programme

The NHS cancer screening programme currently recommends:
- women will be invited for a first test at the age of 25 years (instead of 20 years)
- cervical screening will be offered every 3 years until the age of 50
- women aged 50–64 years will then be offered screening every 5 years

The new method of liquid-based cytology is being introduced over the next few years to replace conventional Pap smears.

NICE requested pilot studies after a systematic literature review indicated that liquid-based cytology might provide substantial benefits but there was a still a lack of evidence to justify its introduction nationwide. The studies from three sites in England (Bristol, Newcastle, and Norwich), showed that the technique led to fewer inadequate tests, i.e. fewer false negatives. In Bristol, for example, the rate of inadequate smears fell from around 9% to 1.5%. It also gives a much quicker reporting time. It is hoped that the new approach will prove cost effective in the longer term, reducing inadequate smears and subsequent retesting.

Recent Papers

GENERAL

The cervical cancer epidemic that screening has prevented in the UK
Peto J, Gilham C, Fletcher O *et al.*
Lancet, 2004; **364**: 249–256

Questions over whether the UK Cervical Screening Programme is effective enough to justify the financial and psychosocial costs involved led to this paper. The authors explain that cervical cancer mortality in England and Wales in women under 35 years rose threefold from 1967 to 1987.

National screening from 1988 reversed this rising trend preventing an epidemic that would have killed about one in 65 of all British women born since 1950. Up to 80% of these deaths, around 5000 per year, are estimated to be prevented by screening, at a cost per life saved of about £36 000. There is strong evidence that early screening substantially reduces the death rate throughout life.

Changes in sexual behaviour also mean that up to half of young women in Britain have been infected with a high-risk strain of HPV by the time they are 30.

Cervical screening
Raffle AE
BMJ, 2004; **328**:1272–1273

This editorial challenges the recent changes in cervical screening protocol.
The author argues that:
- the difference between 3 yearly and 5 yearly screening is too small to measure, which is why we are having to use estimates
- switching to 3 yearly intervals means nine routine tests by age 50 instead of six
- 3-yearly screening costs 60% to 66% more than 5 yearly, and harm from more over-diagnosis and over-treatment increases
- the estimates from the commissioned studies suggest that in the author's own local programme, 3-yearly screening could at best add one extra woman added to the existing 24 annually in whom death from cervical cancer is prevented. Another 1000 would be added to the list of women with abnormal results
- she agrees that screening under 25s is now unethical regarding the harm to benefit ratio
- stopping screening above 50 years is advocated. She estimates that helping one patient over 50 years due to 5-yearly screening takes 420 000 tests, costing over £8m

With limited resources and other pressing issues, how would you spend the money?

Overview of the European and North American studies on HPV testing in primary cervical cancer screening

Cuzick J, Clavel C, Petry KU *et al.*
Int J Cancer, 2006; **119**: 1095–1101

Meta-analysis of 60 000 women in 11 European and North American studies looked into testing prior to cervical smear for high-risk HPV.

- The HPV test was substantially more sensitive (96% overall and quite consistent) than cytology in screening and detecting CIN 2+ changes and above. This was true for all ages and in every study.
- HPV testing is also easier to perform, highly reproducible, easily monitored and gives an objective rather than subjective result.
- Cytology had a sensitivity of 53% overall which was highly variable in the studies, but better in women older than 50.
- HPV testing was less specific (90.7% versus 96.3%).
- The specificity of both tests increased with the age of women tested, probably because there are more transient HPV infections in younger women, the authors said.
- Overall, HPV testing had a positive predictive value of 15.5% compared to cytology's PPV of 20%.

The authors support the principle of using the most sensitive test first and following up positives with the more specific test. They maintain that HPV should therefore be the sole primary screening test. Despite cytology's higher PPV (20%), its low sensitivity leads to a high proportion of cancers being missed and so they claim it should be reserved for women who test positive for HPV.

This is a distinct possibility in the future, but large projects will be needed to trial this approach and illustrate effects on morbidity and mortality.

Lifetime effects, costs, and cost effectiveness of testing for human papillomavirus to manage low grade cytological abnormalities: results of the NHS pilot studies

Legood R, Gray A, Wolstenholme J *et al.*
BMJ, 2006; **332**: 79–85
and

Effect of testing for human papillomavirus as a triage during screening for cervical cancer: observational before and after study

Moss S, Gray A, Legood R, and the Liquid Based Cytology/Human Papillomavirus Cervical Pilot Studies Group
BMJ, 2006; **332**: 83–85

Three centres participating in an NHS pilot for alternative strategies in cervical screening modelled data on more than 10 000 women aged 25–64 who had borderline and mildly dyskaryotic smears on liquid-based cytology.

- They found that performing HPV testing on this group and referring for immediate colposcopy if positive, and repeating cytology (and HPV testing) after 6 months if negative, was an effective strategy.
- Although more expensive than repeat cytology alone, it saved slightly more lives, due partly to earlier and better targeted colposcopy and reduction in loss to follow up.

CLINICAL ISSUES

SCREENING

- The rate of repeat smears fell by 74%, but referral for colposcopy for low grade abnormalities more than doubled.
- The cost of these colposcopies is the major concern with this as a wider approach – the cost to society is estimated as between £7500 and £30 000 per life year saved.

HPV VACCINATION

Cervical cancer, human papillomavirus, and vaccination
Lowndes CM, Gill ON
BMJ, 2005; **331**: 915

At least 95% of cervical cancer results from infection with 15 or more HPV types. HPV 16 and 18 account for 70% on their own.

Large scale trials on several non-infectious HPV vaccines are now in progress in many sites around the world.

The largest concerns a quadrivalent vaccine (for HPV types 6 and 11 as well as 16 and 18). Over 12 000 women up to the age of 26 years in 90 centres in 13 countries participated in this FUTURE II study. Three doses of vaccine or placebo were given over 6 months.

- Of those free of infection after the full vaccination, 100% were still free of infection at 17 months.
- There were no observed cases of high-grade precancerous change or non-invasive cancer in the vaccinated group.
- There were 21 such cases in the placebo group.
- Of those who did not complete the entire protocol for the trial, e.g. by missing an appointment, and who may therefore have become infected in the first 6 months during the vaccination period, 97% were still uninfected (only one case was infected) at review.

These promising results could save a significant amount in screening costs.

Questions remain of course. How much cancer will be prevented? Should we vaccinate boys? Will boosters be necessary? Will vaccination benefit those already infected?

Mortality benefits could take up to 20 years to show due to the long latent period – the very thing which makes screening possible. Screening should of course continue in the meantime. Hopefully we will be in a position to accelerate the delivery of the vaccine throughout the world.

HPV vaccine and adolescents' sexual activity
Lo B
BMJ, 2006; **332**: 1106–1107

Although HPV vaccination is over 90% effective in preventing new infections and precancerous cervical lesions caused by the HPV types that it covers, some have raised ethical concerns.

With sexual activity starting earlier, the vaccine needs to target those around the age of 11–12 in order to catch adolescents before they acquire infection. In the US where this editorial was written, pro-family lobbies like to seek parental choice in anything that might influence sexual behaviour. Informed consent is usually required from parents and children for minors, and advocates of sexual abstinence claim vaccination will condone or promote sexual activity. However, fear of sexual infection is not thought to be a major reason for abstinence.

Vaccination is no problem if the parents agree. Estimates suggest that about 75% will when properly informed. But if an adolescent prefers vaccination and parents refuse there may be a problem. Additionally, in cases of abuse parents do not act in the child's best interest.

Hopefully as the goal is cancer prevention, some of the legal minefields of contraception (which now has legal precedents in the UK) and abortion will be subverted.

Making vaccination routine, i.e. without extensive discussion, could be shortsighted until any concerns about the vaccine are eliminated.

HPV vaccine is also sorely needed in developing countries where cervical cancer takes many lives. The expense is unaffordable and a series of three injections may not be feasible so a global programme of research and assistance is needed.

PSYCHOLOGICAL ASPECTS

Psychological impact of human papillomavirus testing in women with borderline or mildly dyskaryotic cervical smear test results: cross sectional questionnaire study
Maissi E, Marteau TM, Hankins M et al.
BMJ, 2004; **328**: 1293

Testing for HPV has been proposed as a method to stratify risk of developing cervical cancer as it is associated with high-grade pre-invasive lesions and is present in almost 100% of cervical cancers.

The psychological cost is important though and this study found that when smear test results are borderline or mildly dyskaryotic, positive HPV results led to more anxiety, distress and concern. This was worse in the young and where there was a failure to understand what the result meant. This is an opportunity for good communication. Reassurance of the prevalence of HPV may help. Around 20% of young women and about 5% of women over 35 are estimated to be infected at any one time.

Psychological effects of a low-grade abnormal cervical smear test result: anxiety and associated factors
Gray NM, Sharp L, Cotton SC et al.
Br J Cancer, 2006; **94**: 1253–1262

TOMBOLA (Trial Of Management of Borderline and Other Low-grade Abnormal smears) recruited 3500 women with slightly abnormal smears and measured the psychological distress caused by the result.

These were the sort of changes that normally revert to normal by themselves but are kept under review. Those treated later for persisting cervical abnormalities under colposcopy are very unlikely to go on to develop cervical cancer.
- Women reported similar levels of anxiety to those with high CIN grade results.

SCREENING

- 23% were probable cases of clinical anxiety and another 20% were possible cases.
- Symptoms were more severe in the young, those with children, smokers, and those with high levels of physical activity.

The authors conclude that women may not understand what 'pre-cancerous' means and that information strategies with reassurance are much needed to reduce the unnecessarily high levels of anxiety caused by this process.

CHLAMYDIA

What we know already:

- *Chlamydia trachomatis* infection is the commonest sexually transmitted infection in the UK
- Over 82 000 cases were diagnosed in genito-urinary medicine clinics in 2002 – up 10% on the previous year
- The national screening pilot found 14% of patients under 16 years old, 10% of 16–19 year olds, and 7% of 20–24 year olds were infected
- It is the most preventable cause of infertility in women. It is hoped that screening could reduce pelvic inflammatory disease by up to 50%
- Public awareness of chlamydia and its consequences remains inadequate
- Fewer than an estimated 10% of prevalent infections are diagnosed
- Chlamydia screening programmes have been shown to reduce infection and related morbidity. Treatment with a single 1 g dose of azithromycin is simple and has high compliance
- Opportunistic chlamydia screening is being introduced in England, although there is no high quality evidence of its effectiveness
- 'Provider-led' strategies of partner notification (a.k.a. contact tracing) where health providers initiate contact, work better than 'patient-led' strategies where the patient sends their partner in for treatment
- Partner notification carries implications in different cultural settings where power balances in relationships may be very different and could incur risk of domestic violence
- The lack of specificity of many diagnoses can result in high levels of overdiagnosis, and this is a difficult basis from which to start tracing contacts
- It is also unknown what is felt to be acceptable to individuals in terms of tracing, but these answers will be needed to tackle sexual infections effectively around the globe

Recent Papers

Barriers to opportunistic chlamydia testing in primary care
McNulty CAM, Freeman E, Bowen J et al.
Br J Gen Pract, 2004; **54**: 508–514

This qualitative study in UK general practices identified common reasons that hinder the progress of chlamydia screening:
- lack of knowledge of the benefits of testing
- knowing when and how to take specimens
- reticence to discuss sexual health
- particular reticence to discuss screening in a consultation unrelated to sexual health
- time pressures and lack of resources

No earth-shattering conclusions then but the process reflected a general dearth of confidence, which comes out of a lack of central guidance on how to proceed. The

SCREENING

transmission of information needs time and sensitivity to achieve informed consent before testing. Appropriate resources will need to be in place before this extra burden can be placed on primary care.

Incidence of severe reproductive tract complications associated with diagnosed genital chlamydial infection: the Uppsala Women's Cohort Study

Low N, Egger M, Sterne JAC *et al.*
Sex Transm Infect, 2006; **82**: 212–218

This interesting research suggests that the benefits and cost-effectiveness of chlamydia screening might have been overestimated.

Previous studies of hospital and clinic populations imply that up to 40% of cases of untreated chlamydia progress to PID within a few weeks of infection, and that nearly 25% of women with PID will have an ectopic pregnancy or become infertile. This may be an overestimation according to this research in a cohort of 44 000 Swedish women aged 15–24 in the Uppsala study.

The rate of PID was 5.6% in those who tested positive for chlamydia and was 4% in those who tested negative. Lower figures than expected were also associated with ectopic pregnancy and infertility.

Cumulative incidences of hospital-diagnosed pelvic inflammatory disease, ectopic pregnancy, and infertility by age 35 were 2–4% overall, and 3–7% in those with a positive test for chlamydia. This is reassuring for patients, but if the incidence of complications associated with chlamydia have been overestimated, then current screening programmes may not be as beneficial or as cost-effective as hoped.

Additionally, research is beginning to suggest that infection may resolve itself within a year in asymptomatic patients without doing any damage.

Coverage and uptake of systematic postal screening for genital *Chlamydia trachomatis* and prevalence of infection in the United Kingdom general population: cross sectional study

Macleod J, Salisbury C, Low N *et al.*
BMJ, 2005; **330**: 940

Invites went out to 19 773 UK men and women aged 16–39 years to participate in chlamydia screening by posting a urine specimen they collected at home. The authors found that:

- postal screening was feasible but only about 1 in 3 accepted screening
- uptake was lower in the young, in men, in ethnic minorities and in disadvantaged areas
- prevalence of genital *Chlamydia trachomatis* was just below 2.8% for men and almost 3.6% for women
- in those under 25 years, these figures reached around 5% in men and 6% in women
- screening ultimately seems to lead to wider inequalities in sexual health

Partner notification of chlamydia infection in primary care: randomised controlled trial and analysis of resource use
Low N, McCarthy A, Roberts TE *et al.*
BMJ, 2006; **332**: 14–19

Genitourinary medicine clinics are overburdened with workload. This study, a part of the ClaSS project – the chlamydia screening studies project, which is a multicentre randomised trial based on 27 general practices in the Bristol and Birmingham area – looked to see if some of the work involved in contact tracing could be delivered within the practice instead.

Partner notification by trained practice nurses immediately after the diagnosis, with follow up by telephone, was at least as effective as referral to a specialist centre and cost the same amount. This is probably due to the fact that one-third of those referred did not get round to attending the GUM clinic.

This approach could easily be incorporated into the English national screening programme to relieve pressure on overburdened clinics.

SCREENING

SEXUAL HEALTH

What we know already:

- There is a continuing decline in the nation's sexual health with all sexually transmitted infections on the increase
- Attendances at genitourinary medicine clinics doubled in the last 10 years reaching over a million cases a year. Services are overburdened and failing to deliver high quality open access services
- More people have more sexual partners in their lifetime than ever before
- The age of first intercourse gets ever lower and sex education is still patchy and of dubious efficacy
- More teenage girls become pregnant in the UK than anywhere else in Europe
- Over one-quarter of 14–15 year olds think the oral contraceptive protects against infection
- Sexually active adolescents seriously underestimate their risks of sexually transmitted infection
- There has been a decline in safe sex practice particularly among homosexual men
- More men have presented for sexual help since sildenafil was invented
- Estimates of HIV worldwide run to around 38 million cases with 5 million new infections each year
- About 30% of people infected with HIV in the UK are diagnosed late (with low CD4 counts) – less than half of those through routine screening
- Meta-analysis in the 11–18 year age group has failed to find any evidence that preventative strategies were effective in delaying initiation of sexual intercourse in adolescents, in improving use of contraception, or in reducing pregnancy rates

Guidance

Report on sexual health. *House of Commons Health Select Committee*, June 2003.
National strategy for sexual health and HIV. *Dept of Health*, July 2001.

Recent Papers

SEXUAL HEALTH IN THE COMMUNITY

Trends in sexually transmitted infections in general practice 1990–2000: population based study using data from the UK general practice research database
Cassell JA, Mercer CH, Sutcliffe L *et al.*
BMJ, 2006; **332**: 332–334

The national strategy for sexual health proposes that more of the increasing burden is managed within primary care but until this study there has been little investigation of the size of the contribution from primary care.

Pick up of such cases in primary care has increased significantly in recent years.

They treated 23% of chlamydia cases in women but only 5.3% in men. They also treated half the cases of non-specific urethritis and urethral discharge and 5.7% of cases of gonorrhoea in women and 2.9% in men. Men tended to be treated for what are presumed to be symptoms of sexual infections.

Problems with sexual function in people attending London general practitioners: cross sectional study
Nazareth I, Boynton P, King M
BMJ, 2003; **327**: 423

This study in around 1500 men and women belonging to London general practices assessed prevalence of sexual problems in the community.

They found that sexual dysfunction was more common than you might think from the medical notes. However, controversy exists about the medicalisation of these 'disorders' making diagnosis tricky. Is dysfunction disease?

- The most common problem in men was erectile failure and lack/loss of sexual desire.
- Predictors of a problem in men were higher consultation rates and being bisexual.
- In women, failure to orgasm or lack/loss of sexual desire was most common.
- 30% reported seeking sexual advice but records of this appeared in the notes of only 3–4% suggesting doctors may be reluctant to record sensitive material.
- 22% of men and 40% of women had a sexual problem (diagnosed by ICD-10 criteria). This reduced to 16% and 27% if you don't accept lack/loss of sexual desire as a serious problem.

An accompanying paper found persistent sexual problems, defined as lasting over 6 months, to be much less common. They had a prevalence of 6% in men and 16% in women. In men it was mainly premature orgasm and in women lack of interest in sex (*BMJ*, 2003; **327**: 426–427).

The making of a disease: female sexual dysfunction
Moynihan R
BMJ, 2003; **326**: 45–47

This article is written by a journalist and describes the 'corporate sponsored creation of a disease'.

Close ties to drug companies have allowed certain researchers to develop and define a new type of disease – female sexual dysfunction. The potential market for this became apparent with the multi-billion dollar profits from Viagra (sildenafil) launched in 1998 for erectile dysfunction in men.

Defining a disease in women takes a little more guile. An erection may be all or nothing, one or zero, measurable, you might say. But for women the researchers have had to get together at meetings heavily sponsored by interested drug companies to define characteristics of the new condition in order to facilitate credible trials. The definition was broad to say the least as the most commonly cited prevalence of 'female sexual dysfunction' disturbingly comes in at 43%, a figure now widely quoted in the media.

The overmedicalisation and oversimplification has caused concern. Changes in

CLINICAL ISSUES

SEXUAL HEALTH

sexual desire are the norm – a healthy response to patterns of stress, tiredness and relationship difficulties. According to some, use of the term 'dysfunction' is misleading. Difficulties become dysfunction become disease. Doctors treat disease and they like to do it with drugs. It is quicker than paying attention to aspects of causality.

So the area will be highlighted which may be a good thing but as soon as women escape the ever-narrowing definitions of what is normal, the drug-peddlers will be ready to allow doctors to prescribe away everyone's problems.

HIV

Preventing HIV
Ammann AJ
BMJ, 2003; **326**: 1342–1343

For two decades we have known how to prevent every method of spreading HIV and for two decades we have failed to do it.

This editorial argues that priorities need to change. We need worldwide agreements on testing blood donors for HIV, challenging high-risk cultural practices and widespread testing for HIV. Partner notification needs to avoid discrimination and stigmatisation. Measures should be taken to protect underage girls from the risk from infected older men.

A single dose of nevirapine can reduce perinatal HIV infection by 50% but it is massively under-utilised. Those who subtly undermine methods of prevention such as the 'condoms-don't-work brigade' – should desist. Educational programmes promoting monogamy, abstinence, delayed sexual intercourse and condoms should be financed and manned. Behaviour at all levels needs to change – from government, through schools and community leaders, to the individual.

Is this editorial anything new? Not really. It's just that we are not doing it.

Uptake of HIV screening in genitourinary medicine after change to 'opt-out' consent
Stanley B, Fraser J, Cox NH
BMJ, 2003; **326**: 1174

The national strategy for sexual health and HIV recommended that all people attending GUM clinics should be offered an HIV test on their first visit. Some patients assume that they will be routinely tested for HIV at a genitourinary medicine clinic. Not so. Screening for syphilis is routine but not for HIV or viral hepatitis. Can we follow the example of 'routine' ante-natal screening for HIV which had a 96% uptake in the rural locale of this study?

Changing from 'opt-in' HIV screening system for those identified as 'high-risk', to an 'opt out' system of routine screening with the opportunity to refuse testing, increased uptake of HIV testing from 35% to 65% in this study.

The practice was acceptable and well on the way to achieving national targets for uptake.

SEXUAL HEALTH

HERPES

Ethics of screening for asymptomatic herpes virus type 2 infection
Krantz I, Löwhagen G, Ahlberg BM *et al.*
BMJ, 2004; **329**: 618–621

Universal serological testing for herpes simplex virus type 2 does not seem to be ethical, especially where there is a low prevalence of infection. Sensitivity and specificity of tests are good at 95% and some experts have advocated screening but:
- many of those infected are asymptomatic
- there is no cure and infection is life long and sexually transmissible
- the psychosocial impact on relationships could be catastrophic
- cost-effectiveness of testing is unproven
- positive predictive values in areas of low prevalence will be very low, with false positives reaching 30–40%. In high prevalence groups, around 10% have a false positive
- even antenatal screening is expensive and the benefits for babies unproven

ADOLESCENTS

Mandatory reporting to the police of all sexually active under-13s
Bastable R, Sheather J
BMJ, 2005; **331**: 918–919

This editorial discusses 2005 government guidance for mandatory reporting of all sexually active young people under 13 to the police and the collection of data in relation to sexually active young people under 16.

These measures have been criticised as insensitive and risk alienating people already in abusive situations by bringing their situation into the realms of criminality. The GMC's guidance is clear: 'confidentiality can be breached without consent only where there is a risk of serious harm to the patient or others'. The legal status of the protocols is unclear but they seem to imply a retreat from the Gillick judgment.

Mandatory reporting may be too blunt an instrument. Young people value the confidentiality. Compromising this could prevent them from asking for help in the first place.

EMERGENCY CONTRACEPTION

Impact on contraceptive practice of making emergency hormonal contraception available over the counter in Great Britain: repeated cross sectional surveys
Marston C, Meltzer H, Majeed A
BMJ, 2005; **331**: 271

Allowing sales of emergency contraception over the counter has not led to unsafer sex according to a study of women aged 16–49 years. In the 2 years following deregulation this study found:

SEXUAL HEALTH

- no increase in use of emergency contraception
- no increase in episodes of unprotected sex
- unchanged use of regular methods of contraception
- more women bought it over the counter rather than attending elsewhere

According to the Office for National Statistics, pharmacy sales doubled again in 2004 to reach 50% of total requests by 2005.

Emergency contraception
Glasier A
BMJ, 2006; **333**: 560–561

Controversies have surrounded the use of emergency contraception.

However, use in most countries is actually pretty low. In the US it is something of an ideological battleground. Supporters claim that 43% of the reported fall in abortion in the US was due to the use of emergency contraception. England and Wales could have expected to prevent 66 500 abortions with the same logic, but in fact the abortion rate has risen and the reduced access to abortion clinics in the US might be a more relevant factor.

In addition, how sure are we that it really works? A high quality trial will always be unethical. When easily available at home, use more than doubled but three studies failed to show a measurable effect on pregnancy or abortion.

You might as well try it if you do not want a baby, but it is hardly as powerful as those both for or against it seem to claim.

SEXUAL HEALTH

ALLERGIES

Guidelines

The provision of allergy services. *House of Commons Health Committee*. London, 2004

Allergy: the unmet need. *Royal College of Physicians Working Party*. June 2003.
This scathing report on the provision of allergy services is a UK blueprint for better patient care in a burgeoning epidemic.

The report claims there has been a national failure to meet minimum standards of care. There is a major shortage of allergy specialists with only six fully staffed clinics in the UK. This has driven people towards the dubious claims of many complementary therapists and unproven techniques of investigation and treatment.

Allergy is increasing in incidence. Latest projections estimate that approximately one-third of the UK will develop allergy at some point in their lives. It is also increasing in severity. Peanut allergy was rare 10 years ago; now it affects one in 70 children and has trebled in the last 4 years. Further, it is complex. Mixed pictures of, for example, rhinitis, asthma and eczema can co-exist as 'multi-system allergic disease'.

ALLERGIES

The report makes recommendations for a 'whole system' approach to allergy led by appropriately trained specialists who can lead a nationwide training infrastructure involving regional allergy centres and training in primary care.

Recent Papers

Should UK allergy services focus on primary care?
Levy ML, Sheikh A, Walker S et al.
BMJ, 2006; **332**: 1347–1348

The marked increase in prevalence of allergic disease has led to calls for updated allergy services. Now is the time to decide whether it should be primary care that is the key provider of such a service to the UK population.

Multiple allergies affect an estimated 10% of people under 45 years and 5% of older people and are problematic to manage.

These patients could easily end up seeing different specialists rather than one person with expertise in multisystem disease. They might be seeing a gastroenterologist for food allergy and a respiratory physician for asthma and attend ENT clinic for rhinitis.

Diagnosis is made more difficult by the questionable availability and interpretation of the likes of skin prick tests and IgE testing.

There is minimal training in the UK undergraduate and postgraduate programmes. In primary care a local practitioner – a GP with special interest or nurse consultant – could be trained to organise a clinic to serve the whole trust. An overhaul like this will need a major input of resources to make a real difference.

Time trends in allergic disorders in the UK
Gupta R, Sheikh A, Strachan DP et al.
Thorax, 2007; **62**: 91–96

This analysis shows that after rising year on year in recent decades, rates of eczema, allergic rhinitis and hay fever seem to have stabilised and may even be falling according to a review of GP data, prescriptions and hospital records. However, admissions to hospital for anaphylaxis have risen by 700%, for food allergy by 500%, and for skin urticaria by 100%. Speculation as to the reasons includes altered sources of allergens as well as changes to medical practice.

Are the dangers of childhood food allergy exaggerated?
Colver A, Hourihane J
BMJ, 2006; **333**: 494–496 and 496–498

This pair of articles debates the question above.

Although a growing problem, Colver argues that, spurred on by the media, the dangers of food allergy are overstated and cause unnecessary alarm for families and schools. We are increasingly frightened of our food and yet the prevalence of severe reactions including death may not have increased.

The author estimates that one death per 830 000 children with food allergy occurs per year and that of serious childhood reactions admitted to hospital, only 10% would have benefited from having an adrenaline auto-injector at home.

Asthma is so strongly associated with fatal reactions that absence of asthma should reassure parents and doctors. (All but one of nine children with fatal or near fatal reactions in one study and all but one of 32 adult patients in another had asthma.)

Diagnostic problems do not help. In another study, half the children who tested positive to peanut allergy on skin prick could eat them quite happily. It is also common for parents to blacklist many potential allergens when their child is confirmed allergic to one allergen. In addition, most children outgrow allergy to milk and eggs and periodic retesting with an oral challenge in hospital will help confirm this.

Auto-injectors deliver a heavy weight of responsibility to parents, most of whom lack confidence to use it. Hourihane argues for them to be made available for those that might need to use them. He argues that there is little evidence of the anxiety that it is claimed these devices cause and that a perception of control for the family might be a good thing.

ALLERGIES

COMPLEMENTARY AND ALTERNATIVE THERAPIES

What we know already:

- The public want complementary therapies and the government is committed to patient choice
- The British market for complementary and alternative medicine is estimated at £1.6 billion a year
- The growth has been possible due to patients contributing to costs – 90% of complementary therapy is privately purchased
- One in ten adults in the UK has visited a practitioner of complementary medicine
- Around 18% of children (in the Bath area of England) have tried some form of complementary medicine and 7% have visited a practitioner – 85% were said to have benefited
- Half of the general practices in England offer some access to complementary or alternative therapy
- In 30% of practices, a primary healthcare team member offers the service, usually acupuncture and homeopathy; 12% use other independent practitioners (often of manipulative therapies) and 27% make external referrals on the NHS
- Homeopathy in the UK encompasses five homeopathy hospitals and as many as half a million UK clients
- Lack of regulation has allowed some disreputable practitioners to practice 'quackery' and put the public at risk
- In one large Taiwanese study, an estimated 24% of Chinese herbal medicines were shown to be adulterated with conventional pharmacologically active medicines. Half of these had two such contaminants
- Parents pursue 'natural treatments' for their children, but toxicity of many herbal medicines is unknown. One Birmingham study of 24 creams for atopic eczema found all but four adulterated with steroids – mainly the very potent clobetasol which in the doses recommended risked adrenal suppression

New regulations

Regulation of herbal medicine and acupuncture: proposals for statutory regulation. *Dept of Health*, March 2004.

The House of Commons Select Committee on Science and Technology recommended statutory regulation for acupuncturists and herbalists in the UK in November 2000.

Proposals for this were issued in March 2004 by the Department of Health with recommendations for a council that sets standards and investigates practitioners.

An estimated 4000 practitioners are not regulated by other bodies. The idea is that they would need to undergo professional development and be up to date with developments in medicine. Voluntary regulation is thought to be sufficient for the likes of aromatherapy and reflexology. Homeopaths may opt for statutory regulation.

The Medicines and Healthcare products Regulatory Agency (MHRA) has published a consultation document on the regulation of unlicensed herbal remedies.

Statutory regulation of herbal medicine and acupuncture: Report on the consultation. *Dept of Health*, February 2005.

This report analysed responses from the debate on the regulation of alternative therapies.

Recent Papers

GENERAL

Characteristic and incidental (placebo) effects in complex interventions such as acupuncture
Paterson C, Dieppe P
BMJ, 2005; **330**: 1202–1205

This excellent overview discusses how it may not be meaningful to split complex interventions into characteristic and incidental elements in order to analyse them with a biomedical model and ideally, a randomised controlled trial.

The authors explain that this will lead to what they describe as false negative results. Complementary treatments contain a spectrum of treatment factors which add 'incidental effects' (placebo effects or contextual factors such as the credibility of the intervention or consultation style of the practitioner) to any 'characteristic effects' of the intervention (specific effects of the actual process).

Unlike the Western biomedical model whereby the diagnosis precedes treatment, Chinese diagnosis is a rolling process buttressed at each of the many patient–practitioner meetings with measures such as pulse and tongue diagnoses and feedback on the effects of needling. This process is likely to elicit a direct effect in terms of a 'meaning response'. It continually reinforces itself and accommodates new concerns whether physical, emotional or social – a trouble shared is a trouble halved. The spell is weaved while self-confidence and self-awareness increases. The difference is not so much a function of the practitioner as a function of the different theoretical models.

A sham control procedure should include all the peripheral effects except for classical needling.

Complex interventions such as physiotherapy lie in a middle ground. The physiotherapist's assessment rather than a biomedical diagnosis starts the ball rolling. This may be explained to the patient in terms of a weakness of a particular muscle or ligament and the care package prescribed around that.

Killing the goose that laid the golden egg?
Coulter A
BMJ, 2003; **326**: 1280–1281

This article provides a useful synopsis of some issues related to complementary therapies.

COMPLEMENTARY AND ALTERNATIVE THERAPIES

They are extensively used throughout the world and there is a growing lobby for increased integration of complementary and orthodox techniques. Some countries even reimburse the costs of many complementary techniques.

Suspicion remains in the medical profession about many of the alternative practitioners and practices but hostility is starting to erode and training has reached the syllabus of many medical schools.

Often alternative treatments are used in addition to conventional treatments for conditions which are difficult to cure such as back pain, arthritis, migraine, menopausal symptoms and anxiety. Those with life-threatening illnesses also turn to them.

People clearly have a desire to help themselves and adopt some responsibility for their own care. In many cases they are willing to pay for it. Clearly the holistic, patient-centred approach of the therapist has a lot to do with it. The greater amount of time available and the apparent personal tailoring of the treatment are well-liked touches.

The need for critical evaluation is greater than ever to ensure safety and avoid wastefulness. There are moves in many countries to regulate these practices properly. The Dutch want to make it illegal for anyone other than trained doctors to be allowed to make a medical diagnosis. We may see the takeover of these therapies by registered medical practitioners depending on the legislation adopted. Orthodox medicine will then control access to alternative medicine and that is bound to be unpopular with the alternative practitioners.

The power struggle may dilute or destroy the effect of the interventions.

Potential health risks of complementary alternative medicines in cancer patients
Werneke U, Earl J, Seydel C et al.
Br J Cancer, 2004; **90**: 408–413

As many as half the US cancer patients in this study used herbal remedies or dietary supplements such as antioxidants as part of their cancer treatment – 11% used higher than recommended doses.

Warnings of adverse effects or interactions were given to 12%. Most warnings concerned echinacea in patients with lymphoma on immunosuppressive therapies. Other warnings included those for the anticoagulant effects of cod liver/fish oil, evening primrose oil, ginkgo and garlic.

Many of the cancer patients were not sure why they were using the remedies. More than half had not mentioned it to their doctor.

More research is needed to quantify risks and medical practitioners need to be well informed and have a high index of suspicion that patients are on extra treatments.

The situation is similar in the UK. A study of rheumatology patients found that almost half used herbal remedies (particularly echinacea, risking hepatotoxicity, or *Ginkgo biloba*, garlic, or devil's claw, risking bleeding disorders with their other medication). Only 5% had mentioned this but only 1% were aware there might be a problem (*Ann Rheum Dis,* 2005; **64**: 790).

COMPLEMENTARY AND ALTERNATIVE THERAPIES

ACUPUNCTURE

Acupuncture for chronic headache in primary care: large, pragmatic, randomised trial

Vickers AJ, Rees RW, Zollman CE *et al.*

BMJ, 2004; **328**: 744

Each week 10% of GPs either perform acupuncture on someone or refer to someone who will.

This large randomised study of 401 patients at 12 sites throughout England and Wales looked at the success of acupuncture in one of its main indications – chronic headache, predominantly migraine.

The acupuncture points were individualised by the practitioners and the control group received usual care rather than sham acupuncture.

A maximum of 12 treatments were used over a 3 month period and results showed persistent benefits:
- reduction in headache score at 12 months
- significant improvement in physical functioning, energy levels and quality of life
- 22 fewer days of headache per year
- 25% fewer GP visits
- 15% less medication
- 15% fewer sick days

Costs were £403 a year (versus £217 for the controls) most of which was the cost of the acupuncturist. Adding acupuncture to standard care was a relatively cheap way of easing a major NHS headache – £9180 per QALY gained, well below the £30 000 limit the NHS identifies. It is also likely to be a conservative estimate as savings in prescription drugs, productivity gains and benefits in subsequent years were not considered in the cost-effectiveness analysis (*BMJ*, 2004; **328**: 747).

The authors claim such a good value intervention should be widely available for NHS patients.

Acupuncture in patients with tension-type headache: randomised controlled trial

Melchart D, Streng A, Hoppe A *et al.*

BMJ, 2005; **331**: 376–382

This large study of 270 patients described the 'sham' intervention of superficial needling of non-acupuncture points as 'minimal acupuncture'.

The credibility of the real and 'sham' acupuncture were both rated very similarly by patients and both these interventions were equally and significantly effective in reducing the number of days with tension headache compared to a further control of no acupuncture of any kind for 12 weeks.

The point locations for traditional Chinese acupuncture did not appear relevant. The possibility for potent placebo effects is heightened where there is an exotic conceptual framework with frequent practitioner contact which includes a repeated ritual and high expectations.

The same team produced similar results for migraine (*JAMA*, 2005; **293**: 2118–2125).

COMPLEMENTARY AND ALTERNATIVE THERAPIES

Randomised controlled trial of a short course of traditional acupuncture compared with usual care for persistent non-specific low back pain
Thomas KJ, MacPherson H, Thorpe L et al.
BMJ, 2006; **333**: 623

Evidence for convincing effectiveness of acupuncture in the long term in low back pain is sparse. This study in primary care continued usual GP care but randomised two-thirds of the patients to 10 sessions of acupuncture. The effect at 24 months was more significant than the effect at 12 months. The acupuncture group had significantly less pain, less concern about pain and reduced use of analgesics. They did not use a sham acupuncture control and recognise that the personalising effect of therapeutic relationships and the widely reported relaxation of the intervention may help.

A cost effectiveness analysis accompanies this paper. Average cost for the acupuncture group was £460 and for the usual care group was £345. They estimate a cost of £4241 per QALY meaning that the benefit is highly cost-effective (*BMJ*, 2006; **333**: 626).

Acupuncture and knee osteoarthritis: a three-armed randomized trial
Scharf H, Mansmann U, Streitberger K et al.
Ann Intern Med, 2006; **145**: 12–20

This study showed a symptomatic benefit of acupuncture in osteoarthritis of the knee in 53%. With over 1000 participants, the study was large and well-designed. All received six sessions of physiotherapy and anti-inflammatory drugs. They also had either 10 consultations with a doctor, 10 sessions of real acupuncture, or 10 sessions of sham acupuncture.

Sham and real acupuncture worked equally well. Each was effective in more than half the patients compared to standard treatment which only helped 29%.

As ever it is not entirely clear whether the needling or the provider contact are the real cause of the benefit.

A randomized clinical trial of acupuncture compared with sham acupuncture in fibromyalgia
Assefi NP, Sherman KJ, Jacobsen C et al.
Ann Intern Med, 2005; **143**: 10–19

This study of 100 patients with fibromyalgia compared twice-weekly acupuncture for 12 weeks with 1 of 3 sham treatments – acupuncture for the wrong diagnosis (irregular periods), needling at non-acupuncture points, or faking it with toothpicks. The three sham techniques were pooled and blinding was adequate.

Real acupuncture fared no better than sham.

COMPLEMENTARY AND ALTERNATIVE THERAPIES

HERBALISM

Regulating herbal medicines in the UK
Ferner RE, Beard K
BMJ, 2005; **331**: 62–63

This editorial points to three important clinical criteria for licensing herbal medicines – efficacy, safety and quality of manufacture. Evidence is hard to come by and we still have treatments from the 16th century whose claims are not proven one way or the other. The European Union takes the view of registering drugs that have a 'long history' of use. In this context, this means 30 years, half of which should have been in the EU. They argue that longstanding use and experience is a plausible surrogate for efficacy and only safety needs to be considered. The US considers these medicines dietary supplements and outlaws unproven claims of therapeutic effect.

The UK seems likely to go down the route of using the Herbal Medicines Advisory Committee to advise government.

Saw palmetto for benign prostatic hyperplasia
Bent S, Kane C, Shinohara K et al.
N Engl J Med, 2006; **354**: 557–566

Saw palmetto is used by 2 million men in the US to treat benign prostatic hyperplasia.

This high quality double-blind randomised trial in 225 men convincingly refuted previous suggestions of a benefit on prostatic symptoms. Over the year long trial it was not found to be superior to placebo for measures such as prostatic size, urinary flow rate and quality of life.

Acute treatment of moderate to severe depression with hypericum extract WS 5570 (St John's wort): randomised controlled double blind non-inferiority trial versus paroxetine
Szegedi A, Kohnen R, Dienel A et al.
BMJ, 2005; **330**: 503

This randomised trial from Germany compared St John's wort (hypericum extract) with 6 weeks of paroxetine in 250 patients with moderate to severe depression. Although there has been some methodological criticism of the paper, the authors found equivalence of efficacy for depression but with fewer adverse effects for the patients on St John's wort.

Interaction of St John's wort with conventional drugs: systematic review of clinical trials
Mills E, Montori VM, Wu P et al.
BMJ, 2004; **329**: 27–30

This systematic review looked at 22 trials on pharmacokinetics related to use of St John's wort (*Hypericum perforatum*). The main finding was that the methodology of most of the rather small studies in this area was of pretty poor quality and much better research is needed. It seems users of St John's wort suffer possible

COMPLEMENTARY AND ALTERNATIVE THERAPIES

decreases in the bioavailability of conventional drugs but there were insufficient data to either quantify the effect, examine drugs individually or relate the effects to mechanisms of metabolism.

This conclusion is an important one though. Clinicians and patients do not currently have enough high quality information to guide the use of herbal products such as this.

Co-ingestion of herbal medicines and warfarin
Smith L, Ernst E, Ewings P *et al.*
Br J Gen Pract, 2004; **54**: 439–441

This UK postal survey looked at the growing use of herbal medicines and sent out 2600 questionnaires. Half the recipients replied.

The authors were particularly keen on assessing use of herbal products suspected of interacting with warfarin – garlic, ginseng, ginkgo biloba, feverfew, ginger and St John's wort. They found that:
- 19% of patients reported taking one or more complementary medicines
- of these, 9% took one or more of the herbal medications specified above
- 5% definitely felt that the herbal medicine could interfere with other prescribed drugs, 23% thought maybe, 53% did not know, 15% thought probably not and 4% definitely not
- only 4% had discussed the use of these products with their GP

Due to the high rate of self-medication with herbal preparations, the onus is on doctors to make active enquiries and patients to volunteer information on use of these products.

HYPNOTHERAPY

Hypnotherapy for functional gastrointestinal disorders
Drug Ther Bull, 2005; **43**: 45–48

About 20% of people in the UK have functional gastrointestinal disorders such as irritable bowel or functional dyspepsia. The role of hypnotherapy for these medically unexplained symptoms is examined in this review.

Although blinding was limited, there is enough evidence in the five available RCTs for the *Drug and Therapeutics Bulletin* to recommend that gut-directed hypnotherapy may relieve symptoms. However, a suitably trained hypnotherapist may be hard to find.

Gut-directed hypnotherapy for irritable bowel syndrome: piloting a primary care-based randomised controlled trial
Roberts L, Wilson S, Singh S *et al.*
Br J Gen Pract, 2006; **56**: 115–121

The alleviation of symptoms with gut-directed hypnotherapy in IBS has been found in the past to be useful in centres of secondary care. This primary care study looked into 101 patients, aged 18–65 years, with a diagnosis of IBS resistant to conventional management for greater than 6 weeks. The intervention was five sessions of hypnotherapy in addition to usual care.

Compared to usual management alone there were significant improvements in pain, diarrhoea and quality of life in the hypnotherapy group at 3 months, but no sustained effect was shown. The authors tell us that the lack of long-term benefit will preclude introduction of this intervention in a more widespread way.

HOMEOPATHY

Are the clinical effects of homoeopathy placebo effects? Comparative study of placebo-controlled trials of homoeopathy and allopathy
Shang A, Huwiler-Muntener K, Nartey L et al.
Lancet, 2005; **366**: 726–732

This review looked into the implausibilities of homeopathy and matched 110 double-blind trials of homeopathy against 110 for conventional medicine for the same condition. Small study sizes and less rigorous methods inflated apparent effectiveness and the authors found evidence of publication bias for both methods.

Unlike conventional medical trials, however, the authors found weak evidence for a specific effect of homeopathy which was consistent with the idea that it functions as a placebo.

MAGNETS

Magnet therapy
Finegold L, Flamm BL
BMJ, 2006; 332: 4

Selling medical magnets is a billion dollar global business. They are advertised to cure everything from pain to cancer. The studies which claim therapeutic effects fall prey to both familiar and unique biases. Specifically, experiments are difficult to blind. Real magnets might stick to keys in your pocket giving the game away or bracelets might feel a tiny drag subconsciously picked up when near ferromagnetic surfaces.

The harm, however, is very real. The neglect of illness which 'proper' medical science has something to offer is serious and financial harm is profound.

The massive magnetic fields of MRI scanners show neither ill nor harmful effects.

Patients should be advised that magnet therapy has no proven benefits.

COMPLEMENTARY AND ALTERNATIVE THERAPIES

DYSPEPSIA AND *HELICOBACTER PYLORI*

What we know already:

- Dyspepsia is a chronic condition endemic in the UK, affecting 40% of people annually and costing the NHS around a billion pounds per year
- The vast majority of cases are self-managed and do not present to the GP
- The term dyspepsia covers a number of indigestion symptoms such as epigastric pain, heartburn and acid reflux sometimes with feelings of bloating and nausea
- Gastro-oesophageal reflux disease (GORD) refers to endoscopically determined oesphagitis or endoscopy-negative reflux disease
- GORD is now looked upon as a family of diseases, focusing attention on symptoms rather than injury to oesophageal mucosa
- Drugs for these conditions account for the largest prescribing costs in the NHS
- Proton pump inhibitors are now available over the counter in the UK
- *Helicobacter pylori* infection causes antral gastritis, with increased acid secretion and heightened risk of duodenal ulcer
- Mortality from gastric cancer in Europe has fallen by around 50% between 1980 and 1999

Guidelines

A NICE guideline, *Dyspepsia – management of dyspepsia in adults in primary care*, was issued in August 2004.

Key recommendations include:

- review medication for possible causes of dyspepsia, such as NSAIDs or nitrates
- urgent referral for endoscopy regardless of age when symptoms are accompanied by 'alarm symptoms' of chronic gastrointestinal bleeding, progressive unintentional weight loss, difficulty swallowing, persistent vomiting, iron deficiency anaemia, or epigastric mass
- for patients without any alarm features, routine endoscopic investigation is not necessary but in those over 55 years, endoscopy is useful if symptoms persist despite initial interventions especially if there has been a previous gastric ulcer, or increased concern about the risk of gastric cancer
- initial therapeutic strategies for dyspepsia are empirical treatment with a proton pump inhibitor (PPI) or 'test and treat' – testing for and treating *Helicobacter pylori*
- NICE recommends *H. pylori* eradication in *H. pylori*-positive patients who have peptic ulcer disease and endoscopically determined non-ulcer dyspepsia
- patients who have GORD should be offered a full-dose PPI for 1 or 2 months. Recurrence of symptoms should be managed by the lowest 'on demand' dose of PPI that is effective

Recent Papers

Who benefits from *Helicobacter pylori* eradication?

Delaney BC
BMJ, 2006; **332**: 187–188

Definitions of dyspepsia and GORD vary and have led to the terms having poor predictive value for pathology. NICE therefore recommends a common pathway for heartburn and epigastric pain.

- We know now that eradication of *H. pylori* is highly effective in reducing recurrence of proven duodenal ulcer with an NNT of 2.
- Testing for *H. pylori* and treating if found is cost-effective for those with dyspepsia.
- According to the CADET–Hp study, test and treat is more effective than just suppressing acid with a PPI. The MRC–CUBE trial reported in 2006 that this strategy is similar in cost-effectiveness to just using a PPI, having equal QALYs and costs, but resulted in a small but significant improvement in dyspepsia symptoms at 1 year.
- Even when there is no obvious cause to the dyspeptic symptoms and endoscopy is negative for ulcer and oesphagitis, eradication therapy is still pretty effective. The NNT increases to around 15 but no treatment is any better. With the burden of these chronic relapsing conditions, these smaller benefits may be cost-effective and good evidence has at least convincingly refuted early suspicions that eradication might make GORD worse.

What about going one stage further and screening asymptomatic people for *H. pylori* in order to seek and destroy? The study by Lane *et al.* (below) showed benefit with an NNT of 30 to prevent one consultation. Where prevalence is low – only 15% screened positive – accurate tests such as the urea breath test should be used as half of all serology results would be false positives. The cost–benefit is not clear but NICE currently leaves space for eradication as a treatment option in uninvestigated dyspepsia.

Impact of *Helicobacter pylori* eradication on dyspepsia, health resource use, and quality of life in the Bristol helicobacter project: randomised controlled trial

Lane JA, Murray LJ, Noble S *et al.*
BMJ, 2006; **332**: 199–202

This community study looked at the value of *H. pylori* screening in over 10 000 unselected people between 20 and 59 years old.

Positives were given eradication treatment and had 35% fewer consultations for dyspepsia over the next 2 years. They also had 30% fewer regular symptoms. This study showed the effectiveness and feasibility of screening but the increased cost of the medication seemed to make the 'test and treat' approach currently more economically appealing.

CLINICAL ISSUES

DYSPEPSIA AND *HELICOBACTER PYLORI*

Limited impact on endoscopy demand from a primary care based 'test and treat' dyspepsia management strategy: the results of a randomised controlled trial
Shaw IS, Valor RM, Charlett A *et al.*
Br J Gen Pract, 2006; **56**: 369–374

Testing for *H. pylori* has been shown to be an effective replacement for endoscopy in younger patients in secondary care but most dyspepsia is managed in primary care.

This trial randomised patients under 55 years old from 47 practices. Serology was the test used. There were 19% fewer referrals in the intervention group, reducing demand for open access endoscopy but by nowhere near as much as hoped. Estimates in secondary care had reached over 70%.

Systematic review and meta-analysis of randomised controlled trials of gastro-oesophageal reflux interventions for chronic cough associated with gastro-oesophageal reflux
Chang AB, Lasserson TJ, Kiljander TO *et al.*
BMJ, 2006; **332**: 11–17

Meta-analysis of 11 studies found that use of PPIs to control symptoms of cough related to GORD had a much lesser effect than anticipated. Guidelines have suggested that treatment for up to 6 months is needed to resolve the cough, but other studies have shown that GORD is associated with but not the cause of the coughing.

Further Research

- Eradication treatment fails in 10–20% of cases, but failure is more likely in smokers according to a meta-analysis of 13 trials. Treatment was twice as likely to fail in those who smoked but it is unknown whether this is a bioavailability or compliance issue. *Am J Med*, 2006; **119**: 217–224.

- An association has been confirmed between acid suppression therapy particularly with PPIs and *Clostridium difficile* infection diagnosed in general practice. According to the General Practice Research Database, less than 1 case per 100 000 in 1994 has become 22 per 100 000 in 2004. *JAMA*, 2005; **294**: 2989–2995.

- Smoking and high dietary salt worsens reflux but tea and coffee do not according to a large study of Norwegians quizzed about their lifestyle habits. Those who had smoked daily for more than 20 years and those who added salt to their meals both increased their chances of reflux by 70%. *Gut*, 2004; **53**: 1730–1735.

UROLOGY

Recent Papers

PROSTATIC SYMPTOMS

Lower urinary tract symptoms in men
Chapple CR, Patel AK
BMJ, 2007; **334**: 2
and
Self management for men with lower urinary tract symptoms: randomised controlled trial
Brown CT, Yap T, Cromwell DA *et al.*
BMJ, 2007; **334**: 25

Watchful waiting has long been established as a safe alternative to resection of the prostate in lower urinary tract symptoms of voiding, storage and post-voiding, such as occur in benign prostatic hypertrophy. Just advising on lifestyle modification, however, is unlikely to do much to improve symptoms.

Self-management has many more components and this study in secondary care showed it to be significantly more beneficial than usual care. It included education about the causes and natural course of lower urinary tract symptoms and also reassurance about prostate cancer, advice on fluid management, toileting and bladder retraining. Crucially, there was a cognitive ingredient to promote behavioural change by teaching problem solving and goal setting in three small group sessions.

Some 140 men, mean age 63 years were randomised.
- At 3 months, treatment failure occurred in 10% of the self-management group and 42% of the standard care group.
- Symptomatic improvements were sustained up to 1 year.
- The effect was twice that of pharmacotherapy compared with placebo in randomised trials.

Possible biases included:
- selection bias – only those with the time and motivation may attend such a trial
- lack of objective assessment of flow rate (as outcome was by symptom score)
- a higher proportion of the self-management group had a university education (45% vs. 24%)

The authors suggest a large multicentre trial to confirm these apparently large benefits.

UTI

Developing clinical rules to predict urinary tract infection in primary care settings: sensitivity and specificity of near patient tests (dipsticks) and clinical scores
Little P, Turner S, Rumsby K et al.
Br J Gen Pract, 2006; **56**: 606–612

Despite the frequency of this diagnosis, independent predictors of UTI are still poorly validated in primary care.

This study of over 400 women with suspected UTI found that only nitrite, leucocyte esterase and blood independently predicted infection. A dipstick decision rule using these three variables was moderately sensitive (77%) and specific (70%) and PPV was 81%. If all three tests were negative, the NPV was 65%.

Response to antibiotics of women with symptoms of urinary tract infection but negative dipstick urine test results: double blind randomised controlled trial
Richards D, Toop L, Chambers S
BMJ, 2005; **331**: 143

A small study in New Zealand randomised 59 women with symptoms of UTI but a negative dipstick after 3 days of trimethoprim or placebo.
- Trimethoprim shortens dysuria in women with symptoms of uncomplicated UTI and negative dipstick result by a median time of 2 days. The NNT is 4.

- A negative dipstick test for leucocytes and nitrites did not predict response to antibiotic treatment.
- These results support the practice of empirical antibiotic use guided by symptoms, meaning that the minimisation of antibiotic use remains a dilemma.
- An infectious cause for the symptoms is likely in these circumstances, which is not being diagnosed with our usual methods.

A nurse led education and direct access service for the management of urinary tract infections in children: prospective controlled trial

Coulthard MG, Vernon SJ, Lambert HJ et al.
BMJ, 2003; **327**: 656

This nurse-led model for managing UTIs in children in primary care involved education of GPs, counselling of families and rapid access to imaging and managed to make diagnosis of UTI in children more successful.

Phase-contrast microscopy was taught and a microscope offered to the practices. More urine was collected and cultured. Children with probable or certain UTI underwent ultrasonography and DMSA scanning. Infants also underwent cystography.

Overall, the diagnosis rate of UTI and renal scarring doubled in the study practices compared to control practices. It quadrupled in infants (who are at greatest risk of scarring) and also in children without specific urinary symptoms where diagnosis is particularly difficult.

Study practices often awaited culture so there were more delays in treatment but they picked up more UTI to make up for it and their diagnosis was therefore more robust.

The study group used nitrite sticks less often because the researchers did not like them, claiming they miss half the cases. This does seem naïve and the authors do seem to regret reducing the opportunity for instant diagnosis as patients with negative results may have been dismissed. They might have encouraged their use followed by culture of 'negative' samples.

'Blind' treatment of infants with antibiotics based on clinical suspicion was encouraged although this approach may have been too controversial for some practices. Prescriptions of antibiotic prophylaxis increased in the study group. The standard of deputising and A&E doctors seemed lower.

The data imply that GPs have been missing three-quarters of UTIs in infants and half in children overall. This model improved the situation and was popular with doctors and families.

HAEMATURIA

Long-term outcome of hematuria home screening for bladder cancer in men

Messing EM, Madeb R, Young T et al.
Cancer, 2006; **107**: 2173–2179

Of 3500 men over 50 who tested their urine repeatedly for haemoglobin over a 19 year period, 16% were investigated for haematuria and 8% of those were diagnosed with bladder cancer.

UROLOGY

Relatively, the numbers of high and low grade cancers found were similar, but for the high grade tumours only 15% of the patients found by screening had muscle invasion compared to 60% of the unscreened group. After 14 years, 20% of these unscreened patients were dead but none of those detected by screening had died. The authors note that testing for haematuria could be a sensitive method for detecting bladder cancers and seems to improve survival.

The diagnostic value of macroscopic haematuria for the diagnosis of urological cancer in general practice
Bruyninckx R, Buntinx F, Aertgeerts B *et al.*
Br J Gen Pract, 2003; **53**: 31–35

How strong a predictor of serious illness is haematuria? Cases of haematuria presenting to general practice were assessed for incidence of urological cancers in this study taking in around 1% of the entire Belgian population.
- The positive predictive value of haematuria for these cancers in patients over 60 years was 22% for men and 8% for women.
- In the under 60s, predictive values were in single figures.
- No urological cancer was found in the age group under 40 years.

The authors conclude that thorough investigation for urological cancer is indicated in men older than 60 years with macroscopic haematuria.

In patients of either sex under 60 years of age, watchful waiting can be justified.

Time to abandon testing for microscopic haematuria in adults?
Malmström P
BMJ, 2003; **326**: 813–815

The paper reviews the controversial significance of microhaematuria by assessing current evidence in this poorly researched area where little consensus exists.
- In several studies, cancers were detected no more often than in controls.
- Microhaematuria is rare in renal cancer making renal biopsy difficult to justify.
- In men with prostatic symptoms due to BPH, one-third tested positive for microhaematuria but this did not correlate with any feature of the condition so was not helpful in assessment.
- The only disease for which microhaematuria might be considered an early stage is bladder cancer.
- Although new bladder cancer often presents with painless macroscopic haematuria, we do not know the time interval whereby we might pick it up at a microscopic stage.
- Cancers referred at the microscopic stage are around 5% of referrals, but there is no evidence that cancers are less advanced when picked up at this stage.
- The preclinical stage may be too brief, leaving primary screening for microhaematuria with too low a sensitivity.

Epidemiology, prescribing patterns and resource use associated with overactive bladder in UK primary care
Odeyemi I, Dakin H, O'Donnell R
Int J Clin Pract, 2006; **60**: 949–958

This study aimed to clarify incidence and prevalence of overactive bladder by analysing cases of 69 000 symptomatic patients in UK general practice.
- Prevalence was 4 per 1000 people.
- 28% were prescribed anticholinergics of which one-fifth tried more than one medication.
- 59% were referred to secondary services.
- 2.8% underwent urinary tests/investigations.
- 0.2% were seen by a continence nurse.

This study indicated that overactive bladder may be underdiagnosed, under-referred and undertreated in the UK.

The sensitivity and specificity of a simple test to distinguish between urge and stress urinary incontinence
Brown JS, Bradley CS, Subak LL *et al.*
Ann Intern Med, 2006; **144**: 715–723

A simple questionnaire called the 3IQ asks two incontinence questions to distinguish between stress and urge incontinence, which is important for deciding whether to recommend pelvic floor exercises or urge suppression exercises.

The first question asks if urine has leaked in the last 3 months (even a small amount). Those answering positively are asked if the leakage occurs when there was physical activity or a sense of urgency or both. The third asks about the circumstances when it occurs most often to get an idea of whether this is stress, urge or missed incontinence.

The tests were fairly accurate in predicting urge incontinence (sensitivity 0.75, specificity 0.77) and stress incontinence (sensitivity 0.86, specificity 0.60) and, although not perfect, could be a useful tool in primary care settings.

Several non-pharmacological, pharmacological, and surgical treatments may be effective in urinary incontinence. *Evidence-Based Medicine,* 2004; **9**: 173
The following paper is reviewed
Management of urinary incontinence in women: scientific review
Holroyd-Leduc JM, Straus SE
JAMA, 2004; **291**: 986–995

This review of 66 studies found that:
- pelvic floor muscle training, comprehensively taught, increases cure in stress, urge and mixed incontinence
- combining this with bladder training was better than pelvic floor training alone
- electrical stimulation was effective for urge incontinence
- anticholinergics were more effective than placebo for improvement in leakage episodes in urge incontinence

UROLOGY

- effective surgical options for stress incontinence include retropubic colpo-suspension and the suburethral sling procedure

---

Clinical and cost-effectiveness of a new nurse-led continence service: a randomised controlled trial
Williams KS, Assassa RP, Cooper NJ *et al.*
Br J Gen Pract, 2005; **55**: 696–703

This UK trial randomised nearly 4000 women and men to input from a continence nurse practitioner or usual care. The 8 week intervention included advice on diet and fluids, bladder training, pelvic floor awareness and lifestyle advice. It showed significant improvement in symptoms of incontinence, frequency, urgency, and nocturia, which were sustained at 6 months. Satisfaction was high and the service is likely to be a cost-effective model in this under-reported condition.

IMMUNISATION

Recent Papers

MMR

Predicting uptake of MMR vaccination: a prospective questionnaire study
Flynn M, Ogden J
Br J Gen Pract, 2004; **54**: 526–530

This study of 511 parents around the Brighton area of the UK centred around parental beliefs and concerns in relation to the MMR. They used a questionnaire which had a response rate of 57%. The findings were:
- parents feared guilt about any adverse consequences of their decision
- they expressed uncertainty whether to trust the media or the medical profession
- higher uptakes were predicted by uptake of previous vaccinations, having more faith in the medical profession and a lower belief that that vaccination is harmful to the immune system

IMMUNISATION

Effects of a web based decision aid on parental attitudes to MMR vaccination: a before and after study
Wallace C, Leask J, Trevena LJ
BMJ, 2006; **332**: 146–149

We now know that the alleged association with autism is totally without evidence to support it. Yet the harm is done.

Accessing a website with a series of questions designed to inform parents about the pros and cons of MMR has been shown capable of improving parental attitude to the vaccine.

Although it encouraged significantly more to be 'pro-vaccination', to a lesser extent it fed the negative attitudes of those who already were against the vaccine. They continued to dwell on outdated concerns and so avoided any risk of guilt in the event of any adverse outcome.

Concerted efforts to broach concerns have led to an apparent contradiction. Despite an information explosion, parents still choose to believe they have inadequate or biased information. This must come down to a mistrust of doctors and/or politicians and the media. We need to look seriously at our communication strategies regarding decisional conflicts such as this. Tools like the one in this study may be part of the solution for a minority to whom it appeals.

Think mumps
Godlee F
BMJ, 2005; **330**: 1132–1135

This editorial reminds us of the many vaccine scares over the years and the devastating impact of antivaccine activism.

With the mumps outbreak continuing in 2005 as it did in 2004, the author notes that the epidemic is ironically indicative of the success of UK vaccination policy. Cases are mainly in 19–23 year olds who were not exposed to mumps as children due to the success of MMR introduction in 1988, and who missed out on the second dose for various reasons (the second dose was introduced in 1996).

Mumps must now be part of the differential diagnosis for a generation of doctors who have never seen a case. There is no treatment, however, beyond isolating the infected and vaccinating the susceptible.

HAEMOPHILUS INFLUENZAE TYPE B

Trends in *Haemophilus influenzae* type b infections in adults in England and Wales: surveillance study
McVernon J, Trotter CL, Slack MP *et al.*
BMJ, 2004; **329**: 655–658

Haemophilus influenzae type B (Hib) infection rates in the UK fell dramatically after the introduction of childhood immunisation in 1992. However, since 1998 there has been a marked resurgence with cases in children, most of whom were fully vaccinated, doubling every year. Cases in adults kept pace reaching pre-1992 levels.

Reasons include lower than anticipated direct protection from infant vaccination, use of less immunogenic combination vaccines and wearing off of the initial promotion push.

This report measured the associated fall in adult Hib antibody levels, which had fallen by 1994 and stayed steady from then on. This lowered population immunity reflected the reduced transmission from vaccinated children leading to fewer chances to become naturally immune. Most liable to infection were those of ages most likely to mix with children such as parents and grandparents – an older unimmunised group.

The importance of high quality surveillance is underlined by this study. The problem has been picked up, resulting in withdrawal of poorly immunogenic vaccines and implementations of a booster campaign for children under 4 years which should permit herd immunity and prevent further increases in infections.

OTHER VACCINATIONS

Stopping routine vaccination for tuberculosis in schools
Fine P
BMJ, 2005; **331**: 647–648

From autumn 2005 the routine BCG vaccination of schoolchildren against tuberculosis stopped. This change comes as notifications of tuberculosis in England and Wales are at their highest level since 1983.

There are good reasons. Changes in epidemiology, unsubstantiated fears of co-infection with HIV and localisation of TB in immigrant communities mean the time is right to come into line with vaccination policy in many other countries. Imported disease declines with time and has not led to increases in the risk for the indigenous population. BCG vaccination will now be offered to infants in communities with an average incidence of tuberculosis of at least 40 per 100 000 and to unvaccinated families from countries of similar incidence.

Most people born in the UK now will not receive BCG. As most will not be exposed to mycobacteria, tuberculin testing will become more efficient in detecting infection.

Rotavirus vaccines moderately reduce rotavirus diarrhoea in children. Evidence-Based Medicine, 2004; 9: 179
The following paper is reviewed
Rotavirus vaccine for preventing diarrhoea
Soares-Weiser K, Goldberg E, Tamimi G et al.
Cochrane Database Syst Rev, 2004

Rotavirus causes one-third of all hospital admissions for diarrhoea and leads to about 600 000 deaths per year – 6% of deaths in children under 5 years. In the UK 1 in 40 children are admitted to hospital for rotavirus infection in their first 5 years. This review shows that vaccines can be very effective in preventing rotavirus diarrhoea.

Lingering safety concerns have benefited from a study refuting previous concerns about an association with intussusception. A large study, with nearly 70 000

IMMUNISATION

participants, failed to confirm any other serious adverse events over a year of surveillance. Similar efficacy now needs to be demonstrated in developing countries (*Evidence-Based Medicine*, 2006; **11**: 113).

Preventing and treating hepatitis B infection
Aggarwal R, Ranjan P
BMJ, 2004; **329**: 1080–1086

This clinical review suggests it is time to introduce universal immunisation in the UK against hepatitis B. The virus causes more than 500 000 deaths worldwide each year. Although infections are asymptomatic in 70%, 0.1–0.5% get fulminant hepatic failure and the rest get symptomatic acute hepatitis. There are risks of end-stage liver failure and hepatocellular carcinoma. Carrier status affects 5–10% overall.

The complications are difficult to treat but easy to prevent. The vaccine is proven to be very effective and boosters are not routinely required. Universal neonatal vaccination has been successful elsewhere in the world although it might also be done in late childhood.

Those at high risk, e.g. homosexual men, and drug users, must be vaccinated.

Over 150 countries have instituted a universal neonatal hepatitis B programme but the UK is one of the few developed countries to have chosen a selective approach for high risk cases. Data on success and safety elsewhere are forcing a reassessment of this.

Hepatitis B immunisation in Britain: time to change?
Banatvala J, Van Damme P, Emiroglu N
BMJ, 2006; **332**: 804–805

This editorial argues that we may need periodically to revisit our strategy on hepatitis B vaccination. Although we have one of the lowest incidences worldwide, we started to screen pregnant women universally on realising that selective programmes failed to identify 50% of those infected.

There is particular concern about net immigration of a pool of carriers estimated at over 1500 cases per year and cumulative hepatitis B vaccination is now recommended in the Netherlands for children with at least one parent from an endemic country. Changes in populations need fluid global strategies but a full economic evaluation needs to be made to compare vaccination costs of a universal programme with the burden of the chronic disease.

A varicella-zoster virus vaccine reduced the burden of illness of herpes zoster in older adults. *Evidence-Based Medicine,* 2005; **10**: 177
The following paper is reviewed
A vaccine to prevent herpes zoster and postherpetic neuralgia in older adults
Oxman MN, Levin MJ, Johnson GR et al.
N Engl J Med, 2005; **352**: 2271–2284

This double-blind study was the first study to look at a vaccine that avoids reexpression of a latent virus. It found that a single dose of herpes zoster virus in those over 60 years with a history of varicella, reduced the risk of zoster by 51% and of post-herpetic neuralgia by 67% over 5.5 years.

IMMUNISATION

It was very safe and the commentary argues for a universal immunisation programme as the morbidity saved, particularly in those over 60 years, is considerable. The NNT of 59 looks unappealing but it is explained that even if it was 100% effective the NNT would still be 30.

IMMUNISATION

INDEX